A Nurse's Survival Guide to the Ward

Third Updated Edition

At Elsevier, we understand the importance of providing up-to-date and relevant content. For this reason, we are continuously working on updated editions and new titles for the Series. Please visit our website to find out the latest news and the upcoming publications: https://www.uk.elsevierhealth.com/

A Nurse's Survival Guide to the Ward

Third Updated Edition

Ann Richards BA (Hons) MSc DipN(Lon) RGN RNT
Associate Lecturer,
The Open University,
UK

Sharon Edwards EdD SFHEA NTF MSc PGCEA
DipN(Lon) RN
Senior Lecturer,
School of Nursing and Allied Health,
Buckinghamshire New University,
Uxbridge,
UK

ELSEVIER

Edinburgh London New York Oxford Philadelphia St Louis Sydney 2019

ISBN: 978-0-7020-7831-6

Printed in Poland
Last digit is the print number: 9 8 7 6 5 4 3 2 1

Content Strategist: Poppy Garraway/Serena Castelnovo
Content Development Specialist: Kirsty Guest
Project Manager: Anne Collett
Design: Patrick Ferguson
Marketing Manager: Kristen Oyirifi

Working together
to grow libraries in
developing countries

ELSEVIER   Book Aid International

www.elsevier.com • www.bookaid.org

Contents

Preface

In the preface to the earlier editions of the book we drew attention to the ability to provide good evidence-based care for all patients on our ever-busier hospital wards. We think this is still what all practicing nurses, both pre- and post-qualification, seek to achieve. We hope that this little book will not only continue to be a constant companion during those first early days in practice as a student but also provide answers to some of the many questions you will continue to ask well beyond your qualification and your early years as a staff nurse.

The idea for this book originally came from a student nurse at York who was, at the time, working in a frantically busy medical ward. His pleas for such a book were so heartfelt that Christopher Goodall, a lecturer at York, originally started to write the sort of text that the student felt was needed.

Unfortunately, Christopher was unable to complete the book and we thank him for passing on to us the idea of his student, Jerome Whitfield, together with his enthusiasm for this text to be developed.

The book has been thoroughly revised and updated for this updated edition in response to suggestions from our readers. It is divided into six sections covering aspects of care and management on the ward today. Areas where there have been advances in our knowledge base in the past few years have been expanded. Here, you will continue to find information on emergency situations, assessment, observations and measurements, clinical procedures and investigations and pharmacology, as well as brief descriptions of common medical and surgical conditions using a body systems approach.

However, nurses need knowledge that support and enhance their ability to practice at the bedside so the legal issues, health and safety, professional practice issues and ethics in nursing have been updated to reflect this. Holistic approaches to care continue to be included along with the sections related to fundamental procedures to expand areas of nurse interventions such as oxygen administration, fluid and electrolyte balance and nutrition.

The book is still a compact and pocket-sized companion that we hope will come to be regarded by its users as a friend. The aim is to provide the factual information needed to assist in your provision of holistic care. Although the book is aimed primarily at nurses, we feel sure that its content will be relevant for all those working in healthcare today. However, nursing practice is complex and includes many facets of care. Therefore, this book is not meant to replace all your nursing textbooks but contains material that nurses can refer to while working.

You may need to refer to additional texts (see further reading section at the back of the book) either at home or from the ward, hospital or university library for more detailed information.

In writing this book it has been decided to use the terms she to refer to the nurse, and he to refer to the patient. The writers acknowledge that there are many male nurses and female patients; however, it was chosen to use these terms for brevity and clarity and does not imply anything about the nature of nurses or patients.

We are sure that this book will serve the reader well whilst working in clinical practice. It will give confidence to nurses working in all areas of patient care. We hope that you will continue to enjoy using this little book well beyond your student days and that it will provide the support and practical information needed for you to improve your understanding of disease and, alongside this, your patient care.

If you find areas missing or sections which you feel are not relevant or useful, please e-mail us your suggestions. You can contact us via the publishers. We will both be very glad to read and respond to your comments and incorporate your requests in any future editions of the book.

Ann Richards and Sharon Edwards
Hatfield and Uxbridge, 2018

Section 1

Your job and its organization

Section Outline

1.1 ORGANIZING YOUR WORK

The work of a nurse will vary from day to day and from hospital to hospital but the following factors should be considered in all cases:

- You should have a good working knowledge of all your patients: you should know who they are, where in the ward they are lodged and the principal diagnosis for each patient.
- If you are in charge of the ward, you should make a point of seeing all your patients each day.
- Do not be afraid to ask for advice from the sister, doctor or student. It is far better to ask too often than to struggle on not knowing if you are doing the right thing and feeling more and more inadequate.
- If you are not getting sufficient support, guidance about your role and personal and professional development from management, then you need to discuss with the equivalent person, e.g., human resources (HR).
- Organize your off-duty time so that you get enough rest and sleep and ensure that you cook for yourself properly.
- Keep in contact with your friends; carry on with hobbies and interests, which will maintain your contact with the world outside nursing.

The role of the nurse

Caring for the patient:

- Ensure safe practice at all times, safeguarding of vulnerable individuals
- Provide total individualized holistic patient care
- Psychological/sociological and physiological care
- Nursing assessment and management of:
  - Pain
  - Wounds

A nurse's survival guide to the ward. https://doi.org/10.1016/B978-0-7020-7831-6.00001-2

- Nutrition status
- Intravenous (IV) infusion and other invasive lines
- Risk assessment for:
  - Deep vein thrombosis (DVT)/pulmonary embolism
  - Moving and handling
  - Pressure ulcers
  - Malnutrition
- Prioritizes care
- Care of relatives and significant others
- Record observations/monitoring and documentation of care
- Key role in the checking, administration and understanding of prescribed drugs
- Works with the multidisciplinary team:
  - Medical and surgical teams
  - Physiotherapist
  - Occupational therapist
  - Social worker
  - Pharmacist
  - Radiologist
  - Medical technicians
  - Other departments, e.g., theatres.
- Takes part in ethical and moral decision-making:
- Key role in team building, which involves working together to benefit patient care
- Is open to changing practices and innovations
- Plays a major role in communicating with others
- Undertakes and assists with evidence-based care (incorporating all types of knowledge detailed later)

Personal and professional development:

- Awareness of the need for continuous professional and personal development
- Keeps a personal development portfolio
- Encourages and supports others to attend update days, undertake additional qualifications and courses
- Supports and educates less-qualified colleagues

Areas open for consideration related to the role of the nurse:

- Limitations:
  - Environment – where you work, no natural light/poor lighting on night shifts, confined spaces, busy and noisy ward area, lack of teaching rooms, time pressures and increase in workload.

- Management styles: dogmatic, authoritarian, laissez-faire influences on practice, staff and patient well-being and the influence on patient outcomes.
- Resources available: confined to monitoring equipment, dressings and drugs available, no easy or limited access to technology, e.g., electronic databases.
- Medical practices and doctors: nurses need to express their views so that they are effective advocates for patients.
- Advances in technology: often these can enhance practice when patients are critically ill, and so need to be understood and appreciated but also recognized that they cannot and do not always save lives.
- Knowledge of nurses: confines practice to a level of knowledge/ education.
- Government legislation.
- Ambiguous protocols, policies and procedures guidelines.
- Multi-skilling:
  - Increased autonomy — professionalism of nurses (PSA, 2015)
  - Diversions of the nurse's role, e.g., taking of bloods, increase in IV drug administration and cost-effectiveness of nurses' time, is it economics rather than caring for patients?
  - Specialist nurses: nurse consultants, pain nurse, wound care nurse, stoma nurse, outreach nurse or diabetic nurse (these roles will vary depending on the work environment and patient group)
- The legal implications in practice, e.g., litigation of the extended role
- The scope of professional practice — the rules governing healthcare professionals (NMC, 2015; PSA, 2015)

! It is important to remember and be aware of outside influences that often govern how we practice and how we would like to practice.

The role of the nurse as a mentor

Personal and professional learning is about learning from colleagues, peers and groups with whom nurses associate (Edwards, 2017). It is the role of all nurses to provide a role model and support for juniors and show by example the relevance and importance of learning from others. When under guidance from more experienced individuals or in collaboration with other students they can come to realize their potential development better. Thus, nurses of all levels should take the role of a mentor seriously, as it is an integral part of nursing students' and qualified nurses' development. The role of the mentor is demanding and there are pressures that can make the support of learning for and from others difficult. Duffy et al. (2016) identified that because of the difficulties presented with taking on the mentor role, sometimes students experience substandard levels of mentoring. There are mentoring preparation programmes as well as suggestions of a supportive network or community of mentors. However, despite the discussion around the mentorship role, the barriers and difficulties, there is little doubt that mentors can greatly influence nursing students' learning in and from clinical practice.

The multidisciplinary team

Medical staff

- Overall responsibility for patient treatment and management.
- Generally, each patient is under a specialist consultant related to the patient's condition.
- A physician's associate may be involved in the patient's care and management under the supervision of a qualified doctor.

Physiotherapist

- Assist with patients' respiratory function.
- Preserve existing motor skills, restore mobility and consider the role of all limbs whether strong or weak.
- Work towards reducing stiffness, contractions and spasticity.
- Reeducate motor function, coordination and balance.

Occupational therapist

- Restore patients' ability to perform activities of daily living − relearn practical skills if necessary.
- Evaluate patients' perceptual and cognitive functions.
- Adapt objects that improve daily living activities.
- Assess the need for modifications to the home.

Speech and language therapist

- Assess patients' swallowing and gag ability.
- Provide specialized speech therapy, communication advice and aids to assist speech, if required.

Dietitian

- Advise on nutritional and fluid requirements − whether it should be liquid, thickened or pureed food.
- Advise regarding enteral or parenteral feeding requirements and regimens.

Social worker

- May discuss long-term or short-term care options with patient and family.
- Support families and patients by assisting with social and financial issues.
- Arrange benefits.
- Provide careers with home adjustments.

Other staff

- Secretarial support may be required.
- Porters may be involved in transporting patients' specimens day and night.
- Local chaplains, priests or relevant officials of all religions, when there is a need for their services.
- A designated ward clinical pharmacist is invaluable but may not be available in all areas.
- Technicians responsible for the equipment to service, repair and develop equipment.

Working as a team

Teamwork is vital if care is to be carried out expertly and efficiently in any clinical area. The team consists of not only the doctors and nurses and those above-mentioned disciplines but also many other personnel from both within and outside the hospital. These may include:

- the police,
- security,
- specialist hospitals,
- laboratories, e.g., technicians, laboratory staff,
- support staff, e.g., phlebotomists, ECG technicians,
- theatres,
- specialist nurses, e.g., diabetic, wound care, resuscitation, pain,
- other wards/departments. e.g., pharmacy, X-ray,
- community carers,
- helping agencies,
- primary healthcare teams,
- relatives and friends,
- patients,
- ambulance personnel.

Liaison and effective communication within the team are essential to ensure optimum patient care.

Communicating with other team members (multidisciplinary)

Communication is recognized as an important aspect of healthcare with far-reaching effects. It is an essential and integral part of the care nurses provide. Communication needs to be clear and it involves verbal and nonverbal messages that convey feelings and information.

Do not be afraid of discussing patients' illnesses with them or their relatives in as much detail as is appropriate (remember that it is unethical to disclose sensitive information, such as a diagnosis of cancer, to the relatives without telling the patient). Effective communication makes a positive contribution to an individual's recovery by acting:

- as a buffer against fear and confusion,
- as a relief of anxiety and stress,
- to help decrease pain and reduce the number of complications and side-effects,
- to improve compliance,
- as a way of improving coping ability,
- to enhance convalescence.

When you go off duty do not forget you must tell the nurse responsible about any problems a particular patient may have or any care that you have been unable to achieve on your shift.

The nursing handover

At the beginning of each shift, in most wards, a general nursing handover takes place whereby all staff from that shift are present. At the end of this general handover, a nurse will be allocated to a particular group of patients for that shift. At the patient's bedside, the current nurse may give additional information about their care, treatment, drug therapy, next of kin, etc., the purpose being able to ensure that information relevant to that patient's care is provided and thus minimize any disruption in patient care and uphold continuity of care. Typically, during this process, the bedside nurse uses a universally applied structure that reiterates the care plan format, thus incorporating the patient bedside observation, nursing, drug and medical charts. This may be provided on a handout and a copy provided for each member of staff on that shift (this needs to be kept confidential and should not be shared).

At the initial phase of each handover, the nurse begins by giving a basic overview of the:

- patient's age,
- past medical history (PMH),
- reason for admission,
- length of stay in the ward,
- major events that have occurred during admission,
- physical, psychologic and social handover.

Care planning and documentation

When caring for patients, a daily nursing care plan is produced. This involves a systematic patient assessment which is carried out at the beginning of the day shift or on patient admission; goals of care and a report is then written at the end of the shift regarding whether the goals of care have been met or further interventions need to be considered. The night staff will reevaluate the patient's planned care and write a report at the end of their shift. The structure and choice of care plan may vary depending on the clinical practice area in which you are based; however, many clinical practice areas follow the *Roper, Logan and Tierney model*.

In conjunction with care planning, other structures may be applied as follows:

- Standardized care plans are available for a variety of patient conditions
- Integrated care pathways — structured multidisciplinary guides to good practice, placed in an appropriate timeframe, which detail anticipated steps in the care of patients with common clinical conditions, e.g., chronic obstructive airways disease (COPD)/asthma, diabetes
- Care bundles — a set of 3—5 evidence-informed practices that when performed collectively can improve quality of care (Lavallee et al., 2017) and improve clinical outcomes (Borgert et al., 2015)
- Medical algorithms — decision tree approaches to healthcare treatment, e.g., if a patient has a condition or symptom A, B or C, then use intervention X

It is important to note that whichever care plan or additional structure is used, as a healthcare professional, you must familiarize yourself with, understand and implement your care accordingly.

Computers on the wards

The application of computer technology within a ward setting can be an important support tool for healthcare practitioners and is now widespread and diverse. They are as follows:

- Clinical decision support systems
- Automated dispensing devices
- Medication systems and procedures
- Computer physician order entry
- Healthcare information systems
- Electronic medical records

The ward is sometimes a complex environment with rapidly changing patients, personnel, policies and procedures. Ward care can be a demanding environment and may require an enormous amount of data collation, report writing and auditing, with much of this information undergoing repeated transcription. Therefore, it is apparent that one of the vital reasons for computerizing a ward environment is to minimize duplication of data entry and allow the healthcare professional to focus upon the patient. Computers within a ward setting can:

- detect variations in physiologic parameters,
- identify important aspects of care or service,
- monitor and report the important aspects of care by collecting and organizing the data for each indicator,
- assess the action and document improvement,
- communicate the relevant information in report form,
- process correlations in a short period of time and store results.

Yet, resistance to adopting these technologies includes the expense to implement and maintain, and there are issues with patient privacy. It is also worth noting that these technologies are reliant on user input to ensure patient data are accurate and complete.

These technologies may be seen to initially reduce nurses' time in documentation, ordering of medication and risk to patients but may create new problems such as 'alert fatigue' and it can be easy to override the safety systems put in place if alarms begin to irritate the nurse working with the new technology. There is also a danger of the possibility of professionals' over-reliance on technology and the danger of putting too much trust in the ability of systems to provide clinical decision support rather than their own judgement.

1.2 EMERGENCY SITUATIONS

National early warning scoring (NEWS 2)

Patients often have abnormal physiologic values present in the period before deterioration or more seriously have a cardiac arrest; most commonly observed prior to deterioration are changes in six physiologic parameters. Combining these with basic observations of the airway, breathing, circulation, disability and examination (ABCDE), measure of fluid balance and neurologic status forms the basis of this simple system of early detection as follows:

- A + B − Respiration rate (per minute)
- A + B − Oxygen saturation (%):
  - SpO_2 scale 1 used if target range is within normal limits
  - SpO_2 scale 2 used if target range is 88%−92%, e.g., in hypercapnic respiratory failure
  - Air or oxygen?
- C − Blood pressure (BP) mmHg score uses systolic BP only
- C − Pulse beats/min
- D − Level of consciousness or confusion
- E − Temperature in °C

Deviations from the normal score points a total is calculated. There are four trigger points that determine a clinical response (RCP, 2017) as follows:

- A low national early warning score (NEWS 2) (1—4) should prompt assessment by a registered nurse
- A single (red score) (3 in a single parameter) is unusual but should prompt urgent review by a clinician
- A medium NEWS 2 (5—6) is a key trigger and should prompt an urgent review by a clinician or acute team nurse
- A high NEWS 2 (7 or more) is a key trigger and should prompt emergency assessment by a clinician/critical care outreach team

These levels should alert the nurse to deterioration in the patient's condition and those that require additional clinical assessment (Fig. 1.1). These parameters form the basis of the NEWS 2 scoring system. It is used to aid early detection of patients' deteriorating conditions on acute general or surgical wards. The NEWS 2 is a simple scoring system to be used at ward level utilizing routine observations taken by nursing staff. Nurses are identifying those patients at risk of deterioration and then scoring according to their physiologic parameters.

The development of outreach

The increased cost of critical care and a national nurse shortage prompted the Government publication 'Comprehensive Critical Care' (Department of

Physiologic parameter	Score						
	3	2	1	0	1	2	3
Respiration rate (per minute)	≤8		9–11	12–20		21–24	≥25
SpO₂ Scale 1 (%)	≤91	92–93	94–95	≤96			
SpO₂ Scale 2 (%)	≤83	84–85	86–87	88–92 ≥93 on air	93–94 on oxygen	95–96 on oxygen	≥97 on oxygen
Air or oxygen?		Oxygen		Air			
Systolic blood pressure (mmHg)	≤90	91–100	101–110	111–219			≥220
Pulse (per minute)	≤40		41–50	51–90	91–110	111–130	≥131
Consciousness				Alert			CVPU
Temperature (°C)	≤35.0		35.1–36.0	36.1–38.0	38.1–39.0	39.1	

FIGURE 1.1 The national early warning scoring system. *Before making any clinical use of the NEWS2 chart, please download the high-quality, full-colour version from the Royal College of Physicians website: https://www.rcplondon.ac.uk/projects/outputs/national-early-warning-score-news-2.*

Health, 2002b). The report prompted hospitals across the country to concentrate on introducing early warning scores. This was a directive as there have been concerns regarding the capacity problem in the provision of critical care facilities in acute care trusts. Therefore, there was growing concern about the management of critically ill patients outside the intensive care setting. Attempting to reduce what was often referred to as suboptimal care prior to admission to critical care areas, it was decided to provide expert advice in the management of these patients.

The comprehensive critical care (Department of Health, 2002) report recommended that critical care services should provide for those patients who were critically ill and patients at risk of critical illness and those recovering from it. This stimulated the setting up of a number of critical care outreach programmes across the country. Currently there are a number of courses that HCP can undertake to facilitate their development in identifying a deteriorating patient and instigate the necessary interventions as follows:

- Acute life-threatening events recognition and treatment (ALERT)
- Awareness why anticipating and responding is essential (AWARE)
- Bedside emergency assessment course for healthcare staff (BEACH)

The wards are given criteria based on the ABCDE initial assessment of physiologic abnormalities similar to the NEWS 2. If a patient meets the criteria for deterioration, early interventions can be initiated. By using the A-E assessment, ward nurses are prompted to inform the doctor or contact the outreach team to attend the patient.

Ward staff are able to call the outreach team for patients with abnormal physiologic variables or specific conditions such as shock, excessive bleeding or upper respiratory obstruction. The aim of this using the A-E initial assessment is that it prompts early recognition, intervention and treatment of those patients at risk of deterioration from any cause or a cardiac arrest.

A majority of hospital trusts provide early recognition courses for ward-based staff. Hospitals use the ALERT course to provide education for ward nurses and junior doctors (Smith et al., 2012) and to improve their knowledge of vital signs and identification of patients at risk, in an attempt to reduce the number of patients requiring admission to critical care.

ABCDE initial assessment of the acutely ill patient

When a patient's condition is deteriorating, it is important to consider the A-E assessment (Table 1.1) in conjunction with the above-mentioned medical emergency guidelines as follows:

- Airway:
  - Is it clear (if the patient can speak, it is likely the airway is open); obstructed or protected; can the patient speak in full sentences?

TABLE 1.1 Underlying principles of the ABCDE approach to determine a deteriorating patient

A = airway	B = breathing	C = circulation	D = disability	E = exposure
Talking in full sentences	Using accessory muscles	Blood pressure	AVPU or GCS	Remove clothes for a head to toe examination
Look, listen and feel	Colour, e.g., cyanosis, oxygen saturation	Pulse rate – radial and femoral	Optimize ABC	Look for injuries, bleeding, rashes, etc.
Distress, choking, suction if required	Respiratory rate, depth, pattern of breathing	Colour, e.g., pale; Capillary refill >2 s	Treat cause with Naloxone for opioid toxicity	Avoid heat loss
Sounds, e.g., gurgling or inspiratory stridor	Auscultate the chest, e.g., expiratory wheeze	Urine output	Blood glucose, if < 3 mmol/L give glucose	Maintain dignity
Patient's condition should guide direction	Look, listen and feel Treat underlying cause, support if inadequate, administer oxygen	IV access, treat cause, drugs if appropriate	Pupil reaction	Past medical history

ABCDE, airway, breathing, circulation, disability and examination; *AVPU*, Alert Verbal Painful Unresponsiveness; *GCS*, Glasgow Coma Scale.

- Use the look, listen and feel approach to determine air entry
- Is there any noise heard during breathing, such as snoring (partial obstruction by the tongue); gurgling, which indicates secretions, vomit or blood is in the upper airway; inspiratory stridor, which is an indication of an obstruction above the larynx?
- Breathing:
  - Look for chest movement, listen for air entry and feel if the chest is moving
  - Is the patient distressed or using their accessory muscles?
  - Is the respiratory rate high or low (12–15 normal), include pattern and depth of breathing?
  - Colour – is the patient cyanosed?

- What is the oxygen saturation?
- Is the patient using their accessory muscles?
- Is the chest and abdomen moving in the same direction?
- Is there an expiratory wheeze (collapse during expiration)?
- Listen to the patient's chest, are there any rattling noises (indicating secretions)?
- Is bronchial breathing absent or reduced (may indicate a pneumothorax, a medical emergency) or pleural effusion?
- Is air entry equal on both sides?
- Circulation:
  - Is the patient pale or cyanosed (may indicate peripheral vein collapse and may be difficult to cannulate) or haemorrhagic?
  - What is the patient's urine output?
  - What is the BP; it may be normal because compensatory homoeostatic mechanisms increase peripheral resistance in response to reduced cardiac output, so it is not a good indicator of shock (see later); more significant is pulse pressure, which is the difference between systolic and diastolic, and should be between 35 and 45. If increased, it is suggestive of arterial vasoconstriction and if reduced, it is indicative of vasodilatation and sepsis.
  - What is the heart rate (HR); is the pulse bounding (sepsis) or weak (reduced cardiac output)?
  - Check the capillary refill time should be less than 2 s.
- Disability:
  - Check A = if the patient is spontaneously alert, V = responding to verbal stimulus, P = responding to painful stimuli, U = unresponsive.
  - Check BM level
  - Pupil reactions to light (bilateral pin point drug overdose, opiates, brainstem involvement, stroke). Unilateral dilated unresponsive to light (brainstem death, cancer, lesion, cerebral oedema)
  - Glasgow coma scale if time.
- Examination:
  - Get a full medical history from the patient, relatives or friends
  - Undertake a thorough head to toe physical examination after correction of any compromise to ABCDE is secured
  - Temperature if not taken elsewhere — hypothermia from theatre
  - Blood results — creatinine, urea and electrolytes, K+, Na, haemoglobin (Hb)
  - Fluids — fluid balance chart, input and output, increase in weight
  - Gastrointestinal tract (GIT) — abdomen, surgery, drains, blood loss, wound infection, bowel habits sounds
  - Haematology — clotting, Hb, white blood count

- Lines — source of sepsis, IV, drains, catheters, etc.
- Medication — prescribed drugs given, nephrotoxic drugs given, monitored digoxin/vancomycin, drug interactions, allergies

Provide appropriate interventions A-E (Table 1.2). Return to NEWS 2 to recognize any further deterioration and review if score improves or deteriorates.

Cardiac arrest

This is the cessation of cardiac mechanical activity with no clinical cardiac output. If immediate cardiopulmonary resuscitation (CPR) is not started, death or serious cerebral damage will result. Nursing staff should promote CPR training and be the driving force behind a hospital's resuscitation team.

Cardiac arrest may be primary or secondary.

TABLE 1.2 ABCDE appropriate action/interventions

ABCDE assessment	Appropriate interventions
A	Airway obstruction is an emergency; obtain help immediately; airway opening; airway suction, insert airway, intubation may be required. Provide high flow oxygen
B	Provide appropriate oxygen administration considering subgroups of patients, e.g., COPD If respiratory rate inadequate consider bas mask, noninvasive ventilation, intubation Consider appropriate medication/treatment for respiratory disorder depending on cause bronchodilators, chest drain insertion
C	Insertion of IV cannula is required, take bloods for routine investigations; fluids should be commenced, consider smaller volumes for patients with heart failure (closer monitoring, check for fluid overload) If chest pain — early 12 Lead ECG; Aspirin; Nitroglycerin; Morphine
D	If changes in level of consciousness is thought to be drug induced — check drug chart — consider antidote if appropriate Nurse unconscious patients in the lateral position
E	If full exposure of the patient is necessary for a proper assessment respect the patient's dignity

ABCDE, airway, breathing, circulation, disability and examination; *COPD*, chronic obstructive airways disease.

Primary: sudden cessation of cardiac function

- Myocardial infarction (MI).
- Heart disease.
- Electric shock.
- Drugs, e.g., potassium.

Secondary: nonintrinsic cardiac causes

- Asphyxia, hypoxia, hypercarbia.
- Exsanguination.
- Central nervous system (CNS) failure.
- Metabolic/electrolyte disorders.
- Temperature extremes.
- Toxins.
- Acute anaphylaxis.

  Cardiac arrest is usually associated with one of four rhythms:

- Ventricular fibrillation (VF).
- Pulseless ventricular tachycardia (VT).
- Asystole.
- Electromechanical dissociation — absent mechanical activity despite a coordinated ECG waveform; this is diagnosed infrequently.

Basic life support

The instigation of resuscitation in the event of a cardiac arrest occurring on the ward is critical to save lives.

The sequence of basic life support

First ensure you are safe, check the environment for spillages or wires, check the victim's response by gently shaking their shoulders and ask loudly 'Can you hear me' or 'Are you alright'. If there is no response, call for help. Assess the airway, breathing and circulation before initiating active interventions:

! The ABCDE approach when determining a cardiac arrest is slightly different to that of assessing a deteriorating patient.

- A — Airway maintenance, open the airway and ensure it is secure and insert a Guedel's airway if available

- B − Breathing, look, listen and feel for normal breathing for no more than 10 s, if available, maintain breathing using appropriate shield or bag and mask.
- C − Circulation, start chest compressions

In a hospital situation, call the resuscitation team; if outside, dial 999.

The purpose of basic life support is to maintain adequate ventilation and circulation until help arrives. Airway, breathing, circulation is always the priority order. The sequence of action is as follows:

1. Ensure the safety of yourself and the patient.
2. Check responsiveness of the patient. Ask 'are you alright?' give a verbal command and gently shake the shoulders.
3. If the patient responds by answering or moving, leave in position (if safe), assess condition and get help. If she or he does not respond, shout for help and then open the airway by tilting the head and lifting the chin.
4. Keeping the airway open, look, listen and feel for breathing for up to 10 s before deciding that breathing is absent.
5. If the patient is breathing, turn into the recovery position, check for continued breathing, get help. If she or he is not breathing, turn her or him on to her or his back and remove any visible obstruction from the mouth.
6. Assess casualty for signs of circulation.
7. If no signs of circulation, start compressions at the centre of the sternum mid nipple line; depress 1.5−2 inches or 4−5 cm at a rate of 100 times per minute.
8. Combine compressions and rescue breathing at a ratio of 30:2.
9. Continue resuscitation until the casualty shows signs of life and/or help arrives.

Intermediate cardiopulmonary resuscitation

- Many calls in practice are peri-arrests, which have implications for survival and soon will take over from cardiac arrest calls.
- The chain of survival includes four key interrelated steps to optimize survival as follows:
  - Early recognition and call for help as most cardiac arrests are predictable:
    - A drop in BP and reduced oxygen saturation.
    - When these signs occur, a precardiac arrest call can be given.
    - If these are not picked up, the patient could go on to a cardiac arrest.
    - The areas of BP, heart and respiratory rate and oxygen saturation need to be tracked to determine changes in physiology to incorporate early warning systems.
  - Early CPR − the reasons patients arrest, see Table 1.3:
    - Treat life-threatening problem

TABLE 1.3 Reasons for respiratory and/or cardiac arrest

Airway problems	Cardiac problems	
	Primary	Secondary
Central nervous system	Coronary syndrome	Asphyxia
Blood	Dysrhythmias	Hypoxaemia
Vomit	Increased blood pressure	Blood loss
Foreign body		Hypothermia
Trauma	Heart disease	Septic shock
Infection	Valve disease	
Inflammation	Drugs	
Laryngospasm	Hereditary	
Bronchospasm	Electrolytes	
Inhalation/burns	Acid-base changes	
Drugs (suppression)	Electrocution	
Pain (breathing inadequately)		
Pneumothorax/haemothorax		
Chronic obstructive pulmonary disease		
Pulmonary embolism		
Adult respiratory distress syndrome		

- Reassessment
- Assess effects of treatment
- Call for help early — concentrate on this
- Personal safety
- Patient responsiveness
- Vital signs (breathing deteriorates first and so changes first)
- Early defibrillation
- Early advanced life support and standardized postresuscitation care

---

! Adult tidal volume is 500 mL; dead space (air not involved in gaseous exchange) is up to 250 mL. Ventilation using bag and mask should reflect this, and breaths given (adult) need to be greater than 250 mL to be effective.

During CPR consider potential reversible causes (4 Hs and 4 Ts).

- The 4 Hs:
  - Hypoxia
  - Hypothermia
  - Hypo/hypokalaemia
  - Hypovolaemia.
- The 4 Ts:
  - Tamponade
  - Tension pneumothorax
  - Toxins
  - Thrombosis.
- Check electrode position.
- Airway/oxygen.
- IV access (variable rates of absorption from sites, e.g., radial, CVP).
- Give uninterrupted compressions.
- Follow the CPR algorithm.

Advanced life support

The Resuscitation Council (UK) recommends guidelines and protocols to manage shockable rhythms such as VT and VF, and nonshockable rhythms, e.g., asystole and pulseless electrical activity. The protocol stresses early defibrillation and advanced care. Advanced life support involves:

- following the guidelines set out by the Resuscitation Council (UK),
- giving 1 mg adrenaline and sequences of 2:15 compressions/ventilation,
- advanced airway care (intubation) after the first DC shock; once achieved, ventilation can proceed.
- gaining venous access.

Intubation

Advanced airway management involves endotracheal intubation, which allows for spontaneous and positive pressure ventilation.

Endotracheal tubes (ETTs) are usually the first choice in managing a patient's airway. This is a device with an inflatable cuff that is inserted into the patient's trachea via their mouth or nose. It passes through the larynx, and the cuff is then inflated with air to seal the trachea. This is to protect the lungs from aspiration; it does not hold the ETT in place. The ETT is secured in place with ties (either a special holder or ETT tape) and a note taken of the length of the ETT at the patient's lips. This is important because tracheal tubes can move and slip further down, entering the right main bronchus so that the left lung is not ventilated. They can also slip upward, passing back through the larynx, which means that the patient can no longer be ventilated through them.

Indications for intubation are as follows:

- Acute airway obstruction.
- Facilitation of tracheal suctioning.
- Protection of the airway in those without protective cough reflexes.
- Respiratory failure/arrest requiring ventilatory support and high inspired concentrations of oxygen.

Direct laryngoscopy is the most common method used in an emergency, either in the mouth or through the nose. The tip of the tube may require direction with a Magill forceps to enter the glottis. Confirming correct tracheal tube placement is essential, and therefore arterial blood gases need checking for expired carbon dioxide levels.

Complications of intubation include those that occur during intubation are:

- trauma
- cardiovascular response to laryngoscopy and intubation
- hypoxaemia
- aspiration
- oesophageal intubation

And those that occur after the tube is in place are:

- blockage
- dislodgement
- damage to larynx
- complications of mechanical ventilation

Oesophageal tracheal airways are types of supraglottic airways that keep the patient's airway open during anaesthesia or unconsciousness. There is a range of these type of airways available as follows:

- Laryngeal mask airway
- iGel supraglottic airway
- Extraglottic airway device
- Oesophageal tracheal combitube

These devices are an effective alternative to ventilation mask or endotracheal intubation. They are easy and quick to insert and may be inserted blindly. These tubes isolate the lungs from the oesophagus and so prevent aspiration during surgery or unconsciousness.

Shock

Shock is a condition in which the cardiovascular system fails to perfuse the body tissues adequately, thereby causing widespread disruption of cellular metabolism, which results in functional disturbances at an organ/tissue level (for more detail see page 23). There are three stages of shock, each progressively worse, as follows:

1. Compensated (nonprogressive) stage, where compensatory mechanisms stabilize the circulation.
2. Continuing hypoperfusion and deteriorating organ function mark the progressive stage.
3. Refractory (irreversible) stage, where severe cellular and therefore organ dysfunction leads to general decline and death.

There are many causes of shock, including any factor, which affects blood volume, BP or cardiac function. One classification of shock states that according to BP, there are two forms as follows:

- Hypotensive shock — further subdivided into:
  - low cardiac output shock characterized clinically by cold skin
  - high cardiac output shock characterized by warm skin
- Normotensive or hypertensive shock — BP is compensated.

Another classification is recognized by type and aetiology as follows:

- Distributive: septic, neurogenic, anaphylactic, drug and toxin-induced shock
- Cardiogenic: cardiomyopathy, arrhythmic, mechanical
- Hypovolaemic: haemorrhagic, nonhaemorrhagic
- Obstructive: pulmonary or vascular

A more traditional classification categorizes shock according to the primary defect that produced it. With this system there are five forms of shock: anaphylactic, septic, neurogenic, cardiogenic and hypovolaemic.

Anaphylactic shock

Anaphylaxis occurs when a sensitized person is exposed to an antigen to which she or he is allergic. The antigen enters the body and combines with immunoglobulin E antibodies on the surface of mast cells and basophils, primarily found in the lungs, small intestines, skin and connective tissue. An antigen-antibody reaction occurs, which induces the release of histamine and prostaglandin into the blood, leading to the following:

- Increased cell permeability, leading to oedema.
- Vasodilatation in some areas (β-1 receptors) and reduction in BP.
- Vasoconstriction (β-2 receptors) in others (breathlessness).
- Third-space fluid shifts, increased sodium in the intracellular and intravascular space; this fluid loss from the circulation may lead to circulatory collapse.

This results in reduced cardiac output and low arterial pressure. Cellular perfusion fails to meet the metabolic demands, resulting in acidosis, coagulopathies and capillary pooling.

Septic shock

The main organisms responsible are gram-negative enteric bacilli such as *Escherichia coli*, *Pseudomonas*, *Klebsiella, Proteus* and *Enterobacter* or gram-positive organisms such as staphylococci, streptococci and *Clostridium*. These organisms enter the vascular system and release endotoxins, which cause an interstitial fluid leak, increased vascular permeability and vasodilatation, which leads to shock.

A great hazard for the development of sepsis is parenteral nutrition (PN).

- The PN solution is an ideal medium for bacterial growth if contaminated. All care of the feeding line must be aseptic.
- The feeding line may become infected (the catheter must be used for feeding only, not for taking blood or drug administration). The most common infecting organisms are *Candida albicans* and *Staphylococcus epidermidis*, which are part of the skin flora.
- The practice of bypassing the gut and delivering nutrition directly into the blood can lead to problems, as the gut not only plays a major role in the digestion and absorption of nutrition but also acts as a protective barrier against the translocation of bacteria and endotoxins to the bloodstream.

The results of septic shock are as follows:

- Tachycardia.
- High cardiac output — maintained at a normal/high level by the increasing tachycardia.
- The patient feels warm and has a high temperature.
- A low circulating volume owing to venous pooling, increased capillary permeability and third-space fluid shift.

If volume loss is not corrected, hypovolaemia will persist, cardiac output will decrease and the skin will become cool. As in all other types of shock, the primary problem is tissue hypoperfusion; consequently, nutrients and oxygen fail to be delivered to cells. Sepsis can be treated with antibiotics.

Treatment guidelines have been produced to improve survival from sepsis as follows:

- The Sepsis Six standardized by the inclusion of three ins and three outs, which need to be completed within the first hour following the recognition of sepsis:
    - Three ins are administration of oxygen therapy, IV fluid administration and IV antibiotics
    - Three outs are blood measure of lactate, blood cultures and urine output

- Quick sepsis organ failure assessment (QSOFA) is used to determine the extent of a person's organ function or rate of failure as follows:
  - Heart failure − fluid balance chart positive balance, increase in weight, changes in vital signs, coughing up frothy sputum
  - Renal failure − changes in blood results increase in urea and creatinine, reduced haemaglobin; fluid balance chart reduced urine output, positive balance, increase in weight; urinalysis contains protein
  - Liver failure − changes in liver function tests; urinalysis contains bilirubin, jaundice
  - Respiratory failure − changes in respiratory rate, pattern and depth, oxygen saturation, arterial blood gases
  - Neurological abnormalities − confusion, disorientation, changes in Glasgow coma scale
- Sepsis survival campaign (SSC) is around interventions that may need to be included in addition to the Sepsis Six as follows:
  - Consideration of the family/initiate palliative care
  - Blood analysis
  - Intubation/ventilation
  - Continuous monitoring of blood glucose levels
  - Prevention of stress ulcers; DVT/pulmonary embolism and pressure ulcers
  - Renal replacement therapy
  - Sedation/analgesia
  - Nutrition such as enteral feeding

! These standardized treatment guidelines are mainly for medical practitioners, but there is no reason why nurses cannot consider these areas in the management and care of their patients with sepsis.

Neurogenic shock

Neurogenic shock causes changes to smooth muscle tension in the walls of the circulatory vessels through nervous system action, leading to an imbalance between parasympathetic and sympathetic stimulation. There is a loss of sympathetic tone, causing peripheral vasodilatation and resulting in severe hypotension. There is decreased vascular tone and systemic vascular resistance (SVR), inadequate cardiac output, reduced tissue perfusion and impaired cellular metabolism.

Neurogenic shock may be the result of the following:

- A severe brainstem injury at the level of the medulla.
- An injury to the spinal cord.
- Spinal anaesthesia.

It may mask signs and symptoms of other types of shock.

> **!** If neurogenic shock is present, there should be a heightened suspicion for an undetected source of haemorrhage.

Cardiogenic shock

Cardiogenic shock occurs when the heart, due to impaired myocardial performance, cannot produce an adequate cardiac output to sustain the metabolic requirements of body tissues. MI is the most common cause of cardiogenic shock, as the area infarcted becomes dysfunctional and, depending on the size of the infarction, stroke volume and cardiac output may decrease with a concurrent increase in left ventricular end–diastolic pressure.

Compensatory mechanisms are stimulated by the decrease in BP and catecholamines are released. This causes an increase in HR and contractility, BP and SVR to maintain arterial pressure.

The compensatory mechanisms improve blood flow for a time, but more oxygen is required by the already ischaemic cardiac muscle to pump blood into the constricted systemic circulation, consequently increasing cardiac workload. The heart becomes more ischaemic and cardiac failure worsens, jeopardizing potentially viable tissue and increasing left ventricular work. As cardiac output continues to decline, BP and tissue perfusion decrease, which results in cardiogenic shock and ends with the patient's death.

Hypovolaemic shock

Hypovolaemic shock is the most common type of shock and occurs due to a decrease in the circulating fluid volume so large that the body's metabolic needs cannot be met. The decline in blood volume is produced by the following:

- Continued bleeding
- Plasma loss
- Bleeding disorders
- Water or fluid shifts
- Dehydration
- High temperature

This decreases venous return and cardiac output, primarily affecting tissue perfusion.

The degree of shock depends on the amount of blood lost, the rate at which it was lost, the age and general physical condition of the patient and the patient's ability to activate compensatory mechanisms. Numerous compensatory mechanisms to increase venous tone are activated when the circulating volume and venous return are decreased. As a result, venous capacity is decreased to match the smaller blood volume and adequate transport of oxygen and nutrients is maintained.

If the fluid loss exceeds the ability of homoeostatic mechanisms to compensate for the loss, the central venous pressure (CVP), diastolic filling pressure, stroke volume and systemic arterial BP will fall. As the severity of shock increases, blood pools in the capillary and venous beds, with further impairment of the effective vascular volume available for oxygen transport and tissue perfusion.

Patients in shock will often have components of more than one of the forms of shock. For example, patients in cardiogenic shock may also be hypovolaemic due to loss of fluid into the tissues as a result of high venous pressures or increased capillary permeability. Hypovolaemia is also frequently a complication of septic shock, and in the late stages of hypovolaemic shock patients usually have some degree of cardiac failure and vasomotor collapse, complicating their shock picture.

The stages of shock

Shock from whatever initial cause always has the same end result, e.g., the tissues fail to receive oxygen and nutrients and to rid themselves of waste products. It is inadequate tissue and cell perfusion which causes widespread disruption to cellular metabolism.

It is the responsibility of the nurse for preventing the development of shock. This includes early interpretation of observational and measurable data to recognize its early development. For easy understanding and recognition of shock, it can be divided into three stages: compensated, progressive or uncompensated and irreversible. These stages are not distinct and should be regarded as a continuum.

The initial stage

Some of the new literature on shock proposes an initial stage whereby cellular metabolism switches from aerobic to anaerobic and produces lactic acid (Garretson and Malberti, 2007). However, this stage can be asymptomatic and does not show visual clinical signs; therefore some disregard the existence of the initial stage (Richards and Edwards, 2014). Some of the literature that describes an initial stage of shock includes processes that are more likely to be clinically evident during the progressive stage of shock, e.g., anaerobic metabolism and the production of lactic acid. There is limited evidence that this stage has clinical significance, as the compensatory stage of shock will be recognized almost immediately before any signs of the initial stage can be determined.

Compensatory shock

The body's compensatory stage begins as the body's homoeostatic mechanisms attempt to maintain cardiovascular dynamics and stabilize the circulation, in the face of whatever defect is causing the shock. The compensatory mechanisms involved are as follows:

- Sympathetic nervous system (SNS)— initiated by the decrease in arterial pressure that releases noradrenaline (norepinephrine) and adrenaline (epinephrine) and stimulates baroreceptors.
- Renal autoregulation — with the release of renin-angiotensin-aldosterone system (RAAS)
- Arterial central chemoreceptors — sensitive to changes in carbon dioxide and pH; a reduced carbon dioxide will cause vasoconstriction
- Osmoreceptors — sensitive to a decrease in osmolality and stimulate the release of antidiuretic hormone (ADH)
- Capillary dynamics — when compensatory mechanisms cease to respond to stimulus, BP will start to drop leading to a change in capillary hydrostatic pressure compared with colloidal oncotic pressure (COP) in the capillaries, and fluid will be drawn from the intracellular fluid spaces to bring up BP. In a well-hydrated patient, this can maintain BP for a longer period of time.

! Elderly patients are not usually well hydrated with ICF content, as a consequence, is reduced, thus this group of patients will deteriorate much quicker when in a state of shock.

Generally, the clinical picture of a patient in the compensatory stage of shock is as follows:

- Tachycardia, narrowing pulse pressure, a slight increase in temperature and blood glucose level due to the effect of catecholamines.
- Pale skin colour, cool to cold skin due to the redistribution of blood away from the skin, and clammy due to the activation of sweat glands by the SNS.
- Decrease in urine output, due to selective vasoconstriction of the renal bed and the actions of ADH and aldosterone.
- Absent bowel sounds due to reduced GIT motility from the action of noradrenaline
- An increase in BP and rate and depth of respiration.
- Mental state alterations ranging from restlessness to coma.
- Complaining of thirst.

> **!** These protective mechanisms, observed in the compensatory stage of shock, can maintain circulation and BP. These mechanisms will eventually cease to function and circulatory failure will ensue. If the metabolic acidosis, circulatory failure or volume is not corrected or treatment instigated, progressive shock will occur in a short space of time.
> Therefore, in this phase, decreased BP is not a good indicator of shock.

Progressive or uncompensated shock

Once shock has developed, the course it takes is complex. Certainly, the prognosis in some forms of shock, particularly hypovolaemic shock, is excellent if treated in the early compensatory stage. Once shock has progressed into this stage, the outcome is no longer as predictable. As shock progresses, deleterious changes occur as follows:

- There is an increase in oxygen demand over the ability of the respiratory system to supply sufficient amounts for organ function and respiratory failure may ensue.
- Cellular energy production − adenosine triphosphate (ATP) reduces and lactic acid is produced as a result.
- Cellular membrane disruption occurs as a result of a lack of ATP.
- The role of calcium − which accumulates in cells destroying them from the inside.
- The role of lysosomes − these are destroyed and the toxins within them further destroy the cell from the inside.
- Cellular fluid shifts − inflammatory immune response (IIR).
- Coagulation defects − as clotting factors are used up due to the stimulation of the IIR.

The progressive stage of shock is predominately marked by continuing hypoperfusion, cellular changes and hypoxia, leading to a reduction in BP and deteriorating organ function. How far the deterioration in organ function goes will vary from person to person, but organ function will largely determine the course and outcome. However, some organs bear the brunt of the body's effort to compensate for a decrease in systemic pressure, and as a result, these organs will suffer damage, and dysfunction will appear early in the shock syndrome. The point at which organ dysfunction becomes irreversible is not clear. The major organs affected are the kidneys, liver, GIT, heart, lungs and brain.

Refractory (irreversible) shock

This is the final stage of shock and is where severe cellular and organ dysfunction leads to general decline and death.

In this stage, it may be possible to return arterial BP to normal for a short while, but tissue and organ deterioration continue, and no amount of therapy will reverse the process.

So much tissue damage and necrosis has occurred, so many IIR mediators and toxins have been released into the systemic circulation, and acidosis is so profound that even a return of normal cardiac output and arterial BP will not reverse the downward progression.

At this point there is an almost total depletion of ATP stores, which are very difficult to restore once they are gone. There is usually vasomotor failure due to CNS ischaemia. The vasomotor centres become so depressed that no sympathetic activity occurs. The vascular bed is generally dilated owing to the CNS depression, acidosis and toxins. Deterioration will continue and death will ensue.

Other considerations

There are a number of variables that affect the course of shock, such as:

- age,
- general state of health,
- medications, e.g., polypharmacy,
- pain,
- hypothermia.

Fluid overload or hypervolaemia

An increase in circulating volume can occur for many of the following reasons:

- PMH of MI
- Circulation problems prior to admission, e.g., heart failure, peripheral vascular disease
- Kidney problems, e.g., renal failure
- Cirrhosis of the liver
- Following IV fluid replacement therapy (FRT) given after surgery or shock
- Too much salt
- Sluggish arterial and venous circulation caused by a stagnant flow of blood through the circulation due to continued bed rest or immobility

Prior to problems being observed (cyanosis, pale skin) or measured (BP, CVP) in the patient's condition, these processes activate compensatory mechanisms to maintain homoeostasis, e.g., atrial natriuretic peptide.

Factors that can precipitate fluid overload

There are many specific conditions, which can precipitate fluid overload, by:

● reducing the body's ability to maintain homoeostasis in the event of an increase in circulating volume,
● stimulating control mechanisms that accelerate the symptoms of fluid overload, e.g., the RAAS,
● causing the flow of blood to become turbulent, increasing SVR and BP.

All of these conditions may hasten fluid overload during or following an IV infusion. The most common of these are hypertension, heart failure and peripheral vascular disease.

In all cases of hypervolaemia, there is an increase in circulatory volume. Cardiogenic shock is severe circulatory failure due to a primary defect in the pumping activity of the heart. The circulatory collapse becomes so profound that myocardial contractility is decreased and the body is unable to adequately compensate as cardiac output drops.

When the body is functioning normally, it is almost impossible to produce an excess of total body water. However, this can occur during IV treatment with either a crystalloid (normal saline, Hartmann's solution, 5% dextrose) or colloid (blood, gelofusine, albumin solutions, haemaccel).

The following are the principal aetiologies of fluid overload.

Blood transfusion

In this situation, blood velocity reduces and blood flow becomes slow, leading to pooling of blood in the peripheries, lungs, liver, kidneys and possibly the brain. The heart can no longer pump the increasing amount of volume around the circulation. As the signs of heart failure increase and the kidneys become swamped with fluid and start to receive a lower blood supply, renal failure ensues. The complications of pulmonary oedema, cardiac failure, renal failure, ascites, cerebral oedema and peripheral oedema can be very serious if not treated quickly.

In the majority of cases when a blood transfusion is being administered, a diuretic is generally given with each or every alternate unit. This is even more important in patients who have problems with maintaining an adequate circulation.

Salt/water overload

A fluid overload can occur with both crystalloid and colloid similar to those observed when giving whole blood as follows:

● Crystalloid fluid − The effects can be an overload of both salt and water (isotonic volume excess) or just salt (hypertonic volume excess) or a dilutional low sodium (hypotonic volume excesses).

> **!** Hypotonic volume excesses can lead to a dilutional hyponatraemia, whereby all blood contents are reduced. This is a life-threatening state, and if a patient has had a significant amount of FRT, blood results need to be monitored for any signs of reducing values.

- Colloid fluid — The effect is an increase in COP drawing water/fluid from the ICF space into the circulation leading to a fluid overload.

> **!** Colloid fluid should be used sparingly. If the cause of fluid overload is due to the overuse of colloids, the excess fluid cannot be removed by diuretics, as protein does not appear in urine and cannot be off-loaded by the kidney.

Trauma

Patients with severe multiple trauma require care and attention to their primary injuries. This may include surgery; dressings; IV fluids, e.g., blood, crystalloid or colloid; oxygen; drugs and/or resuscitation. However, there is now a sophisticated understanding of the complex metabolic response of the human body to traumatic injury. Following trauma, the initial physiologic responses that occur are neuroendocrine response; oxygen supply and demand; alterations in metabolism; IIR; and post-trauma capillary leak. These physiologic responses are initiated to protect the body from cell/tissue/organ damage.

Neuroendocrine response to injury

One of the earliest responses to injury is neuroendocrine activation, which is intimately linked in the control of tissue function. Neuroendocrine activation occurs in response to cytokine release from the site of injury and stimulates the SNS, hypothalamus, pituitary and adrenal glands. The nervous system generates biochemical agents that act as hormones, and the endocrine system produces substances that mediate activity within the CNS.

Following an insult, activation of the neuroendocrine system stimulates the release of numerous substances into the circulation, including the following:

- Catecholamines (adrenaline and noradrenaline) via the SNS and adrenal cortex, causing tachycardia, increased cardiac output and BP, rate and depth of respirations, blood flow redistribution, glycogenolysis, gluconeogenesis and lipolysis.

- Glucocorticoids via the hypothalamus release corticotrophin-releasing hormone, while the anterior pituitary gland secretes adrenocorticotrophic hormone. The adrenal cortex then releases cortisol, a glucocorticoid, which causes gluconeogenesis, proteolysis and lipolysis, anti-inflammatory and cell-protective effects to prevent damage from excessive activation of the metabolic response.

The effect of catecholamines occurs almost immediately, effecting change in target organs with extreme rapidity and intensity. Heart rate can double in 3–5 s, cardiac output can increase fourfold and selective vasoconstriction and vasodilatation occur to redistribute the circulating volume to vital organs (heart, brain).

The neuroendocrine response in injury protects the body from the effects of injury. However, it causes the following:

- An increase in oxygen consumption and myocardial work.
- Redistribution of blood flow away from the 'nonvital' gut, which may result in translocation of bacteria and endotoxins into the circulation, resulting in septic shock.
- High catecholamine levels, which can lead to arrhythmias, causing cardiac arrest in a compromised heart.

Therefore, if this response is prolonged, it is believed to contribute to shock and multiple system organ failure (MSOF).

Inflammatory/immune response

The wound or injury site plays a role in the systemic response as the wound produces extensive inflammation by attracting nutrients, fluids, clotting factors and large numbers of neutrophils and macrophages to the damaged site. These are activated to:

- protect the host from invading microorganisms,
- limit the extent of blood loss and injury,
- promote rapid healing of involved tissues.

This activation is known as the IIR and represents a major physiologic event in the body, which leads to an increased capillary permeability causing the swelling, redness, pain and oedema often observed in inflammation and stimulation of coagulation and fibrinolysis. The IIR is initiated to protect the host and to promote healing and is necessary for survival, but it can lead to an uncontrolled intravascular inflammation that ultimately harms the host. This can be observed in conditions such as the following:

- Adult respiratory distress syndrome.
- Systemic immune response syndrome.
- Disseminated intravascular coagulation.
- MSOF.

Therefore, trauma requires immediate intervention as the process outlined earlier can lead to serious, irreversible consequences and death. The nurse's immediate role is in the following:

- The administration of oxygen.
- The instigation and administration of adequate nutrition.
- The maintenance of an adequate circulating volume.

For more information related to trauma, see Section 5.

Chest drain insertion

Chest drains are used in many different clinical settings; however, all personnel involved with the insertion of the chest drain should be adequately trained. The use of premedication, unless contraindicated, to reduce the patient's anxiety and stress levels are often supported, as the procedure can be somewhat distressing to the patient.

Indications

- Pneumothorax − trauma, CVP insertion.
- Tension pneumothorax after initial needle relief.
- Persistent or recurrent pneumothorax after simple aspiration.
- Large secondary spontaneous pneumothorax in patients over the age of 50 years.
- Malignant pleural effusion.
- Empyema.
- Pleural effusion.
- Traumatic haemopneumothorax.
- Postoperative, e.g., cardiothoracic or thoracic surgery.

Risks associated with chest drain insertion

- There is a risk of haemorrhage, therefore, where possible, any coagulopathy or platelet defect should be corrected prior to chest drain insertion. For elective chest drain insertion, anticoagulants should be stopped and time allowed for their effects to resolve.
- The differential diagnosis between a pneumothorax and bullous disease requires careful radiologic assessment so as to give the appropriate treatment. Similarly, it is important to differentiate between the presence of a collapse and a pleural effusion when the chest X-ray shows a unilateral 'whiteout'.
- Lung tissue densely adherent to the chest wall throughout the hemithorax is an absolute contraindication to chest drain insertion.

The patient's position

- The preferred position for drain insertion is on the bed, slightly rotated on their side, with the patient's arm on the insertion side, placed behind the patient's head to expose the axillary area.
- An alternative is for the patient to sit upright leaning over an adjacent table with a pillow or in the lateral decubitus position.

Insertion

- Aseptic technique should be employed during tube insertion.
- Confirming drain site insertion − if fluid or free air cannot be aspirated with a needle at the time of local anaesthesia, then a chest tube should not be inserted without further image guidance.
- Imaging should be used to select the appropriate site for chest tube placement.
- Position of chest tubes − the most common is in the midaxillary line, minimizes any risk to underlying structures, e.g., internal mammary artery, and avoids damage to muscle and breast tissue resulting in unsightly scarring.
- Securing the drain − large-bore chest drain incisions should be closed by a suture appropriate for a linear incision: 'Purse string' sutures must not be used
- Two sutures are usually inserted, the first to assist later closure of the wound after drain removal and the second, a stay suture, to secure the drain
- Large amounts of tape (sleek) and padding to dress the site are unnecessary, and concerns have been expressed that they may restrict chest wall movement or increase moisture collection
- A transparent dressing allows the wound site to be inspected regularly by nursing staff for leakage or infection.

Closed system drainage

- All chest tubes should be connected to a single flow drainage system, e.g., underwater seal bottle or flutter valve.
- The tube is placed under water at a depth of approximately 3 cm with a side vent, which allows escape of air, or it may be connected to a suction pump. This enables the operator to see air bubble out as the lung reexpands in the case of pneumothorax or fluid evacuation rate in empyemas, pleural effusions or haemothorax.
- The continuation of bubbling suggests a continued visceral pleural air leak, although it may also occur in patients on suction when the drain is partly out of the thorax and one of the tube holes is open to the air.

- The respiratory swing in the fluid in the chest tube is useful for assessing tube patency and confirms the position of the tube in the pleural cavity.
- The use of a Heimlich flutter valve system allows earlier mobilization and the potential for earlier discharge of patients with chest drains.

There are other emergency situations such as seizures, asthma, diabetic emergencies, and these are dealt with under the appropriate body system in Section 5. In addition, there are other situations that require administration of FRT and/or oxygen, and these are considered under essential interventions in Section 4.

Section 2

Principles of adult nursing

Section Outline

2.1 LEGAL ISSUES

Property

In the rush and excitement of care, it is vital not to neglect or mislay any patient's property. Often the patient/family does not realize something is missing until discharge, which could be some weeks later, and difficulties can arise unless accurate records are kept. The following principles might help:

- It is always wise to keep a patient's property together and list it in detail as soon as possible in the property book on the ward (check hospital policy). Make a specific note of valuables such as money or jewellery.
- Note, too, if the patient is wearing or not wearing a watch or carrying any money so that there is a written record should any confusion arise.
- If the patient is unfit to make a decision, any valuables should be stored in a safe place in accordance with the hospital procedure (generally hospital property).
- If patients wish to remain in custody of their valuables, they need to sign a disclaimer form that the trust cannot take responsibility for the loss of personal property and that it should be deposited in the hospital safe.
- A duplicate copy of the patient's belongings list sent to the property office should always be given to the patient.
- Property should not be handed to relatives other than at the patient's specific request and written documentation of this should be kept.
- When patients leave the department, all personal property should go with them, preferably in one large bag clearly labelled with name and destination. Receipts for any items taken into safe custody should be firmly attached to the notes or given to the patient if s/he is in a fit state.

A nurse's survival guide to the ward. https://doi.org/10.1016/B978-0-7020-7831-6.00002-4

Patients' complaints

All patients have the right to make a complaint if they feel that their rights have been infringed, and such complaints must be taken seriously. A formal complaint is usually made in the first instance to the person, e.g., consultant or organization providing the service, e.g., hospital or community service involved. Alternatively, patients can make a complaint to the commissioner of that service — either National Health Service (NHS) England or the area clinical commissioning group (CCG). This can either be verbally or in writing, and is immediately reported to the senior manager who is responsible for investigating it.

The patient and liaison service (PALS) offers confidential advice, support and information about the complaints procedure, including how to get help. PALS will listen to patients' concerns and make suggestions.

The patient and any staff involved are kept informed of any steps taken. Clinical complaints should be referred to the consultant in charge of the case who will discuss how it is to be handled with the senior manager.

Most complaints can be dealt with at a local level. When a complaint is likely to involve litigation, the health authority will seek legal advice and the staff concerned should be made aware of the help that is available to them through their professional association or trade union.

The complaints procedure usually involves the following steps:

1. The complaint will first be examined by the hospital or community services management before a decision is taken as to whether to refer the case to the nurse's council.
2. The board decides whether the case should be referred to the Professional Conduct Committee for nurses namely the Nursing and Midwifery Council (NMC).
3. The health service ombudsman may be involved when a patient feels the health authority has not dealt with a case satisfactorily.
4. The health service commissioner publishes an annual report.

Incident reporting

Incident reporting helps institutes ensure a safe and secure working environment (NICE, 2012). Incident management is a process of identification, reporting, investigation and learning to minimize the risk of reoccurrence. All incidents are reported to National Reporting and Learning Systems when any patient could have been harmed or suffered some level of harm. It is important that all incidents are reported to ensure the following:

- Keep patients safe
- Protect patients from harm
- Learn from mistakes

- Take action to prevent emerging patterns
- Alert practitioners to risks and prevent avoidable harm

It is important to record all details of incidences when they occur on a ward; this should include completion of the relevant form that might include the following:

A description of the incident:

- The patient's response
- Your action or reaction to the incident
- A list of all personnel who were aware of the details of the incident
- Have relatives/carers been informed

Current organizations involved in health services

The key organizations of health services in England changed in April 2013 and are placed under the following:

- Department of health (DH) — the priorities of the DH and agencies for 2015–20 are outlined in the shared delivery plan (DH, 2018). This report has six objectives: to keep people healthy, transform primary, community and social care, support the NHS, support research and innovation, ensure accountability, create value.
- NHS, which incorporates the following:
  - NHS England
  - CCG
  - Public Health 2010

2.2 HEALTH AND SAFETY

Moving and handling

While on the wards caring for patients, you will be involved in moving and handling. Moving and handling will be a key part of working and caring for patients at the bedside. It is important the practice of moving and handling is undertaken safely, and the correct hospital policy or procedure is undertaken. Any manual handling operation must meet the following two objectives:

1. The handler needs to employ minimal effort.
2. The patient must experience minimal discomfort.

These objectives can be achieved and the risk of injury reduced by undertaking a comprehensive assessment of the task's requirements. Poor technique when handling patients can result in injury to the mover(s) and the patient, accidents leading to injury to both mover(s) and patient, discomfort and a lack of dignity for the patient being moved. Risk assessment must be undertaken when manual handling cannot be avoided and there is a risk of injury.

> **!** When moving and handling people there is a risk of causing harm, therefore a risk assessment needs to be undertaken as to the possible severity of that harm.

People handling risk assessment is the likelihood of a particular situation causing harm, taking into account the possible severity of that harm. People handling risk assessment should include the following and uses the acronym TILEE:

- **T**ask — the job to be undertaken, e.g., sit the patient up in the bed, walk the patient to the toilet, bed bath a patient etc.
- **I**ndividual — the nurse, and includes the skills/experience of the person(s) who is going to be involved and takes into consideration the height of nurses involved in the task.
- **L**oad — the patient is the load; involves ascertaining details of the patient's weight and abilities as follows:
  - Ask the patient to raise their legs while sitting.
  - What does the patient understand by simple commands?
  - Why is the patient in hospital?
  - Do they require analgesia before moving?
  - Are there any drains, catheters, cardiac monitoring trailing flexes?
- **E**nvironment — consider the area surrounding the patient, what are the constraints, consider safety and trailing flexes.
- **E**quipment — what is the most appropriate equipment to use, have the staff been trained in using it, what safety checks need to be carried out before using the equipment?

Ward staff undertaking a moving and handling procedure need to do a risk assessment prior to the moving and handling event. This must be documented, which is part of the professional duty of care. It is important to remember that safe moving and handling impacts on all nursing activities, e.g., making a bed, wound dressings, taking a patient's blood pressure and stocking shelves.

When suitable equipment such as hoists, small handling aids and electronic profiling beds are provided, these should be used, well maintained, serviced, in good working order and placed close at hand.

Training and education in the use of manual handling equipment and practices should be an ongoing process with yearly updates for all staff. The aim is to have fewer nurses injured and to increase comfort and safety for patients. Factors that contribute to safer handling are as follows:

- Trained, fit staff
- Adequate supervision

- Ergonomic assessments
- Planned maintenance
- Repair and replacement of equipment
- Control of purchasing
- Suitable and sufficient handling aids
- Influencing attitudes of patients and relatives
- Reporting and investigation of incidents
- Competent agency staff
- Sufficient staff

Many patients may be able to move themselves or assist nurses while being moved and should be encouraged to help in ways compatible with their capabilities or health status.

The principles of safer manual handling are as follows:

- Assess unavoidable handling tasks and update assessment regularly.
- Channel the effort through your legs to protect your back.
- Move your feet in turn, not your body. Turn feet successively in the direction of movement (rather than twist at the waist).
- Bend your knees when appropriate but avoid overbending.
- Keep close to the load (when safe to do so).
- Maintain the natural curves of your spine and avoid twisting.
- Wear a uniform that allows unrestricted movement at shoulders, waist and hip, with nonslip shoes that provide support.
- Try to vary your tasks (so that different muscle groups are used in turn).
- Relax and move smoothly; avoid sudden movements.
- Remember to look after yourself with enough rest, suitable exercise and a healthy diet.
- If in doubt, seek advice. **Do not risk it.**

Violence, bullying and harassment in the workplace

Violence

Violence towards staff members is any incident in which a health professional experiences abuse, threat, fear or the application of force arising out of the course of their work, whether or not they are on duty. The management of violence is necessary when the person:

- shows a predisposition to violence,
- makes a physical attack on another person or object,
- becomes disturbed to the extent that their behaviour is considered a threat to their own safety and the safety of others.

The principles underlying the management of violent persons are as follows:

- Prevention of violent incidents is the foremost principle. This may not always be possible if the following physiologic causes are the reason for the violence:
  - Brain tumours
  - Endocrine imbalance
  - Hyperthyroidism
  - Hyperglycaemia
  - Convulsive disorders
  - HIV encephalopathy
  - Dementia
  - Neurologic impairment
  - Alcohol/substance abuse
  - Pain
  - Side-effects of medication
- Restraint is always therapeutic, never corrective, and where a one-to-one violent confrontation arises, the best method is to use a breakaway technique.
- The risk of physical injury should be minimized; any restraint should be appropriate to the actual danger or resistance shown by the person.
- In all situations of violence, the locally agreed procedure for the nursing management of care of violent patients should be adhered to.
- Restraint may be necessary in certain situations, but it is always therapeutic, never corrective.

! When restraint is necessary, the risk of physical injury should be minimized; any restraints should be appropriate to the actual danger or resistance shown by the person.

- The policy for violence should include:
  - environmental and organizational factors,
  - anticipation and prevention of violence,
  - action following an incident.

Workplace bullying and harassment

The issue of bullying in the workplace is extremely prevalent yet remains underresearched in literature (Edwards and O'Connell, 2007). Although bullying appears to be categorized under the classification of violence, numerous studies do appear to adopt it as an individual issue (Edwards and O'Connell, 2007). Bullying is a form of violence. Without denial, bullying exists in all areas of society, from toddlers to the very aged. It is not specific to gender, race, age or profession. Bullying takes many forms and can be subtle, indirect, direct or completely explicit. Regardless of its format, the consequences of bullying behaviour can be detrimental to nurses' psychologic and physiologic well-being. Unfortunately, bullying is rife in the healthcare sector, especially in the nursing profession.

The impact of bullying on the victim can have an enormous range of consequences, including psychologic and physical effects on the victim, impacting on his/her personal and professional life. Individual responses include people giving up their jobs to avoid the perpetrators, victims experiencing psychologic stress, recurring nightmares, reexperiencing the trauma and moodiness, to name but a few.

> **!** As professionals, it is important to support colleagues if situations occur and follow the processes in place to discourage a workplace bullying culture.

Violence and bullying legislation, policies and guidelines

No employees of the NHS should have to experience any form of violence, aggression or bullying behaviour. There are various national and governmental policies, guidelines and legislation from 1974 to current day to protect them from such horrifying ordeals. The Government has developed guidelines (ACAS, 2014)) directed at employees and employer's responsibilities for preventing bullying and harassment in the workplace. There are also resources available for employers in order for them to effectively prevent and reduce the incidence of bullying and harassment. Procedures for dealing with aggressive patients, withholding treatment, developing local policies, development of counselling services for victims, dealing with complaints, methods of staff training and education against violence, how to record and monitor harassment and relevant legislation are all outlined in detail in the zero tolerance for workplace violence website. Employers and employees of all trusts should have access to this information, and members of the public should be made aware that any form of aggressive behaviour would not be tolerated.

Although in theory with all of the published guidelines available, there should be a reduction in violence, bullying and harassment in practice. However, violence and bullying against staff still occur. The reasons why these policies are not working need to be further explored. Perhaps NHS staff are not aware of their existence or employers are choosing not to implement them in their trusts. Regardless, the issue of violence and aggression against healthcare professionals will not be reduced until it is dealt with appropriately.

In order for a change in the working environment to occur, various actions must occur. Primarily, nurses must accept that there is a need to alter practice and have a shared vision of a healthier working climate as follows:

- The ethic of caring for each other — staff will function more profitably in a happy, teamworking environment.
- Education and training — the greatest method for overcoming change is through education: the need for education and training on how to manage and deal with abusive/violent patients and bullying.
- Provide policies, protocols and guidelines of workplace violence that exist within the hospital, including management of intrastaff bullying and abuse.

Standard infection precautions

The problem with identifying infected patients has been acknowledged and is incorporated into all areas of care to prevent the transmission of blood-borne pathogens. Standard precautions are employed to protect healthcare workers against infection by using handwashing and appropriate protective clothing (plastic aprons, goggles gloves) to prevent exposure of skin and mucous membranes to blood or body fluids.

Patients who are admitted to a hospital may already be immunologically vulnerable and invariably have a reduced immune response. This may be due to the individual patient's general condition, their inability to take nutrition or fasting practices in hospital. It might also be due to prescribed treatments or drug therapies. Therefore, the healthcare professional must be vigilant in relation to infection control practices as the patient's immune system can be severely reduced and, therefore, put the patient at risk of obtaining a hospital-acquired infection. Listed below are a number of areas where nurses may take measures in addressing the patient's potential vulnerabilities of having a reduced immune response:

- Nonsteroidal anti-inflammatory drugs (NSAIDs) — prescribed to relieve pain and work by reducing the release of prostaglandin during the inflammatory response. NSAIDs are acidic and increase the acidity of the stomach and can lead to the formation of ulcers, and strict adherence to administering these drugs after meal times is essential (Richards and Edwards, 2014). Patients taking NSAIDs should not take other protein-bound anticoagulants such as aspirin, as these displace high-protein-bound drugs from protein sites causing more free anticoagulants. These drugs reduce the inflammatory response and as such the healing mechanism may also be delayed.
- Broad-spectrum antibiotics — do not only destroy the invading bacteria but also devastate the normal flora present in the mucous membranes, destroy resident flora living in the mouth and vagina, allowing pathogens

(commonly *Candida albicans*, which causes thrush) to colonize leading to fungal infections.

- Antacids — neutralize acidity of the gastric juice and can give rise to an increase in the production of bacteria living in the stomach, small and large intestine, which can lead to diarrhoea.
- The administration of chemotherapy and radiotherapy — can depress the bone marrow and lead to increased risk of patients becoming neutropenic, which leads to an increased risk of septicaemia.
- Steroids — synthesized by the adrenal cortex as cortisol is the naturally occurring hormone. Corticosteroids are anti-inflammatory and suppress the immune response, which aids healing and can result in an increased susceptibility to infection and impaired wound healing (Galbraith et al., 2007).
- A reduced nutritional intake — for wound healing (see Section 3) requires an adequate protein intake as they supply the amino acids necessary for repair and regeneration of tissues and produce many of the proteins involved in the immune responses. Fibrous tissue is protein-based and hence scar tissue will have poorer tensile strength in those who are protein-depleted. Vitamin A is necessary for reepithelialization and vitamin C is required for collagen synthesis and capillary integrity. Zinc deficiency is thought to be associated with delayed wound healing. Zinc supplements have been shown to promote venous ulcer healing in those who were zinc-depleted. Nutrition affects the body's ability to fight infection, and a patient admitted to the hospital may have suppressed nutrition before admission or obtain poor nutritional support while in hospital (Richards and Edwards, 2014).
- Changes associated with ageing — body processes deteriorate due to age, and the innate immune system is no different: therefore, the elderly are at greater risk from developing complications due to the following:
  - Increased risk of infection — fibroblast activity reduces with age, slowing healing; the elderly have a reduced innate immune system and do not take an adequate diet
  - Reduced healing processes — collagen fibres in the skin decrease in number, and the skin becomes wrinkled and loses its elasticity, loss of subcutaneous fat, skin becomes thinner in areas not exposed to sunlight and less resistant to trauma, bruising may result from minor injuries, mitosis in the basal layer of the epidermis is slower
  - Reduced ability to maintain body temperature — due to an impaired ability to sense changes in the ambient temperature, impaired hypothalamic mechanisms and decreased metabolic processes, together with problems with mobility and exercise, compound the problem.

While in hospital patients may have a reduced innate response to an invasion of the body by bacteria and/or viruses, therefore infection control practices are imperative. Continuous audit is needed to ensure every effort is being taken to prevent the spread and multiplication of microbes.

These simple precautions should be included as part of the routine care of all patients. This level of precaution (e.g., gloves for contact with excreta, and handwashing) could prevent the transmission of many pathogens and make a major contribution to the reduction of hospital-acquired infection.

Hazards on the ward

On the wards there are particular risks to patients, staff and visitors; it is therefore important that nurses are vigilant in relation to safety on the ward as follows:

- Doors to the ward should remain closed, and strangers who are not recognized as a visitor or staff member are challenged.
- Bulky items such as noninvasive ventilation, drip stands and IV pumps have a designated storage area, as these may obstruct walkways, doorways and fire exits or cause a trip hazard.
- Slips, trips and falls from trailing wires and liquid spills are all avoidable hazards.
- Raise cot sides.
- Never leave a patient unattended in the bath, use a nonslip mat if available, check the temperature of the water and never run a bath with hot water only.
- Medical equipment, drugs, lotions and other potentially hazardous items should be kept in a locked cupboard.

! There are particular risks in clinical areas where patients are cared for, and all practitioners should carry out risk assessments within their own clinical environment.

Health issues

A definition of health is subjective and depends on an individual's life experiences. Therefore, healthcare professionals need to acknowledge that a patient's interpretation of health is highly individual and is affected by self-esteem, social support and social status. Facets of health and its management are centred on the following:

- Health promotion — this describes an approach to encouraging lifestyle changes amongst individuals and communities. It encourages people to increase their control over their health, enhancing health and its determinants.

- Health protection — is concerned with the prevention of disease and associated risk factors, achieved through vaccination, immunization, sanitation, sexual health and maternity. Surveillance is about ensuring certain diseases, e.g., infections, which are communicable, are notifiable.
- Health education — a vital aspect of both health promotion and protection and is described on three levels as follows:
  - Primary — prevention of the onset of illness, e.g., immunization
  - Secondary — shorten episodes of illness and prevent progression of ill health through prompt diagnosis, e.g., screening
  - Tertiary — limit complications from irreversible conditions, e.g., cardiac rehabilitation.
- Public health — outlines the government's strategy for reducing inequalities in health. It examines health from a political, social, environmental, economic and psychologic perspective.
- Health policy — is determined by government papers, some of which are detailed in the previous section.

Safeguarding adults

Nurses have a responsibility to safeguard the patients in their care. Safeguarding is ensuring that adults are safe and free from abuse and neglect. It includes working together to identify those at risk from abuse or neglect.

The number of areas that constitute abuse (RCN, 2015) is as follows:

- Domestic violence
- Sexual abuse
- Psychologic abuse
- Financial or material abuse
- Modern slavery
- Discriminatory abuse
- Organizational abuse
- Neglect and acts of omission
- Self-neglect
- Poor professional practice
  - Poor care standards
  - Lack of positive responses to complex needs
  - Rigid routines
  - Inadequate staffing and insufficient knowledge base within the service
- Unacceptable treatments
  - Withholding food and drink
  - Seclusion
  - Unnecessary and unauthorized use of restraint
  - Inappropriate/overuse of medication

There are also patterns of abuse as follows:

- Serial — a person seeks out/grooms a vulnerable individual
- Long-term — domestic violence
- Opportunistic — theft as money or valuables are lying around
- Situational — due to pressure of work
- Neglect — due to stress outside of work, e.g., debt, alcohol or mental health problems.

Summary

All nurses must respond if there are any concerns about safeguarding as follows:

- Be aware of what constitutes abuse/engage in training
- Recognize any signs of abuse
- Share any safeguarding concerns
- Report/document any concerns
- Refer to other agencies
- Share relevant information with other agencies/teams
- Participate in investigations
- Reflect on the incidences and learn from them

2.3 PROFESSIONAL PRACTICE ISSUES

Professional practice

This ensures that nurses can practice according to the philosophic underpinnings of their profession, creating a culture of excellence. It is about recognizing the importance of empowering the nursing workforce and improving the quality of patient care. Promoting professionalism and trust is integral to The Code (NMC, 2015) and the National Patient Safety Agency (NPSA, 2012).

Codes of practice

The NMC makes explicit a set of values and performance expectations to which all nurses can subscribe and that influences practice behaviour (NMC, 2015). A Code (NMC, 2015) outlines professional standards of practice in four areas as follows:

- Prioritizing people
- Practice effectively
- Preserve safety
- Promote professionalism and trust

The code gives direction and cohesion to registered nurses for which it has been designed. The Code has become the basis for most major guidance documents (www.nmc-uk.org) and is the template against which misconduct is judged.

Hence it is important to be familiar with the code and to discuss cases and events at ward, departmental and community levels, as well as in classrooms and study groups. All of the NMC publications can be found on their website www.nmc-uk.org.

> It is important to be familiar with the NMC code and to discuss cases and events at ward, departmental and community levels, as well as in classrooms and study groups.

Clinical supervision

Clinical supervision is an exchange between skilled practicing professionals to come together to enable them to reflect upon their practice to enhance development and improvement in their knowledge and skills. It is about exploring nursing practice and becoming more effective through helping nurses to think about and begin to reflect on their practice to improve care. Thus clinical supervision provides opportunities for the following:

- Reflection and review of practice
- Discussion of patient individual cases
- Implementation of change or modification of practice
- Identification of training and professional development needs

Clinical supervision is a dynamic, interpersonally focused experience, which promotes the development of therapeutic proficiency. One of the primary reasons for all supervision is to ensure that the quality of therapeutic work is of a consistently high standard in relation to the client's needs.

Clinical supervision is an important part of taking care of oneself and staying open to new learning, ongoing self-development, self-awareness and commitment to learning. It focuses on the essence of professional nursing practice and is linked to the process of guided reflection, which is necessary to increase effectiveness as a practitioner in today's healthcare climate.

Clinical supervision should be viewed as a way of increasing effectiveness through the provision of high challenge and high support, not as a means of monitoring and surveillance. The outcomes of using clinical supervision are suggested as follows:

- Achieving therapeutic competence, professional skills and knowledge
- Ensuring the quality and effectiveness of work with clients

However, central to clinical supervision is guided structured reflection.

Reflection

Reflective practice involves practitioners paying attention to significant aspects of experience in order to make sense of them within the context of their work. By reflecting on and taking action to resolve the contradictions that occur in practice, practitioners come to know themselves and, as a consequence, learn to become increasingly effective. Schon (1983) developed two key concepts as follows:

1. Reflection-in-action − the reflective thinking one is doing while one is doing the action.
2. Reflection-on-action − occurs, in contrast to reflection-in-action, after the experience has taken place.

Edwards (2017a,b) developed this further, which identifies a four-dimensional process to give access to improved professional practice and includes the following:

● Reflection-before-action, which requires learners to reflect before entering into clinical practice work
● An expansion of reflection-in-action and the moment-to-moment decision-making that takes place during caring for patients at the bedside
● Reflection-on-action requires looking back on a situation after it has occurred
● Reflection-beyond-action looking further forward with regard to the value of reflection, using it to facilitate self-exploration and lifelong learning

Reflection is essential for self-evaluation and improving one's clinical competency. It is argued that to reflect effectively and to practice reflectively are now requisite skills for all pre- and postregistration nurses. Reflection has become so integrated into mainstream nursing that it is easy to forget its radical origins. The root of reflection is as a source of knowledge. Reflection offers a challenge to technical rationality, the straightforward application of context-free prepositional knowledge to practice.

Reflection is a way in which professionals create new understandings of knowledge in practice; it pulls together disparate thoughts, attitudes and opinions and gives them focus (Rolfe, 2000). The use of reflection can result in new learning, development of thinking about different angles and encourage further reading to improve and develop knowledge. Therefore, there is a potential to write down and use reflection as a means of developing unique nursing knowledge.

Approaches to guide reflection and writing

There are many reflective practice tools available to assist nurses more on their reflection-on-action, from simplistic models, e.g., Gibbs (1988) (Fig. 2.1), Driscoll (2007) to the more complex ones, e.g., Johns (1994) (Box 2.1).

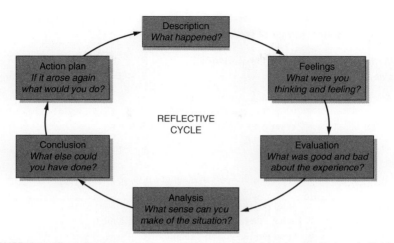

FIGURE 2.1 The reflective cycle. *From Gibbs, G., 1988. Learning by Doing: A Guide to Teaching and Learning Methods. Oxford Polytechnic FEU, Oxford.*

Gibbs' reflective cycle (1988) (Fig. 2.1) is as follows:

- Description
- Feelings
- Evaluation
- Analysis
- Conclusion
- Action plan

Driscoll's model of reflection (1994) is as follows:

- What — returning to the situation providing an account of what happened
- So what — understanding the context, identifying feelings and effects of actions
- Now what — modifying future outcomes and detailing the implications

Johns' model for structured reflection (2000) (Box 2.1) is as follows:

- Description of the situation
- Detailing issues that are significant
- Aesthetics — achieve, response, consequences, others' feelings and knowledge
- Personal — exploring feelings
- Ethics — was actions for the best
- Influencing factors

BOX 2.1 Johns' model of structured reflection

Write a description of the experience
Cue questions

Aesthetics	What was I trying to achieve? Why did I respond as I did? What were the consequences of that for: The patient? Others? Myself? How was this person feeling? (or these persons?) How did I know this?
Personal	How did I feel in this situation? What internal factors were influencing me?
Ethics	How did I feel in this situation? What factors made me act in incongruent ways?
Empirics	What knowledge did or should have informed me?
Reflexivity	How does this connect with previous experiences? Could I handle this better in similar situations? What would be the consequences of alternative actions for: The patient? Others? Myself? How do I now feel about this experience? Can I support myself and others better as a consequence? Has this changed my ways of knowing?

- Knowledge used to inform a situation
- Reflexivity — links to previous experiences, improvements, consequences of taking alternative actions, feelings about experience and support of self and others

There is a need in nursing for the development of competent practitioners who are flexible, adaptable and reflective. Reflection can highlight the need for competence, as an important consideration for determining the scope of practice. A competent practitioner is deemed to have many attributes, including critical thinking and the ability to problem-solving; a subskill of these is reflection. Continued professional development is essential in nursing, and reflective practice is suggested as one method of achieving this. Given the increased focus on reflection, it is intended within this section to review the implications of these directives.

The limitations of reflection

Reflection, in its many guises, does not always accurately verbalize or artic-ulate the complex activity of psychologically and emotionally processing the issues that trouble us as nurses in everyday clinical practice from time to time. How do we deal with and process psychologically and emotionally, e.g., the telling of a husband whose wife is dying following the birth of their baby daughter? How do you cope with or care for a mother and father whose child is brain stem dead after running into the road? How do nurses address the death of a father of three children and their seriously injured grandfather, as a result of a faceless drunk driver? How do you tell distraught parents that their child died after 2 h of resuscitation? All of these are very real issues, much of which is often left unspoken.

These events often result in a kind of ferocious emotional and psychologic assault on nurses in their everyday work. Can reflection offer a solution? There is no doubt that carefully coached thinking can clearly help and offer thera-peutic respite.

Critical thinking

To deal effectively with rapid change, healthcare professionals need to become skilled in higher-level thinking and reasoning. Critical thinking is relevant to all forms of nursing practice and can be used when situations or problems arise whereby there is no definitive answer or to make it easier to find solutions. There is not always the theoretical evidence to support practice; therefore, healthcare practitioners need to incorporate into their practice critical thinking processes to provide new answers to practical questions, which may not be answered with traditional research methods (Edwards, 2003, 2007). Everyday healthcare practitioners sift through an abundance of data and information to assimilate and adapt knowledge for problem clarification in an attempt to find solutions. Healthcare professionals need to be equipped and ready to find solutions, make decisions and solve unique and complex problems within their clinical environment.

Critical thinking is essential and plays an important part in developing students, both newly qualified and qualified healthcare professionals, to help support and interpret the often-complex issues in relation to practice. The explanations of critical thinking processes outlined in the literature are often complex. Professional bodies are promoting the concept of healthcare pro-fessionals being analytical practitioners, who are able to demonstrate critical thinking in the clinical setting. Similarly, critical thinking is widely recognized as an important part of nursing and equally essential to students and qualified practitioners alike.

The development of these cognitive processes encourages the individual to become open-minded, consider alternative perspectives and respect the right of others to hold different opinions. It is about equipping healthcare professionals with the tools needed for independent and lifelong learning.

Evidence-based practice/healthcare

For some time there has been preoccupation with evidence-based practice (EBP) in the healthcare setting. This term is now being replaced by the phrase evidence-based healthcare (EBH) by some authors. However, there do not appear to be any overarching principles that have been set to guide healthcare professions in the quest for achieving EBP. Any principles would need to take account of the current situation in respect of EBH, and this is linked to the underpinning key concepts. These key concepts include the following:

- Clinical effectiveness, practice development and (clinical) audit
- Problem-solving, decision-making, clinical judgement and expertise
- Research-based practice

EBH brings responsibilities and issues for healthcare professions, practitioners, healthcare organizations and patients alike, which are currently measured in respect of clinical effectiveness and quality. There are two key expected outcomes of EBH as follows:

- Desirable patient outcomes (which generate the necessity for active patient involvement in their care)
- Clinical effectiveness

So as well as needing to take account of all of the key concepts and features, any guiding principles must also reflect the need for patient involvement and the drive for clinical effectiveness and quality.

EBP is a highly complex concept based upon the value judgements for nursing; this will necessarily focus on the patient experience encompassing the development of a wide range of knowledge. Best evidence comes from a variety of sources. The main source is generally considered to be research. In the absence of a gold standard for generating and judging nursing research evidence, other mechanisms are necessary to ensure that best evidence is developed and used in practice.

Nursing knowledge

Nursing knowledge covers those aspects of knowledge that are relevant to nursing (Edwards, 2002b). The different types of knowledge in nursing are many and varied; the generation of knowledge therefore becomes complex. Carper (1978) identified four ways of knowing: practical, scientific, personal (including experiential and intuition) and ethical.

Aesthetic knowledge

- The importance of the art of nursing − it is expressive and viewed through action.
- Aesthetic knowledge is about expert practice and the motivation to care − the desire to care for someone and to enable them to cope with their illness or disability or to recover fully and perhaps enjoy an increased level of wellness and quality of life.
- It is about the understanding of human experience, insight into the dimensions of the human condition and the lived experiences of illness, suffering, dying, healing, pain and disability.

Empirical knowledge

- This includes empirical research, scientific enquiry, reductionism and positivism.
- This is often viewed as the only 'true' or 'valid' knowledge as it has been subjected to rigorous empirical testing utilizing mainly quantitative approaches to research.
- It includes theoretical knowledge from books, journals and conferences and draws on traditional ideas of science, including biology, sociology, psychology and pharmacology.

The use of empirical knowledge means that skill and knowledge of a particular situation must be supported by well-litigated scientific knowledge. This implies EBP and highlights that empirical knowledge needs to inform practice. Empirical knowledge is often broadened to include inductive methodologies, e.g., qualitative research.

Personal knowledge

- Is about becoming self-aware.
- It does not emanate from books, journals, lectures or academic conferences. It is also about 'we know more than we can say' or 'understanding without rationale'.
- It can be as valid as scientific knowledge and nurses can be confident in using it as a justification for actions.
- It includes both experiential knowledge and intuition.

Experiential

- Experiential includes gaining inner personal meaning from life experiences. Healthcare professionals have personal experiences such as having a baby, bereavement or a close family member spending a period of time illness in the hospital.

- These experiences develop experiential learning, which can form part of an individual's knowledge base so that they may draw upon clinical situations in the future.
- It is also knowledge that is gained from the experience of professional practice. Healthcare professionals have many clinical experiences during their years in practice, and it is these that can inform future practices when similar situations are met.

Intuition: 'just knowing'

- Intuition or tacit knowledge is widely accepted within healthcare.
- Intuition has been cited as an integral part of clinical practices.
- It helps to develop creativity and often it is not directly communicable in language.
- This type of knowledge is just a hunch, gut feeling

Ethical knowledge

- It is often thought to include questions about when to withdraw treatment, when to and when not to resuscitate a patient, allowing relatives to be present during resuscitation.
- It is also about making everyday clinical decisions, such as should you take the patient requesting to go to the toilet first or change and clean the patient who has been incontinent in the bed.
- It is about moral knowledge, decision-making and prioritizing. It includes what is good, right and responsible and involves confronting conflicting values.
- In ethical knowledge, there may be no satisfactory answer to the dilemma.

2.4 ETHICS IN NURSING

Ethical principles

Accountability

Accountability can be exercised in a number of different ways. The NMC highlight the following principles:

- The interests of the patient or client are paramount.
- Professional accountability must be exercised in such a manner as to ensure that the interests of the patients or clients are respected and are not overridden by those of the professions or their practitioners.
- The exercise of accountability requires the practitioner to seek to achieve and maintain high standards.

- Advocacy on behalf of patients or clients is an essential feature of the exercise of accountability by a professional practitioner.
- The role of other persons in the delivery of healthcare to patients or clients must be recognized and respected, provided that the first abovementioned principle is honoured.
- Public trust and confidence in the profession are dependent on its practitioners being seen to exercise their accountability responsibly.
- All registered nurses, midwives and health visitors must be able to justify any action or decision not to act in the course of their professional practice.

Responsibility

Responsibility takes three major forms as follows:

- *Responsibility for self* is often captured in a professional practice code (www.nmc-uk.org). Wilful failure to adhere to these responsibilities usually results in action to exclude the individual from the right to practice.
- *Responsibility for others* is a much more complex issue which varies according to position, degree of authority delegated and the nature of accountability to be exercised. It includes the following:
  - Concern for the safety of all in the shared work environment
  - The need to be explicit with all colleagues about authority and accountability issues as they affect both yourself and others
  - Working only within your levels of knowledge and ability.
- *Professional responsibility* entails the legitimate freedom to choose one course of action or intervention over another, combined with the responsibility for making correct choices in each clinical circumstance.

Professional responsibility is an important issue as all professionals can be required to provide service in areas in which they are not adequately prepared. This can occur because of pressure of work and because individual clients have a particular relationship with certain practitioners and seek help from someone they know and trust rather than a more appropriately prepared person. Being open about such limitations is not a sign of weakness but rather a key indicator of mature and caring practice.

Confidentiality

The nurse is under legal obligation not to disclose confidential information without the patient's consent. Disclosure of information occurs in the following ways:

- With the consent of the patient/client
- Without the consent of the patient/client when the disclosure is required by law or order of a court
- By accident

- Without the consent of the patient/client when the disclosure is considered necessary in the public interest

The NMC have published an advisory paper on confidentiality, and a summary of the principles on which to base professional judgement in matters of confidentiality is as follows:

- A patient/client has a right to expect that information given in confidence will be used only for the purpose for which it was given and will not be released to others without his/her consent.
- Practitioners recognize the fundamental right of their patients/clients to have information about them held in secure and private storage.
- Where it is deemed appropriate to share information obtained in the course of professional practice with other health or social work practitioners, the practitioner who obtained the information must ensure, as far as is reasonable, before its release that it is being imparted in strict professional confidence and for a specific purpose.
- The responsibility to either disclose or withhold confidential information in the public interest lies with individual practitioners, and they cannot delegate the decision and cannot be required by a superior to disclose or withhold information against their will.
- A practitioner who chooses to breach the basic principle of confidentiality in the belief that it is necessary in the public interest must have considered the matter sufficiently to justify that decision.
- Deliberate breach of confidentiality other than with the consent of the patient/client should be exceptional.

Advocacy

Advocacy is defined as the act of pleading a cause for another. It is a process of acting for or on behalf of someone. The word *advocacy* is not specifically used in The Code (www.nmc-uk.org), but it is implied in the first clause where nurses, midwives and health visitors exercising professional accountability must: 'Serve the interests of society and above all safeguard the interests of individual patients and clients'.

Advocacy is an important principle in nursing adult patients because it makes it clear that, generally, adults are rational. Adults are capable of making choices and decisions; however, some illnesses and specific situations may mean they lose a certain amount of autonomy and need a person to speak for them. That person might be a nurse.

Freedom, autonomy and informed consent

Autonomy

Autonomy relates to independence of action, meaning that one can perform one's total professional function on the basis of one's own knowledge and

judgement. It consists of making decisions and acting on them. To be autonomous, one must be accountable. Autonomy means the following:

- Self-rule.
- A patient is free to make up his/her own mind and act on his/her own
  decisions.
- A patient has the right to be given all the information required to make an
  informed autonomous decision about care or treatment received.
- Ethical principles of self-determination and self-governance with
  concomitant responsibility for one's own actions.

The ethical principle is important as no one has the legal right to impose
his/her will (however well intended) upon another, and everyone has the right
to determine his/her own actions and what is done to and for him/her. All
surgical interventions and delivery of nursing care, in a legal or ethical sense,
are possible solely because the client or patient has consented to them.

The principle of autonomy underlies concerns about informed consent for
surgical, medical and nursing interventions. Patients have a right to be
respected as autonomous beings capable of making decisions for themselves
and responsible for their own actions. Therefore, they need to know their
healthcare rights and responsibilities and what to expect when in hospital and
even from individual nurses, doctors and other healthcare professionals whom
they may encounter.

Consent

Consent can be defined as the 'voluntary and continuing permission of the
patient to receive a particular treatment based on an adequate knowledge of the
purpose, nature and likely risks of the treatment, including likelihood of its
success and alternatives to it. Permission given under any unfair or undue
pressure is not consent'.

In order for consent to be obtained lawfully, the patient must:

- be competent,
- be conscious,
- be mentally capable,
- have the relevant information to give consent,
- have understood information given,
- have given consent voluntary.

In the absence of consent all, or almost all, medical treatment and all
surgical treatment of an adult is unlawful, however beneficial such treatment
might be. A patient has the fundamental right to give or withhold consent prior
to examination or treatment. Sometimes it is difficult to give a patient all the

facts needed to make an informed decision. The following must be borne in mind when giving information:

- Is something being withheld so the patient makes the decision as the doctor or nurse desires?
- If all the information were given, might the patient decide not to cooperate?

Information is withheld to persuade the patient to undertake a procedure, truth telling and honesty are compromised, trust is lost and individual autonomy cannot be exercised.

Most consent is implied, such as holding an arm out for a blood test or opening the mouth for an inspection or treatment. But such consent should not be taken for granted. It is not a signature which counts but respect for the other person. When consent is not sought, for whatever reason, that person's life is devalued (see informed consent, discussed in the following section).

A person is regarded in law as able to give consent if s/he is able to understand what is being said and to make a decision based on that information. Sixteen years is generally regarded as the minimum age for consent to hospital treatment, although a 1985 House of Lords ruling established that a child could give consent to treatment if s/he fully understood the nature and purpose of the proposed treatment and the likely consequences.

Most procedures require written consent from the patient following detailed explanation by a doctor whose responsibility it is to ensure that written informed consent is obtained. For children under the age of 16, consent is generally obtained from an adult/parent who should be contacted and asked to come to the department as soon as possible.

In an emergency a doctor may decide to do the following:

- Treat a minor having received verbal consent over the telephone from a responsible adult.
- Accept the child's own consent.
- Assume consent for any treatment necessary to save life or limb or to alleviate great pain.
- Act despite refusal of consent from a patient's relative in some circumstances.

Failure to gain the consent of a mentally competent adult before touching him/her or even intending or threatening to touch may lead to legal action on charges of trespass, assault or battery. Consent may be implied, verbal or written, although the first two may be difficult to prove at a later date (see Autonomy, p. 54).

The patient who refuses treatment Patients have a full legal right to refuse consent to treatment and to take their own discharge from hospital, unless they are deemed to be of such unsound mind that they cannot be allowed to do so. If patients wish to discharge themselves you should do the following:

- Try to persuade the patient to stay and explain to him/her why the investigation or treatment is necessary.
- Tell the patient that they are leaving against medical advice.
- Contact the doctor, who will get the patient to sign a self-discharge form (discharge against medical advice form).

! Legally, patients are not obliged to sign a self-discharge form, and some refuse to do so. In any case of self-discharge, and especially if the patient has refused to sign the form, you must write a full account of events in the nursing notes.

Mental capacity act 2005 This Act governs the way in which decisions are made on behalf of people lacking mental capacity. It also includes provisions for advanced decisions to refuse treatment. It also sets out a framework in which healthcare professionals can assess the best interest of a patient who lacks capacity, together with provisions relating to medical research. In addition, the Act now makes it a criminal offence to ill-treat or neglect a person who lacks mental capacity, and such a person may be liable to a term of 5 years imprisonment.

This Act is underpinned by a set of five key principles set out in Section 1. These are as follows:

1. There is a presumption of capacity and that every adult has the right to make his/her own decisions and they must be assumed to have capacity.
2. The rights of individuals are to be supported to make their own decisions, therefore all appropriate assistance must be given before anyone may conclude that they cannot make their own decisions.
3. Individuals retain the right to make decisions even if eccentric or unwise.
4. The best interest notion prevails for incapacitated individuals.
5. Only the least restrictive intervention should be performed on an incapacitated individual to minimize their infringement of basic rights and freedoms.

The Act also sets out clear parameters for research as follows:

- Research involving incapacitated persons may be lawfully carried out if an appropriate body (normally research ethics committee) agrees that the research is safe, relates to the person's condition and cannot be undertaken as effectively on people who have mental capacity.

- If the research is to enhance new scientific knowledge, it must be of minimal risk to that individual and carried out with minimal interference or intrusion to their rights.
- Carers or nominated third parties must be consulted and agree that the individual concerned would want to join an approved research project (www.dca.gov.uk/capacity).

Applications to the High Court Applications to the High Court are made by hospitals when the following are present:

- Serious uncertainty about a patient's capacity to consent to treatment or their best interest is being jeopardized
- Serious unresolved disagreement between a patient's family and health professionals

Section 3

Identification of patient problems

Chapter Outline

3.1 HOLISTIC APPROACHES TO CARE

There are a number of elements and principles, which help to identify values and beliefs concerning the nature of nursing. This section introduces nurses to how they can further articulate and understand the full potential of their practice. It is important that nurses do not see patients in a reductionist way as just a collection of parts (brain, heart, lungs, kidneys, etc.) but try to understand their patients as a whole. Patients should be seen as members of communities and with a network of family roles and relationships. This view underscores the values and principles of holism.

The core assumptions of holism are as follows:

- The recognition that patients are whole people and cannot be viewed in reductionist terms.
- Merely isolating and examining its parts cannot understand the whole person.
- That nursing moves beyond disease management and requires that the nurse and patient collaborate to promote health.
- The environment within which individuals live must be included.
- That people live in cultural and social communities.
- People have networks of relationships with others, most notably within the family.
- That individuals have sexual needs as well as physical, psychologic and social needs.

Each health experience is unique for both the person receiving care and for the caregiver. Holism is a concept centred on the needs of the patient and the

A nurse's survival guide to the ward. https://doi.org/10.1016/B978-0-7020-7831-6.00003-6
59

nurse works with the patient from a basis of concern and mutual understanding.

Integrated care pathways

Care pathways map out a process of patient-focused care which specifies key events, tests, interventions and assessments occurring in a timely fashion to produce the best prescribed outcomes, within the resources and activities available for an appropriate episode of care (Campbell, 1998). In practice this describes, in advance, the care of patients within specific case types. The case type may be diagnostic such as hip replacement, procedural such as lumbar puncture or a condition such as pain.

Whatever the case type, there are common strands which are mapped out on the care pathway which is then used as a clinical guideline, with the practitioner using his or her clinical judgement on whether to follow the anticipated care on the care pathway or to deviate from that care. Decisions to deviate from the care may be based on a variety of causes such as follows:

- Patient condition
- Lack of consent by the patient
- Lack of resources
- Inappropriate skills of the caregiver

Such deviations are recorded as part of the care pathway documentation, thus providing a facility by which care may be individualized as appropriate. Such deviations are usually known as *variances*. It is these variances that make the difference between clinical guidelines, protocols or algorithms, none of which has the facility to actually record why the prescribed care was not given. Interventions may have much in common, but patients are different and the skill of the caregiver is to be able to differentiate and make clinical judgements about the appropriateness of the intervention. Care pathways allow clinical freedom in a way that clinical protocols do not. The care pathway has the advantage of being an audit tool. If the variances are completed correctly, an audit of the pathways will show which particular components have the most variances and why. For example, if an item on the pathway is to record the patient's blood pressure (BP), there may be many reasons why this cannot be done. If other types of guideline/protocol are used, then the action is simply not taken.

A pathway of care should, wherever possible, be multidisciplinary, agreed between all professionals and used as a multidisciplinary record of care. This eliminates separate note keeping and has the added advantage that all carers know what interventions have taken place and when, and if they did not take place, why. A clear and stated hierarchy of evidence should support the items and the sources clearly stated. Each patient within an agreed diagnostic group will have exactly the same standard of care at the same time and will not rely on any member of staff having to remember what the care should be and when to provide it. Problems can occur when no evidence is available to underpin practice, and it is recommended that 'local best practice' be used to underpin an intervention.

Research has recently showed that local best practice may be used as a generic term for the provision of care where no discussion on what this may be has taken place. If this method is to be used, then all disciplines should be involved in the decision-making and a transparent process for deciding what an intervention should be and how it was arrived at must be documented.

A pathway may be time orientated — this is over a set period of time — or goal orientated where a particular goal or target has to be reached before the patient moves onto the next. For example, for an orthopaedic patient, it may state that a physiotherapist provide active care on the second postoperative day or it may state that when the patient is pain free then active care is provided.

The pathway must be tailored to each clinical area taking into account local resources, whilst never moving away from the underpinning evidence base. There are many different templates for care pathways and the reader is directed towards Pathways of Care for more details of these and much help in pathway design and writing.

Variance tracking

As described earlier, variances are the lynchpin of care pathways and it is essential that details of such variances are recorded and analysed. The initial part of the planning process must include how variances are to be recorded and who will be responsible for tracking, analysing and reporting back on them. It can be helpful to set up a system of coding, but care should be taken not to exclude any variances from anticipated care by trying to categorize them all.

Care bundles

A care bundle is a set of evidence-based practices that when used together in a reliable way can improve patient outcomes (McCarron, 2011). What is unique about care bundles is they are structured protocols that are agreed upon and the responsibility of each clinical team member. Thus, the MDT work collectively to deliver the best possible up-to-date care using evidence-based research and practices. A simple bundle is a set of 3–5 evidence-based practices or interventions supported by research that are used together. All the elements of the bundle include a series of steps to ensure clinical improvement occurs. There are a number of care bundles available for practitioners; here are some examples:

- Ventilator bundle
- Central line bundle
- Severe sepsis bundles

- Methicillin-resistant *Staphylococcus aureus* bundle
- Stroke and transient ischaemic attack bundle
- Surface, skin, keep patient moving, incontinence, nutrition (SSKIN) care bundle

There is some evidence emerging from a study undertaken by Lavallee et al. (2017) that suggests care bundles may reduce the risk of negative outcomes when compared with usual care.

Nursing process

The nursing process provides a framework for organizing individualized nursing care that focuses on identifying and treating unique responses to actual or potential alterations in health. It consists of five steps: patient assessment, planning care, implementation of interventions and evaluation of the process and patient status:

- *Assessment* − all the patient information is gathered and examined to obtain all the facts necessary to determine the patient's health status and identify problems. This can include assessment strategies such as the ABCDE assessment.
- *Goal setting* takes place after patients have been assessed. Goals are sometimes referred to as aims of nursing, objectives, desired end results or expected outcomes of care. To be useful, goals need to be stated in a clear and precise way. One way of achieving this is to state them in behavioural terms − what you would expect to observe, hear or see demonstrated if the goal is achieved. In other words, you set a measurable response, which would be expected from the person for whom the goal is set and subsequently observed whether it has been achieved. Involvement of patients in goal setting can result in more effective achievement and greater satisfaction for those providing healthcare. However, not all patients are able to make decisions for themselves or to be full partners in setting goals, such as those who are unconscious, confused or mentally handicapped. In these instances relatives or friends may become involved in establishing appropriate goals with nurses.
- *Planning* − once problems are identified, those which need immediate attention are addressed. A plan of action is formulated which includes the following key activities:
  - Setting priorities
  - Establishing goals
  - Determining nursing interventions
  - Documenting nursing care plan
- *Implementation* − putting the plan into action, which involves the following activities:
  - Continuing to collect information about the patient

- Performing the nursing interventions and activities
- Recording the patient's health status and response to nursing interventions
- *Evaluation* – determining how well the plan has worked and whether any changes need to be made.

The purpose of the nursing process is to document information for other members of staff, to initiate support and continue observations and measurements to ensure the effectiveness of interventions.

Observation of the patient

Nurses may not realize it, but they begin to 'assess' and 'make observations' about patients from the very moment they set eyes upon them:

- Are they on a trolley or in a wheelchair?
- Are they walking using a stick or do they have a limp or an unsteady gait?
- Facial colour, pallor, flushed or cyanosed
- Respiratory difficulty, rapid or shallow breathing
- Cool, moist or dehydrated skin
- Ischaemia of the eyelids, lips, gums and tongue
- Facial expression indicating pain, anxiety, fear, anger
- Oedema of the feet, legs or sacral area
- Increased or decreased body weight; loose-fitting clothing or false teeth
- Pulsating neck veins
- Poor posture
- Dry mucous membranes

Observations are made not only of the patient's physical condition but also of indicators of his or her psychologic and emotional state too. An important point to stress is that observation depends not just on sight but also uses the senses of hearing, touch and smell.

These observations will direct the nurse's subsequent, more systematic approach to data collection, which includes further observation of specific factors.

Interviewing the patient

The admission of a patient usually commences with an interview, and it is from this structured discussion that a great deal of crucial information is obtained:

- Assess relevant health history, enquiring if there is any family history, any episodes of fatigue, restlessness, syncope or confusion.
- Ask patients to show you any medications that they are taking or take occasionally and check that the medications are taken as prescribed. If the

patient does not have the medications on hand, ask a relative or friend to bring them in to you.

- Determine any risk factors for disease, such as diabetes, a high-fat/cholesterol diet, does the patient smoke or take any exercise?
- Ask the patient about coping strategies, which may help to determine how well the patient copes with stress.
  - Determine any religious beliefs or preferences, sleeping and eating patterns.
  - Ask about psychologic status, e.g. recent bereavement, eating habits.
  - Determine social status of the patient.
  - Questions about diet, income, family concerns and job status are necessary as all can influence health and recovery.

A good nursing assessment relies heavily upon the nurse's skills in interviewing patients and nurses need to acquire a good interviewing technique. Observational skills also play a part in interviewing because information is forthcoming from patients' 'nonverbal communication', in addition, to what they actually say. Whether the nonverbal cues appear to support or contradict the verbal communication may be of importance. For example, a patient in a postoperative ward might say to the staff nurse 'No, I do not have any pain' but at the same time be showing facial expressions which indicate anxiety, uncertainty and obvious pain.

Nurses should not underestimate the importance of skilled verbal communication in interviewing. The nurse needs to learn to ask the right questions, to know how to encourage the patient to give information and, perhaps most important, to recognize nonverbal cues given by the patient.

Patient communication

Communication can be verbal and/or nonverbal, conscious or unconscious. It is an essential activity of living, which is as important as physical support. Patients often express dissatisfaction with communication during their hospital stay, which relates to the quality and amount of information received and to insufficient, confusing and contradictory information being given by different healthcare professionals.

Nurses, by giving active information, can speed up recovery and reduce the number of complications and the need for pain relief. In the acute care setting, the development of verbal skills, the giving of information and the additional use of listening skills are insufficient on their own. The nurse needs to increase his or her proficiency at monitoring and interpreting nonverbal cues from physically dependent patients who are unable to communicate verbally, due to speech loss or factors affecting speech, such as breathlessness or pain.

Nonverbal communication is the term used to describe all forms of human communication not controlled by speech and can be used therapeutically by nurses. The nonverbal component of communication is five times more influential than the verbal aspect.

Stress can be actively reduced using relaxation, and soothing techniques and caring can be conveyed through touch. Touch is a means of giving and gathering information, but consideration should be given to the fact that people are individuals, so interpretation of tactile communication will differ from person to person.

The communication process comprises five elements:

1. The sender or encoder of the message
2. The message itself
3. The receiver or decoder of the message
4. Feedback that the receiver conveys to the sender
5. The environment in which the message is transmitted

When planning to meet patients' communication needs, there are six essential areas to include:

1. Orientation to the time, day, date, place, people, environment and procedures
2. Specific patient teaching on any aspect of care
3. Adopting methods to overcome patients' sensory deficits
4. Comforting patients who are confused or hallucinating
5. Communications, which maintain the patient's personal identity
6. Helping the communications of voiceless patients

Resources, nursing actions and aids, which can be used in connection with these six areas, are suggested in Table 3.1.

It is important to remember that the information given through communication may not be remembered, especially by acutely ill patients whose drugs may interfere with information processing and storage; the patient may be unable to assign meaning to or organize the information at the time of exposure to it. This can lead to confusion and lack of memory with regard to the event.

Barriers to and interference with communication can occur at any point in the process. A summary of potential problems relating to the patient's reception of messages from the nurse in acute hospital settings is provided in Box 3.1.

3.2 ASSESSMENT

A planned assessment often takes place when a patient is admitted and is an opportunity to collect detailed, specific information in order that the most effective interventions can be offered. It is essential that the focus is not on documentation but on the patient and the importance of communication skills as an essential part of the assessment process cannot be overstated.

TABLE 3.1 Communication aids to meet patient needs
(Richards & Edwards, 2014)

Essential areas of	Resource/aid/nursing planning action

Orientation to time, place, person, people, environment and procedures	• Information regarding:
	  • treatment
	  • care
	  • progress
	  • how patient can help himself
	• Visible clock and calendar
	• Daily newspapers
	• Day and night lighting
	• Positioning near windows
	• Use of glasses, hearing aids (if needed)

Communication which maintains	• Talking about normal life, home, family interests, patient identity preferences, concerns • Offering as many choices affecting the environment as possible • Enable the patient to maintain control of his or her own body — choices, decisions
Special patient teaching	• Rehabilitation programmes after myocardial infarction • Patient information booklets • Breathing/limb exercises
Overcoming sensory deficits	• Has aids he or she usually needs • Aids are functioning and effective • Verbal descriptions of environment if the patient cannot see • Tactile manipulation of equipment
Comforting patients	• Acknowledge and accept the patient's confused or hallucinating delusions or hallucinations while stating that you do not see or believe the same thing
Helping communication of	• Communication bells to attract attention for voiceless patients • Communication cards • Pen and pad • Alphabet cards • Work out a system with the patient and ensure continuity • Speaking appliances for tracheostomy tubes

BOX 3.1 Potential problems relating to communicating in practice

Environment Distortion of the message	• Noise • Poor/bright light • Vibration • Temperature
Distractions	• Other activity • Competing messages
Patient Psychologic	• Perception altered by drugs and/or pathology • Motivation/interest in message • Attitudes/values/beliefs • Anxiety/fear • Emotions/mood • Intelligence • Self-image
Physical	• Conscious level • Sensory deficits: Hearing (impediments, tinnitus) • Sight (short/long sighted, diplopia, hemianopia, blindness) • Movement (paralysis/paresis) • Sensation (loss) • Speech (dysarthria/dysphasia/aphasia) • Constraints to movement (position, infusions, equipment) • Pain
Social	• Language • Culture/lifestyle • Isolation

A health assessment assists nurses in the identification of human responses and provides the basic data necessary to plan holistic care. It should cover areas such as follows:

- Past medical history (PMH), family history
- Episodes of fatigue, restlessness, syncope, confusion, anxiety or depression
- Current medications
- Risk factors, such as diabetes, a high-fat/cholesterol diet, smoking, lack of exercise regime, poor coping strategies
- Religious beliefs or preferences
- Any changes in sleeping and eating patterns
- Social status to determine stress levels, diet, income, family concerns and job status

Autonomic nervous system

To determine the mental state (both physiologic and psychologic), it is necessary to have knowledge of the autonomic nervous system (ANS). The ANS has two subdivisions: the sympathetic and the parasympathetic nervous systems.

The sympathetic nervous system:

- is active in response to stressors;
- is responsible for stimulating smooth muscle fibres to contract (i.e. excitation);
- stimulates the adrenal medulla to release the hormones adrenaline (epinephrine) and noradrenaline (norepinephrine).

The parasympathetic nervous system:

- is active in response to stressors;
- causes relaxation (i.e. inhibition) and is most active during sleep and rest;
- has a conserving effect on body resources.

These responses, under the control of the central nervous system, regulate other areas of the body to maintain homoeostasis. An increase or decrease in either sympathetic or parasympathetic activity in the hospitalized person can often be reflected in other observations such as the BP or heart rate. A general assessment of the patient's ANS may alert the nurse to impending neurologic overstimulation or deterioration.

The Glasgow Coma Scale

The Glasgow Coma Scale (GCS) assesses the ANS via two aspects of consciousness:

Arousal involves being aware of the environment.

Cognition demonstrates an understanding of what the observer has said through an ability to perform tasks.

The GCS was designed to:

- record conscious level and the activity of the ANS or mental state;
- assess consciousness and standardize clinical observations of patients with impaired consciousness;
- monitor the progress of head-injured patients and those undergoing intra-cranial surgery;
- detect any other neurologic disorder (cerebral vascular accident, encephalitis, meningitis);
- minimize variation and subjectivity in the clinical assessment of patients;
- provide a neurologic assessment that might indicate the level of patient dependency and subsequent need for nursing interventions.

It focuses on the evaluation of three parameters: eye opening, motor response and verbal response (Table 3.2). The patient's best achievement is recorded for each parameter. The scores are then added together to give an overall assessment of the patient's neurologic status. A score of 15 represents the best response, a score of 8 or less indicates a comatose patient, a score of 3 means the patient is totally unresponsive.

Painful stimulus

If patients do not open their eyes, obey voice commands, respond to normal interaction or gentle physical stimuli (shaking of the shoulders), spontaneously move limbs the nurse must inflict a painful stimulus and view the response. The brain responds to central stimulation, the spine to peripheral stimulation:

- Central painful stimulation:
  - The supraorbital is the recommended stimulus, but some practitioners prefer the trapezium squeeze as anecdotal evidence from doctors and nurses suggest that supraorbital pressure and sternal rub can lead to bruising.
  - For best results the stimulus should last between 20 and 30 s.
  - The same member of nursing staff, using the same painful stimulus to assess the same patient's neurologic status, should carry it out.
  - When handing over a neurological patient to another member of staff, it is recommended to undertake the GCS procedure together showing how it has been performed during that shift.
- Peripheral painful stimulation:
  - Sometimes used to assess eye opening, as central painful stimuli can often cause eye closure by inducing a grimacing effect.
  - It is applied directly to an unmoving arm or leg.
  - It will initiate a spinal reflex, and the patient will pull the stimulated part away.
  - The best method of peripheral stimulus is to apply pressure on to the nail bed at the side of the finger so as to cause no damage to the structures under the nail bed.

Inflicting a painful stimulus may not always be needed, as the patient may find objects such as nasogastric tubes and oxygen masks irritating and may localize spontaneously to such sources.

It is important to remember that the nurse's goal is to assess the brain's best response to stimulation to catch early deterioration, not to cause pain for no reason.

Pupil size and reaction to light

The normal pupil size in adults varies between 2 and 4 mm in bright light and in the dark 4–8 mm. They should both be the same size and when a light is

TABLE 3.2 The three modes of behaviour used in the Glasgow Coma Scale (GCS) (Edwards, 2001)

Response	Description	Scale
Best eye opening response	Spontaneously: opens eyes spontaneously	4
	To speech: opens to verbal stimuli; not necessarily to command of "open your eyes," a verbal stimulus may be normal, repeated or even loud	3
	To pain: does not open eyes to previous stimuli, opens eyes to central painful stimuli	2
	None: does not open eyes to any stimulus	1
Best verbal response	Orientated to time, place and person	5
	Disorientated and confused to any of the following: time, place or person; ability to hold a conversation but not accurately answering questions	4
	Inappropriate words: uses words or phrases making little or no sense, words may be said at random, shouting or swearing	3
	Incomprehensible sounds: makes unintelligible sounds (moans and groans)	2
	No response: makes no sounds or speech	1
	Other: if the patient is intubated or has a tracheotomy, document ETT or trachea; if dysphasia or aphasic document D or A	
Best motor response	Obeys verbal commands: follows commands, even if weakly	6
	Localizes to painful stimuli: attempts to locate or remove painful stimulus	5
	Withdraws from painful stimuli: moves away from painful stimulus or may bend or flex arm towards the source of pain but does not actually localize or remove source of pain	4
	Abnormal flexion and adduction of arms coupled with extensions of legs and plantar flexion of feet (decorticate posturing)	3
	Abnormal extension, adduction and internal rotation of upper and lower extremities (decerebrate posturing)	2
	No response, even to painful stimulus	1

Pupil sizes in mm

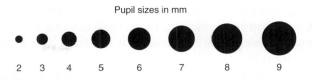

2   3   4   5   6   7   8   9

FIGURE 3.1 Pupil size observed during the Glasgow Coma Scale (GCS) assessment.

shone in one eye and constricts, the other should constrict at the same time. The pupils dilate in the dark and constrict in the light; a failure of this implies the pupil is abnormal.

Shining a torch onto the patient's eye tests pupil size and speed of reaction to light. It is important to note whether the patient has any preexisting pupil irregularities, which are normal for them, e.g. previous eye injury, cataracts, blindness in one eye or a glass/false eye. Check the following factors:

- The pupil size (Fig. 3.1)
- The pupil reaction to light: brisk, sluggish or fixed
- The shape of the pupil − should be round
- If both pupils react equally to light and are equal in size
- When undertaking the pupillary response, the following should be observed:
    - The light should be shone into the patient's eyes to see if they constrict but not directly into the patient's eyes; a torch should be shone from the side into the eye.
    - It is best to carry this out in dim lighting as one sees the eyes constrict better when light is shone on them. Protocols should exist to eliminate any inconsistencies in the patient's score (e.g. discrepancies in dimming the light during the night).
    - Progressive dilatation and loss of pupil reaction on one side occur as a result of pressure on the third cranial nerve on that side, indicating an enlarged intracranial mass (haematoma).
    - Progressive cerebral oedema eventually leads to compression of the third cranial nerve on the other side, so neither pupil then reacts to light (severe brain injury).
    - Some drugs, e.g. atropine, dilate the pupil; opiates, e.g. morphine, constrict the pupil.

Observation of vital signs in conjunction with the Glasgow Coma Scale

The last section of the GCS is the observation of vital signs:

- A high temperature can be due to damage to the hypothalamus, which increases the cerebral metabolic oxygen requirement, an unwanted complication when oxygenation of the brain may already be depleted.

- Control centres for BP, heart rate and respiration are all located in the brainstem, so damage to this area of the brain can lead to:
  - changes in rate, depth and pattern of breathing, due to increases in carbon dioxide;
  - other changes in heart rate and breathing, hypoxia, deterioration of brainstem function (Cheyne-Stokes respirations and/or central neurogenic hyperventilation);
  - increases in BP: when there is an increase in intracranial pressure (ICP), cerebral resistance occurs and in order to maintain cerebral perfusion, BP is raised.
- Neurologic observations should be recorded at frequent intervals, 1 h being the maximum time allowed.

The GCS provides a quick guide for evaluation of the acutely ill patient. The primary purpose of the GCS is to alert medical and nursing staff to deterioration in a patient's neurologic status.

> ! A continued rise in BP and reduction in heart rate in patients with suspected increased ICP are indicative that their condition is worsening.

Anxiety

A person's response to anxiety is due to activation of the sympathetic nervous system, potentiated by adrenaline and noradrenaline from the adrenal medulla. There are many factors in everyday life that provoke anxiety and hospitalization is one of them. Anxiety is difficult to define, mainly because it is often explained as a vague, uneasy feeling, the source of which is often nonspecific or unknown to the individual.

Anxiety may be both positive and negative: positive in relation to learning ability, as a high anxiety level may have a motivating function, negative in relation to particular experiences, e.g. hospitalization.

Coping with the anxiety of hospitalization can sometimes lead to aggressive behaviour as a result of anger and frustration. Alternatively, coping may take the form of escape from the anxiety-provoking situation, resulting in withdrawal, due to the person's feelings of helplessness and the inability to gain control over events.

Anxiety is present in at least some hospitalized patients, so there is a need for nurses to be able to make an accurate assessment. The assessment of anxiety relies on listening and talking to patients, questioning and discussion through interview, observation or the use of tools such as follows:

- Linear analogue scale (LAS)
- Visual analogue scale (VAS)

- Graphic anxiety scale
- Hospital Anxiety and Depression scale (HAD)

  Nurses may already be familiar with their use.

Stress

The concept of 'stress' is seen as an interaction process between the individual and his environment, rather than a single event or set of responses. Stressors make physical and psychologic demands, which require individuals to assess and understand the situation and then to respond to it.

Situations where a person can understand and react to the circumstances in a satisfactory manner are less likely to be perceived as stressful by that individual. However, if the stressor demands new responses or ones, which are underdeveloped (e.g. illness), then it is likely that the experience will lead to stress.

Hence stress is taken to be the absence of or a deficiency in the individual's ability to cope with current environmental demands. The resulting illness caused by stress is linked to increased sympathetic nervous system arousal. The body's response to a stressor is reflected by a reaction, which involves the whole body and generally consists of three distinct response phases:

1. *The alarm reaction* — widespread physiologic response which includes a large outflow into the bloodstream of adrenal hormones in an attempt to defend the body from the stressor.
2. *Resistance or adaptation* — where an attempt is made by the body to reestablish equilibrium and to regain control to maintain homoeostasis. If the body is unable to reestablish homoeostasis because of persistent exposure to the stressor then the third phase will result.
3. *Exhaustion* — ending in death.

The acutely ill individual in hospital is exposed to many stressors simultaneously. These act synergistically rather than cumulatively.

There are a number of events that make significant emotional demands upon the person while in hospital:

- Hearing the initial diagnosis may be a difficult and stressful process; the fear and anxiety generated by the news may be disruptive and debilitating, making it more difficult for the patient to absorb further information or to make informed choices.
- Perception of the situation itself is an intricate concept which may in turn be affected by past experiences, genetic predisposition, values and beliefs, self-concept and the level of anxiety at the time the stressor is perceived.
- Some treatments use powerful drugs, accompanied by side effects which may include nausea and vomiting.

- Continued exposure to stressors can result in the development of stress ulcers, reduced wound healing and cardiac function and a reduced immune response to infection, amongst other physiologic and psychologic sequelae.
- Coping with specific life events — changes which occur through choice (marriage or divorce) or may be totally unforeseen (bereavement, redundancy, accidental injury or long-term illness).

Therefore, the nurse caring for a patient in hospital needs to understand the relationship between the individual and his environment, life events and acute illness and as such take the following into consideration:

- Assessment of recent and current major life events and/or crises, as these may have precipitated the acute illness.
- Assessment of the individual's normal coping mechanisms and support networks, so that these can be enhanced or reinforced.
- Recognition that the present acute illness may cause stress in itself, particularly with regard to:
  - potential impact on employment,
  - dependent family members,
  - financial insecurity, thus making the patient more vulnerable to infection, depression and slower recovery,
  - the need to assist the patient's family members with positive coping mechanisms in a situation that may be them.

The ANS controls many other body functions and the physiologic responses to stress can influence the measurements frequently undertaken by nurses during their daily work. The physiologic responses to stress involve neuroendocrine activation and increased sympathetic activity, which stimulates the cardiovascular system and the adrenal medulla, resulting in the release of numerous substances into the circulation:

- *Catecholamines* — adrenaline increases heart rate, cardiac output, metabolic rate and blood glucose levels and causes dilatation of bronchioles; noradrenaline influences peripheral vasoconstriction, increasing BP.
- *Glucocorticoids* — cortisol from the adrenal cortex leads to gluconeogenesis, glycogenolysis, proteolysis and lipolysis and enhances adrenaline's vasoconstrictive effects.
- *Mineralocorticoids* — aldosterone increases sodium reabsorption in the renal tubules, resulting in the reduction of urine output and increase in intravascular volume, providing compensation for stress and fluid/blood loss.
- *Antidiuretic hormone* (ADH) — targets kidney tubules and inhibits or prevents urine formation. Less urine is produced, blood volume increases and the thirst response will be aroused.

Pain

Pain is one of the main symptoms that cause people to seek treatment. Pain alerts us to damaging forces in and around our bodies. The character of pain differs and can be sharp, burning or crushing. The presence of pain can interfere with obtaining accurate and reliable measurements of vital signs, which can lead to false, inaccurate readings, mask shock and therefore it needs to be assessed early. Pain arises if there is:

- local ischaemia e.g. angina,
- chemical damage e.g. leakage of enzymes in pancreatitis
- spasm of smooth muscle e.g. colic,
- over distension of a hollow organ e.g. the bladder,
- irritation of the peritoneum, pleura or pericardium,
- stimulation of the inflammatory immune response and release of mediators.

Regular assessment of pain contributes to the quality of communication between nurse and patient and regular pain assessment can be a contributory factor in reducing pain.

Before effective treatment of pain, accurate assessment is essential. Because of its subjective nature, only patients can measure their own pain accurately and so nurses should provide simple pain assessment tools to help them assess and communicate their pain:

- *The visual analogue scale* — a straight line, usually 10 cm in length, with one extreme marked 'no pain at all' and the other end marked 'worst possible pain'. Descriptive words may be added.
- *Numerical rating scales* are marked 0–10, with 0 signifying 'no pain' and 10 meaning 'unbearable pain'.
- *Verbal rating scales* or verbal descriptors use 4–5 preset categories and consist of a list of adjectives that describe levels of pain intensity by extremes ('no pain', 'mild pain', 'discomfort', 'severe/distressing pain', 'excruciating/very severe pain').
- *The Bourbonnais pain assessment tool* — two pain assessment tools designed to complement each other, one for the patient and one for the nurse. The tool consists of two parts: a scale ranging from 0 (reflecting no pain) to 10 (reflecting excruciating pain) and a list of adjectives, which describe different perceptions of pain. The person experiencing pain is then asked to match the word or words that describe his pain to the number, which corresponds to the intensity of the pain.
- *The London pain chart* — includes a body outline to record the site of pain, a verbal descriptor scale for intensity and measures to relieve pain.

It is important that the same tool is used throughout and that the tool chosen is the most appropriate for the patient's needs at that particular time. Also, when assessing patients' pain, it is vital to listen to what they are saying about their pain. Nurses persistently rate patients' pain as less than the patients do themselves.

- *The behaviour pain scale* — developed for use in critical care patients who are unable to vocalize their pain, criticized a patients pain varies and may lead to undertreatment.

There are some pain assessment tools that have been devised for specific conditions such as follows:

- Pain assessment in advanced dementia scale (PAINAD)
- Abbey pain scale for those patients who find it difficult to verbalize
- Neuropathic pain scale (NPS) designed to assess distinct qualities associated with neuropathic pain
- Oswestry for low-back pain or back pain functional scale
- Arthritis impact measurement scales (AIMS) for arthritis
- Osteoarthritis symptom inventory scale (OASIS)

Once assessed, it is imperative that the pain is treated, as a failure to relieve pain is morally and ethically unacceptable (see Section 5 for pain relief). Pain can have a detrimental effect on a patient's condition and can significantly slow recovery. The undertreatment of pain can lead to the following:

- Decreased tidal volumes (TVs) and alveolar ventilation, leading to decreased oxygen delivery to organs;
- Avoidance of coughing, resulting in an increase in secretions contributing to atelectasis and chest infections;
- Avoidance of movement, leading to an increased risk of deep vein thrombosis and pulmonary embolism;
- Increased stress response and sympathetic stimulation, resulting in vasoconstriction and tachycardia, raising BP and increasing the workload of the heart.

    Stress interferes with intestinal smooth muscle and leads to an increase in metabolic rate, leading to difficulties in meeting nutritional needs and possible loss of weight.

Ongoing assessment of pain

- Consider the severity of the pain and take into consideration the signs of distress such as follows:
  - Tachycardia, hypertension, restlessness, lack of movement
  - Crying, moaning, screaming, grimacing, cringing, furrowing of brows
  - Less interaction, not cooperating, less eye contact, difficult to gain attention, seeks comfort
  - Not eating, sleeping less or more
- Response to treatment

- Consider the nonphysical aspects of pain:
  - Anxiety about treatment and meaning of the pain
  - Helplessness and depression
  - Social concerns

Undermanagement of pain

Healthcare professionals

- Poor knowledge of pain management
- Inappropriate attitudes (cancer pain is inevitable)
- Poor clinical skills (assessing pain)
- Inappropriate beliefs regarding the management of cancer pain (fears of addiction and tolerance to opiates)
- A lack of appreciation of the nonphysical manifestations of cancer pain

Individual patient

- Low expectations of pain management and a belief that pain is inevitable
- Inappropriate beliefs regarding pain management strategies (fear of addiction and tolerance)
- Beliefs that side effects of medication are inevitable (sedation)

Good pain relief can reduce these responses to pain and lead to a safer and improved recovery.

The use of pain assessment tools in the unconscious patient can prove to be ineffective and inapplicable, as patient cooperation is required to evaluate their degree and level of pain. It is therefore paramount that nurses take pain assessment to the next level of specialized care. Within a ward setting, the bedside nurse must be adequately equipped to take into account and interpret the patient's physiologic parameters as an early indicator of pain, e.g. elevated BP, tachycardia and sweating are all recognized signs of pain.

Pain is a complex and controversial issue; it involves many body structures and much is talked about in relation to its origin and theory. There is no doubt that the nurse plays an important role in the management of pain. Pain can be avoided, leading to better patient satisfaction and quality of life. Nurses must move towards effective care in this important area of clinical practice.

Respiratory assessment

Respiration is an essential body function necessary for the diffusion of gases between the alveoli and blood as well as the maintenance of blood pH. Ventilation is the mechanical movement of gas or air in and out of the lungs. Effective respiration is dependent on many factors, both nervous and chemical in nature, including the chemoreceptors and lung receptors, which control depth, quality and pattern of breathing. Observation of respiration itself can be considered in terms of quality, rate, pattern and depth.

Rate

The normal rate at rest is approximately 14—18 breaths per minute in adults and is faster in infants and children. Changes in the rate of breathing are defined as tachypnoea, an increase in respiratory rate, or bradypnoea, a decrease in respiratory rate.

Depth

This is the volume of air moving in and out with each respiration, normally measured as the TV of about 500 mL, which is constant with each breath. Normal relaxed breathing is effortless, automatic, regular and almost silent. Dyspnoea is breathlessness and an awareness of discomfort with breathing.

Pattern

The pattern of breathing changes in disorders of the respiratory control centre and becomes irregular. The respiratory pattern is normally regular and consists of inspiration, pause, longer expiration and another pause. In certain diseases, the pattern changes:

- *Hyperventilation* is an increase in both the rate and depth of respiration to about 20—30 breaths per minute.
- *Apneustic* is a pattern of prolonged, gasping inspiration, followed by extremely short, inefficient expiration.
- *Cheyne-Stokes* is periodic breathing characterized by a gradual increase in depth of respiration followed by a decrease in respiration, resulting in apnoea.

Undertaking a respiratory assessment

Sight, hearing and touch all play an important part in undertaking a respiratory assessment. In order to carry out an efficient assessment of the respiratory system, a systematic approach should be adopted. The respiratory rate is a good indicator of respiratory function, e.g. if a respiratory rate is >30 or <8, this is indicative of a respiratory problem. In the spontaneously breathing patient, those who are experiencing a tachypnoea >30 bpm or bradypnoea <5 bpm need to be reviewed by medical staff because nontreatment may result in a form of respiratory failure. In ventilated patients who are breathing in a spontaneous mode and are experiencing an increased respiratory rate, this may indicate that they are distressed and struggling to oxygenate effectively.

Apart from rate, the rhythm and depth are also informative indicators of how a patient is breathing. Irregular breathing or the appearance of excessive respiratory muscle effort can both be considered as indicators that the patient is not oxygenating effectively.

Auscultation of the chest

Auscultation is the skill of listening to a patient's breath and heart sounds through a stethoscope. When undertaking the skill of auscultation, you should ensure that you can hear air entry to both sides of the chest. In a normal chest, you are likely to hear three types of air entry sounds as you move around the chest. These are as follows:

- *Bronchial* — These sounds are loud and high pitched and sound like air being blown through a hollow pipe. The expiratory phase is longer and louder than the inspiratory. Normally they are heard only over the upper part of the sternum. They are only heard elsewhere in the lungs when there are respiratory problems.
- *Bronchovesicular* — These sounds are a combination of vesicular and bronchial and are heard mainly in the first and second intercostal spaces near the sternum. The inspiratory and expiratory phases are about equal, and like bronchial sounds they are not normally heard elsewhere when there are respiratory problems.
- *Vesicular* — These sounds are normally described as relatively soft and low pitched, with sighing or gentle rustling sounds heard over the peripheral parts of the lung. Another characteristic is that the inspiratory phase is longer than the expiratory phase and there is no pause between each of these.

Other sounds include the following:

- *Bronchial breathing* — is caused by the transmission of bronchial sounds through consolidated lung tissue to a part of the lung where they are not normally heard.
- *Crackles* — are short, explosive and nonmusical and can be either coarse or fine. They can vary in quantity from scanty to profuse and can occur during either inspiration or expiration and can be heard early or late in the respiratory cycle. Crackles are caused by sputum in the bronchi and trachea or by the uneven opening of the alveoli during inspiration. Coarse crackles are often found in critical care patients with bronchiectasis, while fine crackles are often associated with pulmonary fibrosis.
- *Wheezes* — are associated with musical noises; these can consist of monophonic (single), multiple short or long 'notes' (polyphonic) of a high or low pitch and can occur during inspiration or expiration. Monophonic wheezes start and end at different times and often present in patients suffering with asthma symptoms or pulmonary obstructions, e.g. bronchial tumours, whereas polyphonic wheezes consist of different notes starting

and finishing at the same time and often associated with acute and chronic obstructive airways disease.

- *Stridor* — is a particular type of wheeze which originates from a laryngeal or tracheal obstruction. It is distinctive and can be heard without the aid of a stethoscope, from a distance. It is most commonly heard in patients postextubation who have developed laryngeal oedema, but it can also be heard in patients with a partial upper respiratory obstruction.
- *Pleural rubs* — are present in patients whose normally smooth and well-lubricated pleural membranes have become inflamed or thickened and can no longer pass easily and silently over one another. The sound is often longer and lower pitched, in comparison to a crackle. Pleural rub sounds vary depending on whether a large section of the chest wall is involved and they have the ability to reverse their sounds between inspiration and expiration.

Cardiac assessment

The heart rate and BP are discussed in observations and measurements section, but they are important elements of cardiac assessment. In addition, consider the following:

- Capillary refill time (CRT) is when pressure is applied to a finger or thumb and the time taken for colour to return to an external capillary bed after blanching has occurred, the normal is less than 2 s
- Jugular venous pressure
- Urine output
- Chest pain location, when it occurred, intensity, type, duration, radiation, associated with other symptoms
- 12-lead ECG is measured
- Sweating
- Nausea

The assessment of many of these interventions is dealt with elsewhere in the book.

Assessment of the skin

Loss of homoeostasis in body cells and organs reveals itself on the skin. The skin is an organ from which a great deal of information can be obtained:

- Nutritional status
- Fluid balance
- Circulation
- Emotional state and age

The skin can provide clues leading to the diagnosis of a patient's health problems and to an evaluation of the effectiveness of the patient's care, both nursing and medical. Assessment of the skin involves consideration of the following.

Age

- Skin tends to become drier or more wrinkled with age.
- The general state of grooming gives a clue to the patient's physical or mental state.
- Toenails may be neglected because of arthritis, which makes it difficult for the patient to reach them.

Observation of the skin

- Indication as to the patient's physical condition.
- It may indicate signs of shock, anaemia, high temperatures, reduced oxygen or a particular disease or condition.

Skin colour – great importance in assessment of a patient

- Pallor:
  - Skin is dependent on blood flow through the surface vessels. When blood flow is reduced, pallor will occur owing to the vasoconstriction in response to stimulus.
  - Occurs in other conditions such as myocardial infarction (MI) and exposure to a cold environment.
  - During stress adrenaline causes selective vasoconstriction and noradrenaline causes the blood vessels of the systemic circulation to vasoconstrict.
  - Anxiety and pain may also lead to the appearance of pallor.
- Anaemia:
  - Surface vessel blood flow is adequate, but the haemoglobin concentration of the blood is low.
  - Oxygen saturation monitor is not a good estimate – all haemoglobin present in the blood will be fully saturated giving a normal reading.
- Look at the mucous membranes, e.g. inside the lips or lower eyelid – as blood vessels lie nearer the surface colour can be observed.
- Flushing:
  - An increased blood flow of normal haemoglobin content to the surface of the skin – a red appearance of the skin.
  - In hot weather, cutaneous vessels will dilate to facilitate heat loss from the skin surface.

- In inflammation vasodilatation occurs over the affected area, and redness is a characteristic feature.
- Cyanosis:
  - It occurs when more than 5 g/dL (0.74 mol/L) of Hb.
  - A blue colouration occurs relatively frequently in patients with polycythaemia but is rarely seen in those who are anaemic.
  - It is difficult to assess in black patients whose skin pigments may obscure the condition. The inside of the lips, palms of the hands and soles of the feet may give some indication of the problem.
  - It occurs in individuals suffering from diseases which result in a reduced amount of oxygen being carried by the blood (hypoxaemia), which may be:
    − central and occur over the face or lips.
- Peripheral, where the extremities are affected − usually indicates inadequate or sluggish blood flow in the peripheral tissues.
- Jaundice:
  - An abnormal yellow skin tone − a sign of a liver disorder caused by the accumulation of bilirubin in the blood.
  - Bilirubin is the waste product of red blood cell breakdown by the spleen − 99% is excreted as bilirubin in bile; the other 1% is excreted in the urine as urobilinogen.
  - If bilirubin cannot be excreted in bile owing to an obstruction any excess is excreted in the urine or deposited in body tissues.
  - The earliest sign of jaundice can be detected in the urine.
  - A yellow discolouration of the skin is most easily recognized in the conjunctiva, before leading to changes in skin colour.
  - It becomes evident when plasma bilirubin levels rise above 34 mmol/L (normal less than 19 mmol/L).
  - A slightly yellow appearance may be apparent in the skin in the later stages of malignant disease when cachexia exists.

Scars

- The presence of scars, striae and bruising on the skin can be significant.
- Injection marks may give a clue to drug abuse or to conditions requiring prophylactic medication by injection, such as diabetes or haemophilia.
- Small bruises like dark purple purpura, which are evident in septicaemia, should be considered in relation to the patient's condition.

Palpation of the skin

- The feel of the skin can give information about the patient's fluid balance, state of nutrition and health.

- Moderate and severe dehydration: assessed by gently but firmly pinching up a fold of skin on the back of the hand or on the inner forearm.
- In a well-hydrated person it will immediately return to its normal position.
- In the patient who is in an advanced state of dehydration, the fold of skin may stay pinched for up to 30 s.

Oedema

- Oedema is an abnormal collection of fluid in the tissues — the causes are varied.
- Oedema is a problem of fluid distribution and does not necessarily indicate fluid excess.
- It is usually associated with weight gain.
- Swelling and puffiness.
- Tight-fitting clothes and shoes.
- Limited movement of an affected area.
- Symptoms of an underlying pathologic condition.
- Oedema is recognized by pressing firmly over a bony prominence such as the medial malleolus of the ankle for about 5 s — waterlogged tissue retains the imprint of the finger (pitting oedema).

Obesity

- Skinfold callipers are used to assess superfluous subcutaneous fat.
- Obese skin feels flabby and may wobble when pushed.
- An obese patient who has experienced rapid weight loss may have folds of skin on the abdomen and buttocks.

Temperature

- A relative temperature can be obtained by feeling the skin.
- Will feel warm over an inflamed area — inflammation or over an area of increased blood flow.
- When circulation to a specific area of the skin is increased — swelling and pain in the calf of the leg — a DVT may be provisionally diagnosed.
- Will feel cool or cold over an area of skin that is shut down owing to reduced blood flow.
- It is usual to employ the back of the hand for testing skin temperature — this area has a more constant blood flow.

! The skin can be a powerful observation tool when assessing a patient. It requires no invasive technology, just the experience and knowledge of the nurse undertaking it. The powerful knowledge about a patient's condition that a simple skin assessment can provide requires no further discussion.

Skin care

- Keep the skin clean and well hydrated; dry skin can become rough and scale.
- Wash with warm water using a mild cleansing agent; this will minimize excessive dryness.
- Do not use excessive friction and rubbing during washing, as this can lead to tissue damage through shearing forces.
- Use appropriate manual handling equipment and techniques to prevent mechanical injury to the skin.
- Turning of patients regularly introduces a turning regime and uses pressure relieving mattresses or equipment.
- If the skin becomes soiled, wash quickly to ensure good hygiene.
- Use of a barrier cream or moisturizing agent is recommended.
- Undertake a nutritional assessment if required.

Pressure area risk assessment

Pressure ulcers are an avoidable complication of bed rest and decreased mobility. Patients at greater risk of developing pressure ulcers include:

- Those who are in a poor state of health;
- Those who are malnourished;
- Those with some degree of immobility, particularly the elderly;
- The pathogenesis of pressure ulcers is complex because it is affected by so many predisposing factors. However, there are three major factors identified as significant:
  - Pressure greater than 25 mmHg will occlude capillaries. The tissues are thus deprived of their blood supply, and if the pressure is maintained for a sufficient length of time, the ischaemic tissues die.
  - Friction is caused by dragging patients up the bed, which can seriously damage the microcirculation and lead to pressure ulcers.
  - Strain on structures so great that it tears the muscle and skin fibres from their bony attachments.

A patient suffering from a combination of predisposing factors is more susceptible to developing pressure ulcers. Predisposing factors can be subdivided into two main groups:

1. *Intrinsic factors* − aspects of the patient's condition, mental, physical and medical states, e.g. malnutrition, age, altered consciousness, immobility.
2. *Extrinsic factors* − external effects of drugs, treatment regimens, patient handling techniques, personal hygiene, weight distribution.

Those patients at greatest risk of developing pressure ulcers may be identified using a pressure ulcer prediction scale. There are several pressure ulcer risk assessment tools including the following:

- Waterlow scale
- Braden scale
- Gosnell scale
- Norton scale

The Waterlow scale is the most widely used pressure ulcer risk calculator in the UK but the Braden Scale is often preferred because it is generally more reliable and valid, as the Waterlow scale tends to over predict risk. It is important to note that both scales are overcautious and potentially over predict pressure ulcer risk. Yet it is better to overpredict than underpredict risk, as the cost of treating pressure ulcers is high, while the cost of preventing them is considerably less.

All patients admitted to hospital should be assessed for risk of pressure ulcer development within 2 h of arrival. This requires a comprehensive approach including the evaluation of all risk factors:

- Build/weight for height
- Condition of skin
- Nutritional status
- Continence status
- Neurologic deficit
- Mobility
- Sex/age
- Major surgery/trauma
- Medications

Some patients may have multiple factors and increases their chances of developing a pressure ulcer.

However, it is important to realize that a risk assessment score is not a definitive answer to the question of whether an individual will develop a pressure ulcer, as there are problems associated with risk assessment scores e.g. validity and reliability, appropriate for clinical setting, not familiar with the tool, inconsistent evaluation of patients' risk status and documentation. However, pressure ulcer risk assessment can be an aid to professional and clinical judgement in determining what resources are needed. If used effectively, the calculator can justify a request for resources, e.g. specialized beds and/or efficient moving and handling equipment.

Grades of pressure ulcers and other wounds
Grade I

- Nonblanching erythema of intact skin — red, discoloured area that does not blanch when light finger pressure is applied to it showing damage to the microcirculation

- Observe for change of colour as compared with surrounding skin
- Warm, oedema − an area that is hotter than the surrounding tissue indicates inflammation and is the first stage of pressure ulcer formation
- May be painful

Grade II

Partial thickness of skin loss involves epidermis, dermis or both.

- Blistering or abrasions
- Ulcer formation is superficial without bruising
- Moisture lesions may appear

Grade III + unclassified

- Full thickness skin loss, subcutaneous fat may be visible, but no bone, tendon or muscle are visible
- May develop deep fissures
- Tissue loss may be obscured by slough (yellow/white patches of dead tissue)
- Necrosis − dark area under the skin or black eschar on the skin

Grade IV

- Full thickness tissue loss and exposed bone, tendon
- Can extend into the muscle or other structures

These symptoms can be seen in other wounds not caused by a pressure ulcer. Alongside pain assessment needs to be undertaken, as this will reduce mobility and lead to worsening of the pressure ulcer. Any observation of an infection (excessive exudate, pus, offensive smell) needs to be investigated further, e.g. wound swab.

Wound assessment

Wound assessment is a complex task that provides necessary information before deciding on a strategy for treatment. Using a measurement tool to assess wounds encourages consistent intervention irrespective of who assesses the wound at any time.

A guide to wound assessment should consider the following:

1. Classification of the wound:
   - Mechanical surgical or traumatic wound
   - Chronic leg ulcers, pressure ulcers

- Burns chemical or thermal injuries further classified by depth of the wound
- Malignant primary lesions such as melanomas
2. Information that assists wound assessment age, social, psychologic, nutrition, medical condition, drug therapies
3. Assessment of the wound, a good wound assessment should include the following:
   - A body diagram to record the patient's wound sites; in the case of multiple wounds these should be numbered individually
   - A separate assessment sheet should determine the site of each wound and/or the number identified from the initial body diagram
   - The grade of the wound(s) 1–4 (see pressure ulcer grades)
   - Assessment of the skin surrounding the wound e.g. erythema, excoriation, induration, maceration
   - Consideration of the major areas in relation to the condition of any wound (Box 3.2)
   - The maximum dimensions, traced and recorded, giving the length, width and depth of the wound in centimetres
   - The nature of any wound exudate, clear fluid or pus
   - The pain related to the wound, nature, cause and severity
4. Additional techniques such as technology, the following may be included into the assessment:
   - Doppler ultrasound
   - Duplex scanning
   - Photoplethysmography (PPG)
   - Computed tomography (CT) or magnetic resonance imaging (MRI)
5. Treatment objectives cleaning, debridement/desloughing, exudate control and/or bleeding, reduce risk of infection, wound dressing
6. Documentation and record of progression of the wound

Charting wound healing facilitates accurate recording of observations and wound treatment. Which wound assessment documentation tool used is largely a matter of personal preference, so long as the user is aware of the tool's limitations. It is of paramount importance that the patient's wound(s) are assessed as soon as possible after admission and that the risk is reassessed whenever there is a significant change in his condition.

Nutritional assessment

Assessment of nutritional status is often omitted. However, most nurses are familiar with the use of assessment forms and protocols, including pressure ulcer management and risk assessment scales, which demonstrate how a simple tool employed at an early stage of patient contact can optimize care to produce the best outcome.

BOX 3.2 Major areas that should be included in a wound assessment

Record of wound site	• Body diagram from different angles
	• Back
	• Front
	• Legs:
	  • Front
	  • Back
	  • Medial
	  • Lateral

Condition of wound	• Wound dimensions • Nature of wound bed • Exudate • Odour • Pain (site, frequency, severity) • Wound margin • Erythema of surrounding skin • Condition of surrounding skin infection
Dimensions/drawing	• Length • Width • Depth • Outside tracking • Healthy granulating tissue • Sloughy areas
Documentation	• All these points need to be taken into consideration when documenting nursing observations and wound treatments in relation to wound care

Nutritional assessment can be as simple or as complicated as desired but should be both subjective and objective. Information should be based on nurses' observations of the patient and on the collection of an essential core of material using the ABCDs of nutritional assessment.

A = Anthropometric measurements

One of the most important anthropometric measurements in determining nutritional status is weight and changes in body weight can indicate the severity of malnutrition, a loss greater than 10% being indicative of malnutrition and a loss of 6%−10% being potentially significant. It is important to note that weight is affected by certain disease processes, such as cancer, cachexia and oedema, which minimize its usefulness as a measure of nutritional status. Ideal weight charts must be used with caution, as they do not take into account the effects of dehydration and fluid retention on weight. The charts are designed for the younger population and take no account of varia-tions in weight owing to illness or age.

Height can also be used to determine malnutrition, but it is not always possible to measure height in hospitalized patients, and it may not be an adequate guide in elderly patients. It is sometimes easier to ask the patient how tall he is — most people have a good idea and this is better than nothing.

Height and weight measurements can be used to determine body mass index (BMI), which is calculated by:

$$\text{Weight (kg) divided by height (metres) squared}$$

The normal range is 20—25 and a BMI of less than 20 could be a serious risk to health.

More complicated anthropometric measurements can be used to gain more accurate information and can be useful in oedematous or dehydrated patients where body weight figures are meaningless. Body fat content is quickly and easily estimated from skinfold thickness measurements. Most commonly used is triceps skinfold thickness (TSF) which, in combination with mid-upper arm circumference (MUAC), can be used to calculate mid-arm muscle circum-ference (MAMC) as an absolute index of muscle mass:

$$MAMC = MUAC - 0.3142 \times TSF$$

Body fat percentage is essential to keep you warm; however, too much can lead to a higher risk of diabetes and other health problems; too little can reduce resistance to disease and lack of energy. Body fat percentage can be measured in a number of ways:

- Dividing weight by the square root of height can provide a rough indication of whether a person is underweight, normal or overweight
- Body fat percentage calculators, scales, using callipers

Normal ranges

- Women between 20% and 35% approximately
- Men between 10% and 25% approximately

These measurements can be compared with standards and, if performed serially, will reflect a change in body tissue. These measurements are reliable only if undertaken by a trained operator and are not always accurate or a true prediction of changes in body mass in overweight or elderly patients.

B = Biochemical measurements
Serum albumin

With a level of less than 35 g/L being indicative of protein energy malnutrition, it can be inaccurate as conditions such as stress, nephrosis and burns also exhibit hypoalbuminaemia. Thus the measurement is often misleading and not altogether reflective of nutritional deficiency in the short term. In the chronic situation, serum albumin remains a simple and reliable indicator of malnutrition.

Serum transferrin

Levels could be considered a better marker of acute nutritional depletion. Interpretation of serum levels is complicated by factors such as iron deficiency, which directly affects transferrin production, and so it may not be wholly appropriate as a predictor of malnutrition.

Serum haemoglobin

Measurements will highlight the presence of anaemia, which has been correlated with pressure sore development. Anaemia can occur for a variety of reasons but may be directly related to dietary inadequacy and questioning of dietary intake should always follow this up.

C = Clinical assessment

This includes patient history, psychologic and social status, physical examination, diet history and appraisal of current nutritional intake, anthropometric measurements, biochemical and laboratory data.

Patient history, psychologic and social status

A concise history provides the first clues about existing or potential malnutrition. The following patient factors are important:

- Recent bereavement
- Been ill at home for a long time
- Age
- Is she or he on income support?
- The type of accommodation she or he lives in.

    Observe the patient:

- Does she or he look thin?
- Assess the skin in terms of colour and condition.
- Are his or her clothes loose?
- Do his or her dentures fit properly?

    These factors will all suggest that a problem with nutrition may exist and may also give information about any recent loss of weight.

Physical examination

A physical examination should include the following areas:

- The oral cavity
- The presence of dysphagia, which may cause difficulty in chewing and swallowing, or any physical difficulties with feeding

- Any nausea, vomiting, diarrhoea, which result in reduced absorption and appetite
- Any constipation will affect nutritional intake and can lead to a feeling of fullness, discomfort, depression and confusion, thereby reducing food intake
- Simple respiratory function tests can be recorded, such as vital capacity, maximum inspiration, maximum expiration, to determine respiratory muscle strength

D = Diet history

A diet history should consist of questions about the following:

- Likes and dislikes
- Changes in weight
- Type, quantity and texture of food eaten since the onset of illness, as disease often alters appetite
- Any changes in taste and the ability to obtain and prepare food

All these factors should be recorded in the patient's assessment and nursing care plan.

Undernutrition

Promising results have been demonstrated when nutritional assessment has resulted in initiation of preoperative feeding regimens. This method of identifying high-risk patients results in an optimization of their nutritional status and may help to ensure an uneventful recovery. The patient in hospital not only has an increased demand for energy but also, owing to periods of reduction or cessation of nutritional intake, has a reduced supply of energy-containing nutrients. As a result, undernutrition or, in severe cases, malnutrition may occur.

Undernutrition reduces the body's ability to:

- heal wounds, which increases the risk of pressure ulcers;
- produce haemoglobin, which reduces the oxygen-carrying capacity of the blood;
- produce white blood cells, causing suppression of the immune response and exposing the patient to the risk of infection;
- maintain adequate respiratory drive due to reduction in pulmonary diaphragmatic muscle mass and strength, predisposing the patient to respiratory failure.

All patients should be screened when first admitted to hospital and at regular intervals thereafter. The British Association for Parenteral and Enteral Nutrition (BAPEN) has developed the malnutrition universal screening tool

(MUST), which is a tool that can be used in all adult care settings in both hospital and community settings (Elia, 2003). There are five steps:

Step 1 — measure height and weight and calculate the patient's BMI score.
Step 2 — note the recent percentage weight loss and score using the appropriate table provided.
Step 3 — establish the acute disease effect score.
Step 4 — add the scores from steps 1, 2, and 3 together to obtain an overall risk of malnutrition.
Step 5 — use management guidelines and/or local policy to develop a care plan.

3.3 OBSERVATIONS AND MEASUREMENTS

Obvious examples of measurements are heart rate, pulse rate, respiration, oxygen saturation and mental state, BP, temperature, central venous pressure (CVP) and urine output. These measurements may be carried out to substantiate information obtained from observing, interviewing or assessing the patient.

Heart rate

The heartbeat originates in the sinoatrial node and shortly after the atria contracts. It is followed by a short pause whilst the contraction wave moves down the bundle of His to the Purkinje fibres. The ventricles contract and blood is ejected from the right ventricle into the pulmonary artery and from the left ventricle into the aorta. The ventricular muscle relaxes and the heart returns to its initial position. There is then a long pause, when all chambers are relaxed before the next beat occurs.

The heart beats continuously for the whole of a person's life. Each impact of the heart against the chest wall can be felt or heard with a stethoscope, in the fifth left intercostal space, generally under the left nipple often termed the *apex beat*.

Pulse rate

The rhythmic contraction of the left ventricle transmits a pressure impulse through the arteries. This pulse is customarily palpated at the radial artery in the wrist. The important factors to consider in relation to the radial pulse rate are as follows:

- Rate
- Rhythm
- Pressure (volume)
- Deficits with apex rate

The pulse rate is an important component of cardiac output. Fluctuations of pulse rate in the well individual normally occur together with fluctuations in stroke volume to maintain optimum cardiac output for the activity being performed, for example rest or exercise.

In the resting adult, the pulse rate would normally be about 70 beats per minute. A rate greater than 100 beats per minute is termed a *tachycardia* and a rate less than 60 beats per minute is termed a *bradycardia*.

The rhythm of the pulse may vary normally with respiration, especially in young adults, so that the pulse is irregular, speeding up at the peak of inspiration and slowing down with expiration. This is termed *sinus arrhythmia*. An irregular pulse is commonly categorized as regularly irregular or irregularly irregular. A regularly irregular pulse is most likely to be caused by ectopic beats (a beat originating from a site other than the sinoatrial node), which occurs prematurely. Occasionally odd ectopic beats may occur in healthy individuals. If they are found to persist in an acutely ill person, the medical staff will require notification as they can be indicative of:

- inreased cardiac irritability due to ischaemia or drugs (such as digoxin);
- increased sympathetic activity as a result of stressors (for example, hypoxia);
- potassium imbalance.

All of which require further investigation. An irregularly irregular pulse usually indicates atrial fibrillation where atrial behaviour is chaotic and disorganized and the transmission of impulses to the ventricles is irregular.

The *pulse pressure* is a wave of pressure caused by a sequence of distension and elastic recoil in the wall of the aorta which forces blood rapidly down the systemic arterial system. It determines the strength of the pulse and can be defined as the difference between the systolic and diastolic BPs.

When the pulse pressure is low, the strength of the pulse may be feeble and thready. This may occur when hypovolaemia exists, because the stroke volume ejected by the left ventricle into the circulation is greatly reduced. When the pulse pressure is high, the pulse strength may be bounding and the person experiencing this may feel palpitations or hear his heart pounding.

The *pulse deficit* (radial and apex beat) is the difference between the heart rate counted at the apex of the heart using a stethoscope and the pulse rate counted simultaneously at the wrist. For the majority of patients the heart rate and pulse rate will be the same, but for those who are in atrial fibrillation or who are having multiple ectopic beats, there will be a deficit which is important to monitor by recording both apex and radial rates.

Peripheral pulses

As previously discussed, the pulse pressure is a wave of pressure which can be palpated near the body surface where large arteries are superficially located or where they pass over underlying bone. There are many pulses in the body (identified above) but the pulses of the lower limbs, the poplitaeal pulse located behind the knee and the dorsalis pedis and posterior tibial pulses in the feet, are important in determining adequacy of perfusion to the lower limbs. The pulses in the foot can often be difficult to locate and feel, especially when perfusion to the limbs is severely reduced.

There are many other pulses in the body and measuring and counting these may help to determine the adequacy of circulation and where the problem may be. The main pulses in the body (Fig. 3.2) are as follows:

- Apical
- Radial
- Carotid
- Femoral
- Brachial
- Aortic
- Poplitaeal
- Posterior tibial
- Dorsalis pedis

Measuring pulse rate

The pulse points can be palpated and counted, which can be assessed as to if it is:

- Present
- Absent
- Strong and equal
- Faint and equal

Any changes can give adequacy of perfusion:

- Weakness or a bounding feeling as if there is a great pressure within the artery
- Fast or slow or irregular
- Give clues to the overall circulation of each individual area of the body

Respiration

The respiratory rate is the number of times gas is inspired and expired per minute. The respiratory rate is recorded to:

- determine a baseline respiratory rate for compensation;
- monitor fluctuations in respiration;
- evaluate the patient's response to medications or treatments that affect the respiratory system.

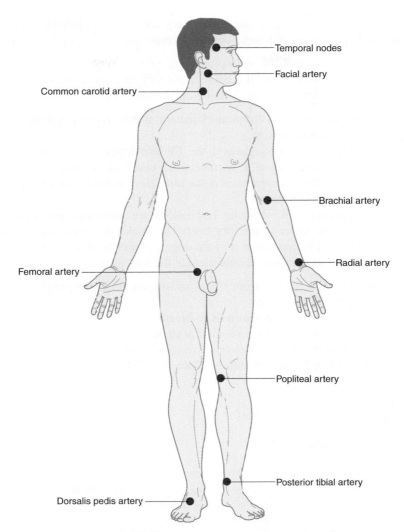

FIGURE 3.2   Pulses around the body.

When assessing respiration there are other important observations to make (in addition to rate) which will help to identify the effectiveness of breathing.

The respiratory rate in adults at rest is approximately 14—18 breaths per minute. Counting of rate should be over a minute and take place when the patient is resting and unaware of the observation because conscious awareness of breathing can lead to alteration in rate and pattern. This is because breathing is under the control of both the involuntary and voluntary nervous system. Changes in rate of breathing are defined as follows:

- Tachypnoea, an increase in respiratory rate e.g. in fever
- Bradypnoea, a decrease in regular respiratory rate e.g. depression of the respiratory centre in the medulla by opiate narcotics

Closely related to rate is respiratory pattern, which changes in disorders of the respiratory control centre.

The depth of respiration relates to the TV. The depth of respiration can be specifically measured using a spirometer or observed by inspecting chest expansion for depth or shallowness at the same time as observing for equality and uniformity of movement.

Noisy, gurgling and wheezing respirations are abnormal and imply an obstruction in the upper respiratory tract. The louder the noise heard at the mouth during inspiration, the greater the degree of airway obstruction present.

In addition, observations should include the following:

- *Cyanosis* — lips, toes, fingers — lack of oxygen, or due to peripheral shut down ($\downarrow$ tissue perfusion)
- *Ability to talk* — due to shortness of breath
- *Use of accessory muscles* — pectoral or sternomastoids are used to increase thoracic size in an attempt to improve ventilation
- *Cough* — effectiveness, sputum production, colour, consistency
- *Chest movement*:
  - Is it bilateral?
  - Can sputum rattle be felt?
  - Is the patient confused?
  - Signs of wheezing?

! In hypovolaemic states, haemodynamic measures, e.g. BP, heart rate and respiration, may initially increase and then decrease, as it becomes more difficult for the body to maintain adequate blood supply.

Blood pressure

Taking the blood pressure (BP) remains one of the most important and widely used assessment tools in hospital, as from this one test much information can be gleaned about the patient's state of health. Nurses generally record BP on admission to hospital to determine a baseline or as a determinant of risk factors for such diseases as cerebral vascular accident, ischaemic heart disease and renal disease, all of which can influence recovery.

The BP should be taken when a patient is admitted, postoperatively, when drugs that alter BP are taken and when the patient's condition has deteriorated. It should also be taken when the patient is hypertensive, neutropenic, pregnant, critically ill, receiving an infusion or has an infection.

The BP is 'the force exerted by the blood on the walls of the arteries in which it is contained'. A number of factors determine it, most significantly cardiac output, peripheral resistance, elasticity of vessels and hormonal and chemical control mechanisms. Two components of BP are evident:

- The *systolic pressure* − the amount of blood which is forced out into the arteries at ventricular contraction
- The *diastolic pressure* − which is the fall in arterial pressure before the next ventricular contraction

There are two methods of taking a BP, direct and indirect:

- *Direct* monitoring of BP is accomplished by cannulating an artery and attaching the catheter to a fluid-filled tubing and transducer, which is connected to a voltage source.
- *Indirect* methods of BP monitoring are more commonly used and fall into two categories: the auscultatory (manual) method and computer-assisted automatic devices.

Two different sphygmomanometers are used for the manual method, the aneroid and electronic.

The traditional oscillatory technique uses a pneumatic cuff and stethoscope, which monitors Korotkoff sounds (Box 3.3). Korotkoff sounds are generated by blood passing through the compressed artery under the cuff and meeting a static column of blood, resulting in turbulence and vibrations. To be detected by a stethoscope, these sounds must be at a frequency within an audible range.

! In low-flow states, such as those associated with hypotension, the auscultatory method has been demonstrated to fail, apparently because of the human ear's inability to appreciate low-frequency vibrations.

The automatic cycling devices have gained increasing acceptance; however, their reliability has been challenged as, like the auscultatory method, many of these devices are blood flow dependent.

Both methods of indirect BP monitoring are subject to error and may be unreliable in the very clinical situations where they are used the most (Box 3.4). This is mainly due to the fact that measuring and monitoring BP are frequently carried out but often performed incorrectly. Recommendations on how to take an accurate BP are given in Box 3.5.

BOX 3.3 Korotkoff sounds

Phase I	The pressure level at which the first clear tapping sounds are heard
Phase II	The time during inflation when a murmur and a swishing are heard
Phase III	The point when the murmur disappears and the louder and more distinct sound is heard
Phase IV	Muffling of sound
Phase V	The sound disappears

Hinchliff et al., 1998. Nursing Practice & Health Care, reprinted with permission from Edward Arnold (Publishers) Ltd.

BOX 3.4 Potential sources of error when taking a blood pressure (BP)

The observer
- Observer bias — prior recording viewed by the nurse or a preference for a specific figure, known as digit preference
- Cognitive deficits — education, inadequate training, no updating on the technique or principles
- Lack of understanding of the correct procedure, e.g. incorrect positioning of the patient, sitting/standing, support of the arm, positioning of the cuff bladder over the centre of the brachial artery, the bladder/cuff not level with the heart
- Lack of concentration
- Hearing problems/deficit
- Sight problems

The equipment
- Cuff/bladder size
- Maintenance — BP machines should be calibrated and assessed every 6–12 months
- The level of mercury not at zero
- Defective control valves caused by leakage, making control of the pressure release difficult

Leaks from cracked or perished rubber tubing
- The stethoscope should be in good condition and have clean and well-fitted earpieces

The patient
- The patient may be suffering from excessive heat or cold, be wearing constrictive clothing, have a full bladder, recently exercised, been smoking,

Box 3.4 Potential sources of error when taking a blood pressure (BP)—cont'd

just had a meal or there may be a distraction, all of which will serve to either increase or decrease the BP.

- Older patients have calcified/rigid arteries or anaemia which can all influence the BP reading.
- A patient suffering from a high temperature may have a low BP due to vasodilatation, causing the BP to fall.
- In all patients the general consensus now is that disappearance of sounds (phase V) is the most accurate measurement of diastolic pressure with the stipulation that if sounds persist to zero (e.g. in pregnant women, children or patients suffering from anaemia), the muffling of sounds (phase IV) should be used.
- In conditions where BP is low there may be distal vasoconstriction and it is common to underestimate the BP.
- In some patients the white coat syndrome affects BP — this is caused when doctors appear at the bedside, giving an inaccurately high BP reading.
- BP does vary during the day — higher systolic in the evening and a low recording in the morning.
- Fear, anxiety, apprehension and pain can all raise the BP and these can be apparent on admission.
- It is recommended in this instance to wait at least 1 h following admission to take the BP.

! Errors in measurement of BP may mean wrong decisions being made in BP management, thus compromising care.

Oxygen saturation measurement

Adequate tissue oxygenation depends on a balance between oxygen supply and delivery and the tissue demand for oxygen. When oxygen demands exceed oxygen supply, hypoxia occurs. Blood flow is closely coupled to the metabolic activity of the tissues and hypoxia results in vasodilatation and an increase in blood flow. The vasodilatation may be due to the release of vasodilator chemicals but may also be due to inadequate oxygen availability for the smooth muscle in the blood vessels to contract. It must be noted, however, that alveolar hypoxia causes pulmonary vasoconstriction. This is called hypoxic pulmonary vasoconstriction (HPV) and redirects blood from the poorly oxygenated alveoli towards those with better oxygenation, thus optimizing gas exchange.

BOX 3.5 Recommendations on how to take an accurate blood pressure (BP)

- If possible the patient should not have eaten, exercised or smoked for at least 30 min before taking a BP.
- The patient should be sitting or lying down in a quiet environment with his arm resting at the heart level on a table or pillow (the antecubital fossa should be level with the fourth intercostal space). An arm that is below this level results in a falsely high reading and vice versa.
- A rest period of at least 3–5 min should be allowed before the reading is taken.
- Measure the circumference of the arm and use the appropriate-sized bladder. However, it is possible with some cuffs to take an accurate BP even if the cuff is not an accurate size by placing the bladder centre over the brachial artery (an arrow on the actual cuff generally marks the spot) (Richards & Edwards, 2014). A gap of 2–3 cm should be left between the antecubital fossa and the bottom of the cuff.
- The sphygmomanometer should be placed near to the observer (no more than 3 ft away) on a flat surface with the mercury level at zero. If the mercury is not at zero, it can produce false high or low readings.
- Locate the brachial artery by palpation.
- Assess the maximal inflation level of the cuff, to prevent causing pain to the patient. This is achieved by inflating the cuff and palpating the radial pulse at the same time; the maximal inflation level will be 20–30 mmHg higher than the level at which the pulse disappeared.
- The patient should not cross his legs, as this will give a falsely high reading.
- Place the stethoscope over the brachial artery, being careful not to use too much pressure, as this lowers the diastolic pressure reading. Release the valve slowly and gently.
- The cuff should be rapidly inflated at 2 mmHg/s and deflated slowly. A slow inflation and a rapid deflation both result in inaccuracies.
- Note the systolic pressure at the onset of the first clear repetitive tapping sound of two beats or more.
- The diastolic pressure should be recorded at the cessation of sound (phase V) for all patients, unless the recording is zero, in which case the muffling of sound (phase IV) should be used. If phase IV is used, it should be documented on the chart.
- The BP should be measured to the nearest 2 mmHg.
- The procedure should take no less than 5 min (Richards & Edwards, 2014).
- If the procedure is rushed, this will result in an underestimation of the systolic pressure and an overestimation of the diastolic pressure.
- The measurement should be recorded on the patient's chart. If it is not possible to achieve optimum conditions, this should also be noted with the blood pressure reading; for example, 'BP 145/95, L arm, phase V (patient very anxious)'.
- If the recording needs to be repeated, at least 1–2 min should have elapsed before reinflating the cuff.

Hypoxia may be due to:

- a blockage, whereby the tissues become hypoxic due to a reduced blood flow, as in arteriosclerosis;
- the loss of red blood cells, which carry oxygen to the cells, often observed in haemorrhage;
- the inability to get oxygen into the circulation, seen in patients with impaired respiratory function.

The nurse is frequently the first to observe the presence of hypoxia and the one who can intervene to correct the problem with oxygenation.

Hypoxia may be observed in a number of ways. There may be changes in behaviour and level of consciousness. This is because the brain needs a continuous, steady supply of oxygenated blood and this is why the brain is a sensitive indicator of a patient's perfusion status. Very early signs of cerebral underperfusion are the inability to think abstractly or perform complex mental tasks, restlessness, apprehension, uncooperativeness and irritability.

Short-term memory may also be impaired. A family member may need to be called upon for information on the patient's normal personality and intellectual status. In addition, there may be changes in BP, pulse, and colour of mucous membranes. This may lead the nurse to extend the assessment for hypoxia by obtaining an oxygen saturation using pulse oximetry (see p. 134) or by the doctor obtaining arterial blood for blood gas analysis.

Oxygen saturation monitoring measures levels of haemoglobin and is widely used in many patient care settings. The normal percentage of oxygen saturated with haemoglobin is 98%. It is important for practitioners to note that the oxygen saturation monitor can give misleading information regarding the true nature of the patient's oxygen status.

The oxygen disassociation curve plots the relationship between the amount of oxygen bound to haemoglobin (oxygen saturation) and the partial pressure of oxygen (PaO_2) in the blood. The steep S-shaped curve highlights that at a normal PaO_2 of 13.3 kPa, oxygen saturation is 100%. If the PaO_2 drops by 5.3–8 kPa the oxygen saturation will remain within acceptable limits at 90%. At a further drop of just 1.7 kPa, the oxygen saturation will drop from 90% to 70%. At this level, breathing is difficult and respiratory arrest may occur, requiring emergency intubation.

An oxygen saturation of 90% may not indicate to the nurse that there is a low oxygen supply in the blood (determined by partial pressure of oxygen). An awareness of these principles will ensure that oxygen saturation monitoring is safe and minimize the potential for unrecognized hypoxaemic episodes.

The oxygen saturation measurement is valuable, as it allows nurses to evaluate the relative state of oxygenation and can help to improve the care the patient receives. However, when using pulse oximetry in practice, other observations should be undertaken in conjunction with it if hypoxia is suspected, e.g. colour, pulse rate, breathing pattern and rate, arterial blood gases (to give partial pressure of oxygen e.g. arterial blood gases).

Temperature

The temperature can affect the circulation if it is abnormally low or high. If the temperature is high, as in infective states, the hypothalamus reflex initiates dilatation of arterioles and veins in the skin, causing a reduction in cardiac output and BP and an increase in heart rate. When the body's core temperature decreases below normal, surface blood vessels vasoconstrict to shunt the blood to the vital organs and prevent excess heat loss from skin surfaces, causing a decrease in oxygen consumption and heart rate and an increase in BP.

There are a number of ways to take the temperature:

● Sublingually for 1 min
● Axilla for 2–3 min
● Rectal temperature not recommended
● Ear temperature

Oral, axillary and ear temperatures are recommended as the most effective ways to take a temperature in the general wards. It should be noted that external variables affect oral temperature readings, including the ingestion of hot or cold substances, recent bathing, recent physical exertion and smoking. For the greatest accuracy, the bulb of the thermometer should be placed sublingually to the right or left and not the area in the middle of the tongue.

Different equipment is available to take the temperature and may influence the temperature reading:

● Electronic oral digital temperature thermometers from the armpit or the mouth with the use of a single-use sheath
● Single-use chemical thermometers – these use a chemical which changes colour with increasing temperature
● Electronic thermometers – a signal indicates when the maximum temperature has been reached, to prevent premature removal of the thermometer
● Tympanic membrane thermometer – uses an infrared light reflectance thermometer that detects heat radiated as infrared energy from the tympanic membrane

The best time of day for temperature recording is important, as there are diurnal variations in human body temperature owing to circadian rhythms and this will affect readings. Temperature is most likely to be elevated at the peak of the circadian cycle, which is between 5 p.m. and 7 p.m.

! Many standard thermometers do not record temperatures below 35°C, so for an accurate measurement of hypothermia a low-reading thermometer is necessary.

Infants and the elderly in relation to temperature control

Infants and the elderly require special attention to maintenance of body temperature:

- Infants produce sufficient body heat but are unable to conserve the heat produced.
- The poor heat conservation is caused by the infant's small body size and greater ratio of body surface to body weight, which gives the infant more surface area for heat loss.
- Infants also have a very thin layer of subcutaneous fat and thus are not as well insulated as adults.

The elderly have poor responses to environmental temperature extremes as a result of the following:

- Slowed blood circulation
- Structural and functional changes in the skin
- Overall decrease in heat-producing activities
- Decrease in shivering response (delayed onset and decreased effectiveness)
- Slowed metabolic rate
- Sedentary lifestyle
- Decreased vasoconstrictor response
- Diminished or absent sweating
- Desynchronization of circadian rhythm
- Undernutrition/dehydration
- Decreased perception of heat and cold

Toe temperature

When the main circulation is impaired, there are changes to the peripheral circulation to the body's extremities. This will be reflected in the peripheral skin temperature, providing good indications of the presence and severity of a circulatory defect. The toe temperature gradient provides a valuable, inexpensive and noninvasive monitor of tissue perfusion.

Skin temperature

Skin temperature can be a useful guide to determining the severity of shock, as during hypovolaemia circulation to the major organs and central temperature need to be maintained. To do this, the body under ANS control improves the circulation through baroreceptor activity, which will cause vasoconstriction and prevent heat loss from body surfaces. The end result is heat conservation, extremities that feel cool to touch, an increase in BP and improved circulation to the body's major organs.

Central venous pressure monitoring

The measurement of the CVP provides important haemodynamic information to guide therapy. The CVP reflects the volume of blood returning to the heart, which exerts pressure on the walls of the right ventricle. This blood will then be circulated through the heart and lungs and around the body.

CVP monitoring determines the following:

- The adequacy of the body's blood volume
- The pumping function of the right side of the heart
- Vascular tone and pulmonary vascular resistance

To determine an accurate CVP, the patient should be placed in the supine position, with the backrest at an angle of up to 30°. It is essential that CVP measurement is made under identical conditions each time so that all possible variables (such as patient position) remain constant.

The most reliable external reference point used to take the CVP is the mid-axilla, using a water manometer. A fall in CVP may indicate the following:

- Moderate hypovolaemic shock, in patients who are bleeding following surgery
- Dehydration
- Extreme vasodilatation, whereby the capacity of the circulation is increased but the circulating volume remains constant, as in patients with pyrexia or from the excessive use of vasodilator drugs.
- Left ventricular failure
- An increase in CVP may represent the following:
  - Exposure to extreme cold, e.g. after surgery, causing severe vasoconstriction, which would return more blood to the heart as the veins are already filled
  - Fluid overload due to blood transfusion, colloid or crystalloid
  - Heart failure

Generally, the value of the CVP reading is overestimated. If a fall in CVP occurs, this is proposed to indicate a moderate hypovolaemia while a consequent rise in CVP is proposed to suggest fluid overload. It is presumed by many that the CVP can be used as a guide to determine severity of fluid loss, measure when too much fluid has been administered and ascertain cardiac instability.

The suggestion is that a normal or reduced CVP will occur in hypovolaemia, during hypervolaemia and left-sided cardiac failure:

- In hypovolaemia due to the loss of fluid.
- In left-sided heart failure due to the left side of the heart generally failing first, causing severe systolic dysfunction of the left ventricle and a consequent reduction in stroke volume and cardiac output. As a result there is a decline in the amount of blood returning to the heart (venous return) and hence a reduction in CVP.
- In hypervolaemia, it may take nearly 24 h for events occurring in the left side of the heart to reflect through the lungs into the right ventricle, atria and superior vena cava and be mirrored as an increased CVP reading.

This implies that CVP levels are not completely reliable in estimating circulatory function. Therefore, a more accurate measure would be that which could determine the pressure in the left side of the heart (see later) via pulmonary artery wedge pressure.

! It is not the single CVP reading that is important but the trend demonstrated by a series of readings over time.

The CVP catheter can also be used for rapid infusion of fluids and blood or to withdraw blood for laboratory samples. The most common complications of a CVP line include pneumothorax, hydrothorax and ventricular arrhythmias, infection and air embolism, all of which should be observed for during the procedure.

Intracranial pressure monitoring

The skull and meninges contain three major components:

- Brain tissue (80%)
- Cerebrospinal fluid (CSF) (10%)
- Cerebral blood flow (CBF) (10%)

The pressure these three components exert in the rigid skull is termed the *intracranial pressure* (ICP). The normal range of ICP is 0–15 mmHg. The brain maintains this normal pressure by compensation mechanisms known as *autoregulation*, which occurs after an insult or injury leading to increased brain, blood or CSF volume. To compensate the following occurs:

- Displacement of CSF from the cranial subarachnoid space, spinal and lumbar space. CSF production decreases and CSF absorption increases.

- Reduction in CBF as venous blood is shunted away from the affected areas. A widespread reduction in CBF to compensate can lead to further brain insult or ischaemia due to the reduced cerebral perfusion.

These compensatory mechanisms may become exhausted and an increase in ICP above 15 mmHg may occur as a result of the following:

- Trauma
- Hydrocephalus
- Infection
- Tumours
- Metabolic disorders
- Cerebrovascular accident
- Encephalopathies

In certain injuries monitoring techniques can be employed to measure the ICP. There are three types of ICP monitoring device, all of which monitor but only one can drain the CSF:

- Ventriculostomy (intraventricular catheter; able to drain)
- Subdural bolt or catheter
- Epidural screw, bolt or sensor

Meticulous records of observations need to be kept, especially of mean arterial pressure (MAP). This is necessary to determine adequate CBF.

Cerebral perfusion pressure (CPP) is the pressure needed to perfuse the brain and the normal range is 80–90 mmHg. It is calculated by subtracting the ICP from the MAP.

CBF is compromised if the CPP is below 60 and reduced CPP may result in irreversible brain damage or death. It is thought that the threshold for mechanical brain injury is an ICP of 20–30 mmHg.

Urine output

The kidney receives about 25% of the cardiac output. Glomerular filtration rate (GFR) is dependent on an adequate renal perfusion. When tissue perfusion is adequate, the production of urine will exceed 0.5 mL/kg per hour. The average urinary output should be between 30 and 70 mL or more per hour. When blood flow to the kidneys is reduced, an increase in vasoconstriction occurs. The overall net effect is that the GFR decreases, reducing urinary output. In contrast, when there is an increase in fluid administration causing hypervolaemia (fluid overload), cardiac failure and pulmonary oedema may occur. In this instance kidney function may also become impaired, due to a reduction in the pumping action of the heart, a reduced cardiac output and blood flow to the kidneys.

In dehydrated or hypovolaemic states, the kidneys play a complex role in restoring extracellular fluid volume and increasing systemic BP. This system is stimulated principally when there is a decrease in BP. This elaborate set of interlinked processes involves the renin-angiotensin-aldosterone system, osmoreceptors and baroreceptors.

If urine output falls below 25 mL per hour, fluid administration may be necessary. This is why urinary output should be measured, either at hourly intervals if a catheter is inserted or from a bedpan or bottle, and accurately recorded. Interpretation of urine output should also consider overall fluid balance (positive or negative over a 24-h period), the quality and colour of urine.

3.4 PROCEDURES AND INVESTIGATIONS

Collecting, testing and sending specimens

The collection of a specimen involves obtaining a required amount of tissue or fluid for laboratory examinations. It is generally performed to:

- isolate and identify microorganisms that cause disease;
- determine antibiotic sensitivity to guide the selection of appropriate antibiotic therapy;
- measure levels of chemicals in blood and CSF to determine diagnosis and treatment.

In some instances nurses should be able to identify the need for microbiologic investigation and, if appropriate, initiate the taking of a specimen. The types of specimens taken are as follows:

- Swabs of the eye, nose, throat, ear, wound, drain site, vagina, cervix, penis and rectum
- One urine sample from a male or female
- Faeces
- Semen
- Blood
- Sputum
- CSF

When obtaining a sample for analysis, the following should be considered:

- Explain and discuss the procedure with the patient and ensure privacy while the procedure is being carried out.
- Wash hands using bactericidal soap and water or bactericidal alcohol hand rub.
- Cleanse the area, if relevant, and collect the specimen, ensuring that no contamination of the specimen has occurred, as this will result in misleading information.

- Place specimen(s) and swabs in the appropriate correctly labelled containers. There are many types of specimen collection tools, e.g. swabs and pots. If you do not know which is the correct container, then seek advice from the microbiology department.
- The greater amount of material and information given to the laboratory, the greater the chance of isolating a causative organism. Therefore, the request form must include the following information:
  - Patient name, ward and/or department
  - Hospital number
  - Date specimen collected
  - Time specimen collected
  - Provisional or diagnosis
  - Relevant signs and symptoms
  - Relevant history, e.g. recent foreign travel, recent toxic therapy
  - Any antimicrobial drugs being taken by the patient
  - Type of specimen
  - Risk of infection for staff
  - Consultant's name
  - Name of the doctor who ordered the investigation, as it may be necessary to telephone the result before the typed report is dispatched.
  - The container should be leakproof and placed in a plastic bag before being sent to the laboratory.
  - Dispatch specimens promptly to the laboratory with the completed request form.

Urine testing

This is a noninvasive technique to monitor the functioning of the kidney and in some instances other organs:

- Fluid balance, acid-base balance and kidney function may be evaluated.
- It can aid diagnosis in diabetes, weight loss, urinary tract infection, liver function, e.g. blockage of flow of bile, cancer of and trauma to the bladder.
- Circulatory status can be monitored.
- It provides valuable clues to the effectiveness of treatment.

The significance of the urine test strip results can be found in the specific gravity, pH or whether blood, protein, bilirubin and urobilinogen, nitrates, glucose and ketones are present.

The specific gravity

As urine is mostly water with a variable quantity of substances dissolved in it, the concentration of these substances will depend on the body's state of hydration and the amount of waste products to be excreted. Testing the urine for specific gravity (SG) can be one way to determine if hydration is adequate.

Dehydration is a common problem in hospital, especially in the elderly, so determining SG may give clues to the physiologic status of the patient. Although inpatient monitoring of fluid balance with intake and output charts is essential, loss of water through the breath, sweat and faeces is not so easily measured. The SG of urine will give a good indication of the net fluid balance and is of particular value in patients where there is an unquantifiable loss, such as in burns cases, breathing difficulties, diarrhoea or fever.

In healthy adults, the SG varies between 1005 and 1035 (pure water is the standard, with an SG of 1000). The SG depends on the state of hydration:

- The first specimen of the morning will tend to have a higher SG than one taken after the subject has had a drink.
- An isolated assessment of SG is of little value, and the test should be repeated on samples taken at known times.
- Urine with a persistently low SG is suggestive of diabetes insipidus or renal damage. As the normal concentration power of the kidneys is lost, the urine passed will tend to be rather dilute.
- An increase in SG will indicate dehydration, perhaps due to bleeding, vomiting, diarrhoea, reduction in fluid intake or fever.

The method for measuring SG is the reagent strip, which measures the ionic strength of a urine sample and expresses this with a simple-to-read colour change. The colour changes on the reagent strips are easier to read than the gradations on the narrow stem of the hydrometer and thus the method is less prone to errors.

The pH

The pH of urine should reflect the acid-base balance of the body, as excess hydrogen or bicarbonate ions are excreted by the tubules to maintain the normal status. Under normal circumstances, the urine has a pH of around 6, but it can range from about 5 to 8.5. Metabolic acidosis arising from starvation, high-protein diets or diabetic ketoacidosis will lead to an acid urine, but diets including a lot of vegetables, mild or even bicarbonate-based antacids can cause an alkaline urine, when the pH will rise.

Urinary pH thus offers an opportunity to assess an aspect of the patient's metabolic state, but it also has therapeutic implications. Renal calculi are formed from insoluble salts and other substances, such as uric acid, found in the urine, which have precipitated out and aggregated into a discrete mass. To help dissolve the stones or prevent recurrence, the pH of the urine can be adjusted to create conditions where the constituents of the stone are more soluble or remain in solution. Knowing the urinary pH can be of use when attempting to diagnose a patient's symptoms. If a urinary tract infection is suspected, proteinuria combined with an alkaline pH is highly suggestive of bacterial infection but less likely if the urine is acid.

Blood

The presence of blood in the urine is a potentially serious sign and needs thorough and rapid investigation. Asymptomatic haematuria is usually the earliest sign of cancer of the bladder which can be treated if detected early enough. It can also be due to trauma, infection or stones. A reagent test strip is available which uses a colour change to blue or green if haemoglobin is present in the sample. Positive results must be followed up to determine where the blood is coming from and appropriate treatment instituted.

> ! False-positive results may occur from containers contaminated with bleach, skin preparation with povidone iodine or from the use of stale urine.

Protein

In early renal disease, the glomerulus and tubules may leak small amounts of protein into the urine. As renal disease progresses, detectable levels of protein will be found in the urine. There are a number of systemic diseases associated with proteinuria including the following:

- Renal disease
- Urinary tract infection
- Hypertension
- Preeclampsia
- Congestive heart failure

Transient positive tests are not always significant and normal urine contains small amounts of albumin and globulin, although generally not enough to give a positive result on a reagent strip. Thus, when testing for urinary protein, a morning specimen of urine is recommended to ensure sufficient concentration. Yet ultimately renal damage may be detected as an asymptomatic proteinuria before any other signs of disease are noticed.

> ! Proteinuria is an early sign as well as a means of monitoring the progress of disease or its response to therapy.

Bilirubin and urobilinogen

In normal health, bilirubin is not found in the urine but is excreted via the bile duct into the gut. However, when the liver is diseased or there is obstruction to the flow of bile into the gut, bilirubin or its metabolites are likely to be found in significant quantities in the urine.

> ! Urobilinogen is normally present in urine, but elevated levels may indicate liver abnormalities or excessive destruction of red blood cells, such as in haemolytic anaemia.

Nitrates

Urine normally contains nitrates from dietary metabolites, and some of the common bacteria responsible for urinary infections will convert these nitrates to nitrites. Nitrites are not normally present in urine but are produced in increasing numbers when gram-negative bacteria such as *Escherichia coli* (*E. coli*) convert dietary nitrates (found in the preservatives in meat products, cheese and smoked food) to nitrites. As *E. coli* is responsible for 80% of urine infection, the presence of nitrites is strongly suggestive of urinary tract infection. A reagent strip that will detect nitrites in urine can confirm a bacterial presence. The following should be considered:

- The specimen for testing should have been present in the bladder for 4 h before voiding, to allow sufficient time for the nitrate/nitrite conversion.
- Visible signs may also be present (for example, is the specimen clear or cloudy?) and should be noted.
- If the specimen is clear and blood, protein, leucocytes and nitrites are not present, you can be sure there is no urinary tract infection.
- If the specimen is turbid and one or more of the four tests are positive, there is a 50% chance that the urine is infected.

It would be appropriate to send the specimen to the laboratory for culture and sensitivity and refer the patient to the doctor for treatment. A short course of low-dose antibiotics and increased fluid intake is recommended.

Glucose

Glucose is not normally found in urine. The presence of glucose may be due to raised blood glucose levels (hyperglycaemia). It can be associated with many medical conditions including the following:

- Diabetes mellitus
- Stress
- Cushing's syndrome
- Acute pancreatitis

There is a case for screening middle-aged and older people when admitted to hospital as they may, at an early stage, be relatively asymptomatic before more serious symptoms present. Once a diagnosis of diabetes is made, urinalysis for glucose can be a valuable method of monitoring the disease, particularly as diabetic retinopathy, kidney disease, peripheral vascular and cardiac disease are secondary to prolonged hyperglycaemia.

There are two categories of urine tests for glucose: the Clinitest and the impregnated test strips. The Clinitest is quite cumbersome but provides an accurate measure. Test strips do not measure the quantity of glucose in the urine so accurately and therefore are probably only adequate for screening purposes.

Ketones

When the body metabolizes fat, breakdown products include ketone bodies, which are excreted in the urine. In good health they are not detectable in urine. Usually ketones may be found in people who are fasting but can also be present in excessive amounts in people with uncontrolled diabetes. There are two tests available for ketones: Acetest, which is a tablet, and a strip test, which is available either as a single test, Ketostix, or incorporated into one of the combined multiple-strip sticks.

Ketones are acidic substances and when present in excess can lead to metabolic acidosis, which, if untreated, can cause death. Early detection is therefore of value.

Appearance

The appearance of the urine should be noted for colour and clarity. Colour changes may be due to endogenous pigments such as haemoglobin (red or red/brown colour), bilirubin (yellow) or intact red cells (smoky red). Exogenous pigments may also cause colour changes:

- A red-coloured urine may be due to eating beetroot or to contamination with menstrual blood.
- Orange discolouration may be due to the pigments found in some laxatives.
- A blue/green colour may be caused by methylene blue in some proprietary medicines.

Odour

The odour of a urine specimen should be noted before further testing:

- Normal, freshly voided urine has very little smell but develops an ammonia-like smell on standing.
- Infected urine smells foul and may have a characteristic fishy smell which worsens on standing.
- Substances such as acetone excreted by diabetics with ketoacidosis or patients who have been starving or suffering from anorexia give urine a characteristic smell.
- Eating fish, curry or other strongly flavoured foodstuffs can also make the urine smell.

The results of ward or clinic testing of urine should be recorded accurately in the patient's records, as soon as possible after testing. Remember, a negative test result may not only point to an alternative diagnosis but it is also a valuable baseline indicator to be referred to later in evaluating the progress of a patient during the course of an illness. A negative result should always be recorded even if at the time it appears unimportant or irrelevant.

Stool specimen

There are a number of reasons a stool sample may be required:

- To test for blood — can be done on the ward to test for occult blood seen in diverticulitis, polyps, cancer, haemorrhoids or ulcers
- Culturing of the stool to determine organisms seen in cases of diarrhoea
- To observe texture, shape, size using the Bristol stool chart types 1—7, with 3—4 being normal, used alongside other tests to diagnosis medical conditions e.g. ulcerative colitis, Crohn's disease, irritable bowel syndrome, constipation
- Consider the colour of the stool:
  - Black stool can indicate old blood and a sign of bleeding high up in the gastrointestinal tract e.g. gastric or peptic ulceration
  - Dark red can be indicative of fresh bleeding, is serious and requires immediate nursing interventions and action
  - Pale looking or white stool can indicate liver disease, as bilirubin (the waste product red blood cell breakdown) is excreted in bile expelled into the large intestines and excreted in faeces and gives it a dark brown colour. Changes occur in stools if there is a blockage of the bile duct by a gall stone or swelling of the liver due to alcohol or hepatitis.

The findings from a stool sample are used alongside patients' symptoms such as abdominal pain, weight loss, fatigue and other investigations to determine causation.

Blood tests

Many early changes that occur in the body may be reflected in the results of a blood sample, well before they become clinically obvious. Blood tests can aid diagnosis, assist in monitoring circulatory status and help provide valuable clues to the effectiveness of treatment.

Blood cultures

Bacteraemia and fungaemia indicate failure of the host's immune system to localize infection and its primary focus. They are associated with significant morbidity and mortality, and therefore accurate and speedy microbiologic detection of infection using blood cultures is essential. The timing of blood cultures is crucial, as most bacteraemias are intermittent. Blood cultures should be taken when the signs of infection are present, e.g. during fever, chills, rigours, changes in mental state and lethargy.

When taking blood cultures, rigorous attention to aseptic technique is necessary as a failure to do so could result in a pseudobacteraemia, e.g. contamination of the culture from outside the bloodstream. A fresh sample of blood is preferred, as obtaining blood from an indwelling central venous catheter can increase the risk of contamination.

Haemoglobin levels

The haemoglobin (Hb) level is the amount of red blood cells in the blood. Hb is contained in the erythrocyte's cytoplasm and is primarily responsible for carrying oxygen to and carbon dioxide from the body's tissues. Hb also plays a major role in blood viscosity.

The normal concentration of Hb in the blood is 12—15 g/100 mL of blood. A low Hb will indicate that red blood cells are being lost. When considering the Hb, it is important to consider the patient's age, general state and the rate of fall of the Hb concentration. An Hb concentration that has fallen suddenly, such as in acute blood loss, is not well tolerated by the body and a transfusion is required to improve the delivery of oxygen to the tissues. A slow reduction in Hb is better tolerated as the body has time to adapt to the fall as it takes place gradually over weeks or months. This occurs in iron-deficiency anaemia, megaloblastic anaemia, renal failure and anaemias associated with chronic disorders.

In addition to determining Hb levels, other signs may be present to confirm findings:

- In white skin the epidermis is nearly transparent and allows the colour of the Hb to show through as a pinkish tinge, as the blood circulates through the dermal capillaries. When Hb is poorly oxygenated, both the blood and the skin of white people appear blue (cyanosis).
- In black people, cyanosis of the skin can be observed in the mucous membranes and nail beds.
- By spending many hours in close contact with the patient, undertaking careful monitoring and observation, the nurse may notice the more subtle changes that occur in the patient's condition (cyanosis) before the physiologic parameter is actually measured (Hb).

! It is necessary to consider cyanosis in relation to the total clinical picture as it occurs in other clinical conditions such as respiratory diseases and heart failure.

Plasma osmolality

Osmolality is a measure of the number of milliosmoles per litre of solution or the concentration of molecules per volume of solution. When solute is added to water, the volume is expanded and includes the original amount of water plus the volume occupied by the solute particles (e.g. sodium, potassium, calcium, etc.). When there is an increase in osmolality, there is a reduction of water in relation to the solutes contained within it, as the solute concentration has not changed.

The osmolality of intracellular and extracellular fluid tends to equalize and so provides a measure of body fluid concentration and thus the body's hydration status. The normal osmolality of body fluids is 280–294 mOsm/L. A serum osmolality of less than 280 mOsm/L will generally indicate an excess of fluids in the vessels, suggesting overhydration or hypervolaemia. An increased serum osmolality greater than 295 mOsm/L indicates a loss of fluid and dehydration or hypovolaemia may be present.

> ! With an increase in osmolality, thirst and a dry mouth are often experienced. The nurse may then consider suggesting that the blood level be investigated.

Haematocrit levels

A factor which influences blood flow is the consistency of the blood. Flow varies inversely with the viscosity of the fluid. Thick fluids move more slowly and cause a greater resistance to flow than thin fluids. The viscosity of blood depends on its red cell content. The greater the percentage of red cells in the blood, the more viscous the blood. This relationship is expressed as the haematocrit, the ratio of volume of red blood cells to the volume of whole blood.

The haematocrit determination is the percentage of a given volume of blood that is occupied by erythrocytes. A high haematocrit reduces flow through the blood vessels, particularly the microcirculation (arterioles, capillaries and venules). Conditions in which the haematocrit is elevated, for example dehydration, haemorrhage, anaemias, leukaemias, cyanotic congenital heart disease and polycythaemia, can lead to an increase in cardiac work as a result of increased vascular resistance.

The viscosity of blood also increases if blood flow becomes very slow or stagnates. This condition is called *anomalous viscosity*. The haematocrit is a useful guide for determining if whole blood or some other intravenous fluid should be used for volume replacement in the haemorrhagic shock patient. Maximum oxygen-carrying capacity is achieved with a haematocrit between 35% and 45%.

Urea, creatinine and electrolytes

The doctor or phlebotomist often takes blood in the mornings. The results of these blood tests have a prime place in assisting the nurse to gain a full detailed assessment of the patient. For further details, see Table 3.3.

TABLE 3.3 Normal blood values

	Values
Haematology	
Haemoglobin:	
• Male	14.0–17.7 g/dL
• Female	12.0–16.0 g/dL
White blood cell count	$4–11 \times 10^9$/L
Platelet count	$150–400 \times 10^9$/L
Serum B_{12}	160–925 ng/L
Serum folate	4–18 µg/L
Erythrocyte sedimentation rate (ESR)	<20 mm in 1 h
Coagulation	
Partial thromboplastin time (PTTK)	35–50 s
Prothrombin time	12–16 s
Serum biochemistry	
Albumin	34–48 g/L
Amylase	<220 U/L
Bicarbonate	22–30 mmol/L
Bilirubin	<17 µmol/L (0.3–1.5 mg/dL)
Calcium	2.20–2.67 mmol/L (8.5–10.5 mg/dL)
Chloride	95–106 mmol/L
Creatinine	0.06–0.12 mmol/L (0.6–1.5 mg/dL)
Glucose	4.5–5.6 mmol/L (70–110 mg/dL)
Potassium	3.5–5.0 mmol/L
Sodium	135–146 mmol/L
Urea	2.5–6.7 mmol/L (8–25 mg/dL)

Liver function tests

These determine how well the liver is functioning and can be obtained by sending a blood sample to the laboratory for liver biochemistry. They look at serum levels of the following substances.

Bilirubin

Normal range <17 μmol/L. Very high levels occur in biliary obstruction and serial measurements are useful in following the progress of some diseases, e.g. primary biliary cirrhosis, or response to treatment.

Aminotransferases

These enzymes are present in hepatocytes and leak into the blood with liver cell damage. Very high levels may occur with acute hepatitis (20–50 times normal). Aspartate aminotransferase (AST) (normal range 10–40 U/L) is also present in heart and skeletal muscle and seen in MI or skeletal damage. Alanine aminotransferase (ALT) (normal range 5–40 U/L) is more specific to the liver than AST.

Alkaline phosphatase

Normal range is 25–115 U/L. Raised levels are seen in cholestasis from any cause. Alkaline phosphatase is derived from bone and is also raised in Paget's disease, osteomalacia, growing children, metastases and hyperthyroidism.

γ-glutamyl transpeptidase

Normal range in males is <50 U/L and in females, <32 U/L. This is a liver microsomal enzyme which may be induced by alcohol and enzyme-inducing drugs, e.g. phenytoin. A raised serum concentration is a useful screen for alcohol abuse.

Serum proteins

Liver synthetic function is determined by measuring the serum albumin and the prothrombin time (clotting factors of the intrinsic pathway are synthesized by the liver).

Drug analysis

Therapeutic drug monitoring by blood analysis is available for a wide variety of antibiotics and some cardiac drugs. This is necessary for drugs that possess a narrow therapeutic range in serum. If the serum levels are too low, the patient is jeopardized by the probable lack of efficacy; if they are too high, the patient may suffer serious toxicity.

The three most common drugs that require regular analysis are gentamicin, digoxin, and phenytoin.

Drug monitoring is time-consuming and costly but leads to improved drug administration by preventing toxicity and improving outcome.

Cardiac enzymes

When myocardial cells are damaged, they release a number of enzymes into the circulation known as cardiac enzymes (Table 3.4). It could be argued that interpretation of these specialist results is the domain of the doctor. However, holistic nursing involves the identification and understanding of all aspects of illness to provide effective and high-quality patient care.

The estimation of myocardial enzymes is of great diagnostic importance in a MI. The enzymes most commonly measured are as follows:

- Aspartate aminotransferase (AST)
- Lactate dehydrogenase (LDH)
- Creatine kinase (CK)
- Troponins

These enzymes are normally present in low levels in the serum of healthy people, but their rise in concentration can be used to determine the diagnosis and severity of an MI. They cannot provide information about the location of the damage and CK and LDH only indicate muscle tissue injury. However, a precise investigation of MI can be made by analysing the concentrations of myocardial band (CK-MB) and isoforms of these enzymes, e.g. LD_1, LD_2.

Arterial blood gases

Blood can be taken from an artery and analysed to determine partial pressure of oxygen and carbon dioxide to understand the patient's acid-base balance. The movement of oxygen from the alveoli in the lungs to the pulmonary blood occurs due to the pressure gradient that exists. The partial pressure of oxygen in the alveoli is 13.7 kPa as compared with 5.3 kPa in the pulmonary capillaries, which allows exchange of oxygen through diffusion. Similarly, oxygen is easily exchanged between the capillaries to the tissues, because of a steep partial pressure gradient.

Measuring these partial pressure and other values in arterial blood can determine the following:

- Whether the patient is acidotic or alkalotic
- The cause of the condition (respiratory or metabolic)
- Whether the condition is being compensated

TABLE 3.4 Cardiac enzymes

Enzyme release	Peak values	Normal values	Other situations
Creatine kinase (CK) • released when cardiac muscle starts to die • is the first enzyme to increase after infarction	Values rise within the first 6 h after myocardial infarction (MI) Reach a peak between 18 and 24 h Values may return to normal after about 72 h as no more cells are dying CK levels should be measured • at the time of patient's admission • 24 h later • at the end of the second and third day	Normal for men is 15–120 U/L Women 10–80 U/L CK values can rise 10-fold to thousands in severe cellular death	• During trauma • In muscle disease • In cerebrovascular damage • After muscular exercise • With intramuscular injections
CK isoforms • MB is the one related to the heart • The presence of CK-MB in the plasma indicates myocardial necrosis	Measurement ensures levels are not confused with other muscle injury Helps to give an idea of the extent of muscle damage LDH level is raised within 8–24 h Peaks in 3–6 days Returns to normal in 8–14 days	If CK-MB levels are greater than 5% of the total CK level, the diagnosis of myocardial infarction is almost certain 240–525 U/l	It is only found in heart muscle LDH release is also found in • liver disease • renal disease • pulmonary embolism • shock • IM injection

Continued

TABLE 3.4 Cardiac enzymes—cont'd

Enzyme release	Peak values	Normal values	Other situations
LDH isoforms • Principally LD1 • A rise in this isoform indicates myocardial necrosis	Has five isoforms denoted as LD1–LD5 The pattern of LD1 level greater than LD2 occurs within 12–24 h after the attack	If the LD1 level is greater than the LD2 level, an MI is indicated	Released by the myocardium
Aspartate aminotransferase (AST) • There are no cardiac-specific isoforms	AST concentrations rise in 8–12 h Approaching peak in 18–36 h Returning to normal in 3–4 days	10–40 U/l	AST is not specific to cardiac muscle and its use in the diagnosis of MI is limited
Troponins (Tn) • Proteins present in striated muscle • Function as regulators of muscle contraction	Has three isoforms: TnC, TnI, TnT TnI is cardiac specific and measured in MI Rises within 4 h and remains elevated for 10–14 days	Lower limit 0.4 ng/mL Upper limit 50 ng/mL Diagnostic level for MI 1.5 ng/mL	This test has improved sensitivity over CK-MB, allowing identification of patients that present 48 h to 6 days after infarction

When attempting to analyse a person's acid-base balance, scrutinize the blood values in the following order:

1. Note the pH. This tells whether the person is in acidosis (pH < 7.35) or alkalosis (pH > 7.45), but it does not tell you the cause.
2. Check the PCO_2 to see if this is the cause of the acid-base imbalance. The respiratory system acts fast and an excessively high or low PCO_2 may indicate either that the condition is respiratory or metabolic or if the patient is compensating:
   a. The PCO_2 is over 5.7 kPa (40 mmHg): the respiratory system is the cause of the problem and the condition is a respiratory acidosis.
   b. The PCO_2 is below normal limits (5.2 kPa, 35 mmHg): the respiratory system is not the cause but is compensating.
3. Check the bicarbonate level. If step 2 indicates that the respiratory system is not responsible, then the condition is metabolic and should be reflected in increased or decreased bicarbonate levels:
   a. Metabolic acidosis is indicated by HCO_3^- values below 22 mmol/L.
   b. Metabolic alkalosis by values over 26 mmol/L.

Notice that PCO_2 levels vary inversely with blood pH (PCO_2 rises as blood pH falls) while HCO_3^- levels vary directly with blood pH (increased HCO_3^- results in increased pH).

If any changes occur in the partial pressures of oxygen or carbon dioxide, e.g. due to respiratory disease (asthma, COPD, ARDS) or metabolic disease (diabetes, renal failure, vomiting, diarrhoea) disruptions in the acid-base balance of the body may result.

Metabolic acidosis ($HCO_3^- < 22$ mmol/L; pH < 7.40)

Occurs in conditions such as follows:

- Severe diarrhoea
- Renal disease
- Untreated diabetes mellitus
- Starvation
- Excess alcohol ingestion
- High ECF potassium concentrations

Metabolic alkalosis ($HCO_3^- > 26$ mmol/L; pH > 7.40)

Occurs in conditions such as follows:

- Vomiting or gastric suctioning of hydrogen chloride-containing gastric contents
- Selected diuretics
- Ingestion of excessive amounts of sodium bicarbonate

- Constipation
- Excess aldosterone (e.g. tumours)

Respiratory acidosis ($PCO_2 > 5.7$ kPa; pH < 7.4)

Occurs in conditions such as follows:

- Any condition that impairs gas exchange or lung ventilation (chronic bronchitis, cystic fibrosis, emphysema)
- Rapid, shallow breathing
- Narcotic or barbiturate overdose or injury to brainstem

Respiratory alkalosis ($PCO_2 < 5.7$ kPa; pH > 7.4)

- Direct cause is always hyperventilation
- Brain tumour or injury

Electrocardiogram rhythm strip (cardiac monitoring)

The electrocardiogram (ECG) rhythm strip records the electrical activity of the heart in one particular lead, generally lead II. Cardiac cells are specialized and are unlike any other cells in the body, as each individual cell can initiate its own electrical impulse. The ECG rhythm strip is a record of the changes in electrical activity occurring within cardiac muscle. Although the cardiac cells involved in the contraction are specialized, cardiac muscle has this special property, hormones and chemical transmitters are important in producing the finer control of the heart and maintenance of homoeostasis.

Bipolar and unipolar electrodes provide an ECG rhythm known as the PQRST waves, which detect the electrical charges within the cardiac cell. The ECG can provide information about the heart rate and rhythm, the effects of electrolytes or drugs on the heart and the electrical orientation of the cardiac muscle. The normal ECG trace should record between 60 and 100 complexes (PQRST) per minute.

The ECG rhythm strip can give information about the following:

- The heart rate and rhythm
- The effects of electrolytes on the heart
- The effect of drugs on the heart
- Electrical orientation of the cardiac muscle

In a normal heart the sinoatrial (SA) node, situated in the right atrium, initiates the cardiac electrical impulse. The SA node is often called the *cardiac pacemaker* as it beats the fastest, between 60 and 100 beats per minute (bpm). Following discharge of the SA node, waves pass through specialized conducting pathways in the atria, each cell acting as stimulus to the next. This process causes atrial depolarization (contraction) and is represented on the ECG as the P wave.

The impulse then reaches the atrial ventricular (AV) node, then passes through the bundle of His and down the right and left bundle branches to finally arrive at the Purkinje fibres. The time it takes an impulse from the SA node to reach the Purkinje fibres is represented as the P-R interval (significant in some heart blocks). The Purkinje fibres give rise to ventricular depolarization (contraction), represented on the ECG as the QRS complex. The T wave soon follows which depicts repolarization (the heart going back to the resting phase) of the ventricles (Fig. 3.3).

The whole sequence of the PQRST portrays the systolic phase of the heart (heart contraction). The space between each beat is known as the repolarization or diastolic phase (resting phase) of the heart, whereby the arteries of the body are perfused with nutrients and oxygen is exchanged for carbon dioxide at cellular level.

What is an ECG?

The action potentials transmitted through the heart during the cardiac cycle can be recorded on the surface of the body. The recording can be obtained by electrodes on the body, connected to an ECG machine. The voltage changes

Waveform	Time	Voltage	
P interval	Not longer than 0.11 seconds or 3–4 small squares	2.5 mm–3.0 mm in any lead	
PR interval	0.12 seconds or 3–5 small squares	Not significant	
Q wave	0.03 seconds	Less than 25% of the R wave	
QRS	0.04–0.11 seconds or 2–3 small squares	Not significant	
R wave	See QRS	The total QRS (above or below the isoelectric line) must be 5.0 mm or greater in leads I, II, III to be considered normal	
ST segment	Not significant	Normally isoelectric but may be elevated 2.0 mm above isoelectric line or depressed 0.5 mm below the isoelectric line	
T wave	Not significant	No more than 5.0 mm in standard leads, 10.0 mm in chest leads	
U wave	Should be in the same direction as the proceeding T wave	Less than 1 mm	

FIGURE 3.3   The PQRST waveform of an ECG. *Modified from Edwards, 2002. Br. J. Nurs. II, 454–468, reproduced with permission.*

are fed to the machine, amplified and displayed visually on a screen, graphically on ECG paper, or both.

Terminology

- Isoelectric line — baseline
- Positive — upward deflection
- Negative — downward deflection
- Voltage — height and depth of a wave
- Time — measured along horizontal axis, one second = 5 large squares
- Cardiac cycle — represented on ECG by P wave, QRS complex, T wave
- Biphasic — deflection which is both positive and negative

ECG leads

The ECG leads provide a variety of views of the heart's electrical activity from different angles. An ECG lead consists of two surface electrodes of opposite polarity either one positive and one negative or one positive surface electrode and one reference point.

A lead composed of two electrodes of opposite polarity is called a bipolar lead and constitutes the standard limb leads (I–III) which represent the axis of the heart; these record the difference in electrical potential between the left arm, the right arm, and the left leg electrodes.

A lead composed of a single positive electrode and a reference point is a unipolar lead, making up the following:

- Augmented limb leads (aVR, aVL, and aVF)
- Precordial leads (V1–V6)

The various leads produce different ECG tracings.

Routine monitoring of ECG is usually obtained in lead II, as it is in the direct line of positive axis.

ECG paper

ECG paper moves at 25 mm/s and consists of small and large squares (5 small squares). ECG measures time and amplitude:

- Time is measured on the horizontal plane.
- Small squares are 0.04 s in time, and 1 mm in voltage.
- Large squares are 0.2 s in time, and 5 mm in voltage.

Amplitude is measured on the vertical axis of the graph paper:

- Small squares equal 0.1 mV.
- Large squares equal 0.5 mV.

Methods of calculating heart rate

$$25 \text{ mm} \times 60 = 1500 \text{ divided by 5 small squares} = 300$$

Count the number of small squares between R waves, divide these into 1500, e.g. 18 small squares divided into $1500 = 83$ bpm.

Count the number of large squares between R waves and divide these into 300, e.g. 4 large squares divided into $300 = 75$ bpm.

During a period of acute illness, the sequence of the ECG can be affected. The rate may increase owing to heart failure, hypertension, blood loss, pain, stress or anxiety or reduce its rate owing to overprescription of certain drugs (digoxin) or a lack of oxygen supply. Abnormal rhythms can occur from heart failure, coronary artery disease, MI (Edwards, 2002), fluid overload (Richards & Edwards, 2014) and fluid and electrolyte imbalance (Edwards, 2001).

Sinus rhythm

The P wave

- Atrial depolarization and it is the first positive deflection seen.
- It should be no longer than 0.11 s, or three small squares; amplitude is normally 0.5–2.5 mm.
- It should always be followed by a QRS complex, unless conduction disturbances are present.

The PR interval

- Measured from the beginning of the P wave to the beginning of the QRS complex irrespective of whether the QRS complex begins with a Q or an R wave.
- It varies between 0.12 and 0.20 s, or 3–5 small squares.
- Dependent on the heart rate and conduction of AV node.
- Normal tracing indicates electrical impulses have been conducted through the correct conduction pathways.

The QRS complex

- Consists of three waves, Q, R and S.
- Should be narrow and sharply pointed.
- Represents ventricular contraction (depolarization), marking the beginning of ventricular systole, and can be predominately positive (upright), predominately negative (inverted), biphasic (partly positive, partly negative).
- Varies between 0.04 and 0.11 s, or 2–3 small squares; amplitude varies from less than 5 mm to more than 15 mm.

The ST segment

- This is the resting period between ventricular contraction and the returning of the cardiac muscle to its resting stage.
- Early repolarization, should always return to the baseline, depressed or elevated in abnormalities.

The T wave

- Represents repolarization of the ventricular myocardial cells.
- Usually slightly rounded.
- Deep and symmetrical inverted T waves suggest cardiac ischaemia.
- T waves elevated more than half of the height of the QRS complex (peaked T waves) could indicate hyperkalaemia.

The QT interval

- This is the period from the beginning of ventricular depolarization (onset of the QRS complex) until the end of ventricular repolarization, or the end of T wave.
- During this period, the heart is fully refractory (the absolute refractory period).
- During the latter period of the interval (from the peak of the T wave onward), the conduction system is relatively refractory.
- Drugs may prolong the QT period.

Normal sinus rhythm

- Rate: 60–100
- Rhythm: regular
- Pacemaker site: SA node
- P waves: normal in shape, upright
- PR interval: normal, 0.12–0.20 s
- QRS: normal, 0.14–0.12 s
- Clinical significance: none, normal rhythm

The rate of discharge of the SA node can increase (*tachycardia* – over 100 beats per minute) owing to the following:

- Disease of the heart, e.g. heart failure, hypertension, MI
- Blood loss
- Pain
- Stress or anxiety
- Haemorrhage, dehydration

The SA node may reduce its rate of discharge (*bradycardia* — less than 60 beats per minute) owing to the following:

- Overadministration of certain drugs (digoxin)
- A lack of oxygen supply
- Myocardial infarction

Abnormal rhythms can occur from the following:

- Heart failure
- Coronary artery disease
- Myocardial infarction
- Arteriosclerosis
- Fluid overload
- Fluid and electrolyte imbalance

The diagnosis of arrhythmias

The following are some of the important features which can be looked for in an ECG in its interpretation:

- Rate of discharge — is the rate 60 or above 100?
- Rhythm or regularity of the complexes
- Duration of the PR interval
- Whether each P wave is followed by the QRS complex
- QRS complex — width, configuration, deep Q waves in leads
- T waves — are they inverted throughout, only in certain leads, or more prominent in others?
- Interpretation

Changes to an ECG rhythm strip can be determined by interpreting changes that occur in time and voltage to the PQRST waveforms (www. ecglibrary.com/ecghist.html) and by using a standardized approach to the diagnosis of arrhythmias. An ECG rhythm strip can identify abnormal rhythms, such as follows:

- Sinus bradycardia
- Sinus tachycardia
- Sinus arrhythmias
- Atrial fibrillation
- Atrial flutter
- Atrial ectopics
- Ventricular ectopics (unifocal, multifocal)
- Ventricular tachycardia (SVT)
- Ventricular fibrillation
- Asystole
- Heart block

The 12-lead ECG

A 12-lead ECG gives 12 readings from 10 leads and is undertaken to confirm diagnosis and determine any other cardiac damage present. It is more useful when diagnosing an MI or other cardiac problems, e.g. heart block. It can be performed simply and quickly and views the heart electrically in a three-dimensional manner. The limb leads are attached to the forearms and calves, with a small amount of conduction gel, and three bipolar leads (I, II, III) and three augmented unipolar leads (AVR, AVL, and AVF) can be recorded. Chest precordial unipolar lead placements are secured again by applying a small amount of conduction gel over the six V lead positions (V_1, V_2, V_3, V_4, V_5, and V_6) and allow the heart to be viewed in the horizontal axis from the chest wall.

The 12-lead ECG produces a representation of what is happening directly underneath the electrode so that a practitioner can determine if the conduction pathway of the heart is normal or damaged. During an MI, changes on a 12-lead ECG over a period of days can be detected. These changes occur if cardiac muscle is damaged, so that the electrical waves within the heart have to travel via an alternative route, and this will alter the pattern of the ECG and identify the affected area.

After only 30−60 s of hypoxia, changes can be observed on an ECG rhythm strip and/or a 12-lead ECG. An ECG is often the first diagnostic procedure to yield results. It is designed to record the electrical impulses produced by the heart with the use of electrodes on the skin and generates a waveform that is described as the PQRST (Fig. 3.3).

- The P wave represents atrial activity.
- The P-R interval represents the period of delay within the AV node.
- The QRS complex is the wave of depolarization down the bundle of His, the left and right bundle branches and the Purkinje network.
- The T wave represents ventricular repolarization.
- The flat line from the end of the T wave to the beginning of the next P wave is the resting or filling phase.

Changes to an ECG rhythm can be determined by interpreting changes that occur in time and voltage to the above waveforms (Fig. 3.3) and by using a standardized approach to the diagnosis of arrhythmias detailed previously.

However, it is a 12-lead ECG that a nurse will undertake when a patient complains of chest pain. It is more useful when diagnosing an MI, despite the problems with interpretation, than the rhythm strip.

The zones of alteration

In the early stages of acute MI, there are at least three zones of tissue damage:

1. The zone of hypoxia
2. The zone of ischaemia
3. The zone of infarction/necrosis

The third consists of necrotic myocardial tissue that has been irreversibly destroyed by the prolonged deprivation of oxygen. It is electrically silent and does not contribute to the ECG. The second zone is hypoxic injury that surrounds the necrotic dead tissue. The myocardial cells may survive if adequate circulation to this area is revived or if not it may progress to necrosis. The third zone is called ischaemia that is adjacent to the zone of hypoxic injury. This zone represents cells that have been deprived of some oxygen but may recover. Ischaemic and injured myocardial tissue causes ST and T wave changes on the ECG (Fig. 3.3). The ultimate size of an infarct may depend on the zones of injury.

ST elevation

ST elevation occurs within minutes of the onset of infarction, pathologic Q waves (>40 ms in duration or $> 25\%$ of the height of the ensuing R wave) may take hours or even days to develop. Elevation of the ST segments indicates the presence of ischaemic tissue, but the range and conductivity may be normal. There may be horizontal ST depression and T wave inversion lasting for $70-80$ ms in V_2 through to V_4, which is also indicative of ischaemia. However, this is controversial and considered by some to be nonspecific. Edwards (2002) suggested that serial ECG changes are more helpful, as changes with time are more likely to indicate acute infarction.

The reason for ST elevation is unclear. It is proposed that it is the result of the following:

- Effect of the electrical current going around the injured site to reach the uninjured muscle which alters the level of the baseline of the ECG.
- Injured cells remaining polarized, but the transmembrane potential is less than normal owing to the loss of cellular potassium.
- Injured tissue conducts more rapidly than normal and a voltage gradient develops between the normal and injured tissue; this leads to an ST elevation over the injured area.

Q waves

An infarct is virtually certain if Q waves appear during the course of the illness. However, there has been identification of non-Q-wave infarctions. Diagnosis of non-Q-wave infarction relies on a combination of the history, increased serum cardiac enzymes and ECG changes. These patients are often considered for angioplasty, for even though associated with smaller amounts of myocardial damage, a substantial amount of heart muscle may still be at risk.

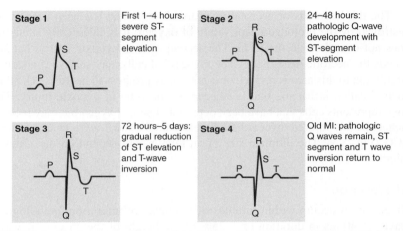

FIGURE 3.4 The four stages of myocardial infarction. *Reproduced from Myocardial infarction: nursing responsibilities in the first hour. Edwards, S.L., 2002. Myocardial infarction: nursing responsibilities in the first hour. Br. J. Nurs. 11(7), 454–468, with permission.*

The four stages of a myocardial infarction

To use a 12-lead ECG as a diagnostic tool for an MI, a sequence of readings need to be taken, as not every change is evident immediately (Edwards, 2002). These are known as the four stages of an MI (Fig. 3.4):

- First 1–4 h; severe ST-segment elevation
- 24–48 h: pathologic Q-wave development with ST-segment elevation
- 72 hours–5 days: gradual reduction of ST elevation and T-wave inversion
- Old MI: pathologic Q waves remain, ST segment and T-wave inversion return to normal

Localizing a myocardial infarction on a 12-lead ECG

The 12-lead ECG can localize the area of heart muscle damage, although indication of the infarction site is not uniformly accurate. An anterior MI may be identified by observing ST elevation, and inverted T waves in particular leads of a 12-lead ECG (AVR, V_1, V_2, V_3, V_4). An inferior MI will have ST elevation in leads II, III and AVF. When looking at a 12-lead ECG, leads II, III and AVF can show signs of an MI most clearly. Often, the infarction involves more than one discrete region of myocardium, e.g. anteroseptal, inferolateral (Table 3.5).

Respiratory investigations

The gas inspired and expired per minute can be measured as lung volumes and capacities:

- Tidal volume (TV) is the amount of gas inspired and expired during normal breathing.

TABLE 3.5 Locating an myocardial infarction (MI) on a 12-lead ECG

MI location	Leads with indicative changes seen in Fig. 3.4
Inferior	II, III, AVF
Anterior	V_1, V_2,V_3, V_4, AVR
Lateral	I, AVL, V_5, V_6
Anterolateral	I, AVL and all chest leads
Anteroseptal	I, AVL, V_1, V_2,V_3
Inferolateral	II, III, AVF, V_5, V_6
Posterior	Tall R wave in V_1, or V_7, V_8, V_9

- Inspiratory reserve volume (IRV) is the amount of gas that can be inspired in addition, to TV.
- Expiratory reserve volume (ERV) is the amount of gas that can be expired after a passive (relaxed) expiration.
- Residual volume (RV) is the volume of gas that cannot be expired and is always present in the lungs.
- Total lung capacity (TLC) is the total gas volume in the lung when it is maximally inflated. It is made up of RV, ERV, TV and IRV.

The lung capacities are always the sum of two or more volumes:

- Vital capacity (VC) is the maximum amount of gas that can be displaced (expired) from the lung and includes IRV, TV and ERV.
- Functional residual capacity (FRC) is the amount of gas remaining in the lung at the end of a passive expiration (RV and ERV). The lungs are at rest or in a state of mechanical equilibrium.
- Inspiratory capacity (IC) is the amount of gas that can be inspired after a passive expiration (from FRC) and includes TV and IRV.

Norms for volumes and capacities are based on age, sex and height and are referred to as predicted values. Changes from predicted or baseline values are taken into account in diagnosing and assessing respiratory disorders.

The volume of air exhaled in a minute of resting breathing is known as the *total minute volume* (MV) and is equal to TV (millilitres per breath) multiplied by the frequency of breathing (breaths per minute). Only about two-thirds of this volume actually reaches the alveoli (this is known as the *alveolar minute volume*). Not all the air entering the airways and lungs participates in gas exchange. The remaining one-third stays within the trachea, bronchus and bronchioles of the lungs. This volume of wasted ventilation is called *dead space ventilation* (VD).

Chronic pulmonary disorders include the following:

- *Obstructive* disorders of the bronchioles (emphysema, bronchitis and asthma), whereby the patient has difficulty moving air rapidly into and out of the lungs
- *Restrictive* disorders of the lungs (fibrosis, adult respiratory distress syndrome)

The measure that is most commonly used in practice is the forced expiratory volume in 1 s (FEV_1) or peak expiratory flow (PEF) rate, which is a useful indicator of a worsening condition.

Chest X-rays

The chest X-ray is by far the commonest type of X-ray to be taken. The different types of chest X-rays are as follows:

- Posteroanterior (PA) — standard department film, the plate is in front of the patient's chest, with the X-ray tube 6 ft behind the patient.
- Anteroposterior (AP) — usually a portable film, the plate is behind the patient's chest, and the X-ray tube is closer to the patient. The positioning of the patient is often inconsistent and often the film will not show full inspiration.
- Lateral — departmental film, difficult to take as a portable film owing to the added difficulties in positioning the patient. Helpful to show specific areas of consolidation.

Examination of a chest X-ray

The examination must be carried out in an orderly sequence, identifying normal anatomical structure and any abnormal shadows.

Normal anatomical structures:

- Labelled to identify left and right, if it is not, the aortic knuckle and the stomach air bubble appear on the patient's left.
- With the correct exposure the vertebral bodies should be visible through the upper part of the heart shadow but not the lower. An overexposed film will appear very dark. The degree of exposure should always be taken into account when comparing successive films.
- Patient in straight position — the medial ends of each clavicle should be evenly disposed on either side of the adjacent vertebral spinous process. If the patient is rotated to the left, the medial end of the left clavicle will be further from the midline than the right.
- Depth of inspiration — determined by the position of the diaphragms and the ribs.

- Soft tissues — in women the breast and nipple shadows should be noted and in men those of the pectoralis muscle. Horizontal lines caused by folds of flesh may be seen in the obese patient.
- Thoracic cage — symmetry of the skeleton should be noted and the width of the intercostal spaces should be equal on both sides. Unilateral crowding of the ribs will be seen in kyphoscoliosis or loss of lung volume through collapse or resection of lung tissue. Rib margins should be examined for irregularities caused by trauma and fractures, etc. It is important to identify the margins of the scapula.
- Diaphragm — each diaphragm should be evenly curved with a clear outline. Both the costophrenic and cardiophrenic angles are clear and sharp.
  - Position — on full inspiration.
    - Right — anterior end of the sixth rib in the mid-clavicular line.
    - Left — 1–2 cm lower than the right.
- Heart shadow — the transverse diameter of the heart should be less than half the maximum diameter of the thoracic cage. The outline should be clear.
- Trachea — this is visible as a vertical translucent band overlying the spinous processes of the upper thoracic vertebrae, should be in midline with the deviation of the lower one-third to the right.

Any abnormal shadow should be analysed for its anatomical site, size and shape of its margins.

- Consolidation — this is the replacement of air in the lung by tissue or fluid of greater density. Often affects part of the lobe, but if a whole lobe is consolidated there will be no displacement of the surrounding structures. Consolidation has the following features: Homogeneous shadowing, confined to segments and bounded by fissures, diaphragm, pleura and chest.
- No loss of lung volume.
- Air bronchograms.
- Relative constancy from day to day.
- Collapse — this is the absorption of air with loss of lung volume. The position of the tissues is often altered with possible displacement of the heart and trachea. The mediastinal outline may be obliterated.
- Pneumothorax — air in the pleural cavity seen as an area of no lung markings, which will result in reduction of lung size. Common features are a white, visible air-lung interface, mediastinal shift to the opposite side (see p. 287).
- Pleural effusion — present as a uniform opacity, which extends up from the costophrenic angle. The upper margin will be concave unless air is present. If air is present in the pleural cavity, there is a horizontal fluid level with

clear demarcation. In the supine position, the fluid will show as haziness over the whole lung, through which normal lung markings may still be visible. A large pleural effusion will cause mediastinal shift to the opposite side.

- Asthma — in asthma the X-ray is often normal except during severe attacks or long-term asthma, then the following will be seen:
  - Overinflation
  - Low but curved diaphragms
  - Vessels remain normal
- Chronic bronchitis — the film may be normal even though the patient is severely disabled. Areas of infection may cause consolidation and/or collapse.
- Pulmonary oedema — may be cardiac or noncardiac in origin, may see upper lobe venous engorgement, fluffy shadows, pleural effusion may be present, cardiac enlargement may develop owing to dilatation of the left ventricle.
- Pulmonary embolism — generally to exclude other pathology, patchy areas of atelectasis are often seen in submassive PE, may be confused with consolidation or collapse. May see some vascular shadowing in the affected areas, other diagnostic procedures are more reliable, e.g. nuclear imaging or pulmonary angiogram.
- Positioning of invasive devices to observe the tip and position during movement or following insertion:
  - Endotracheal tubes
  - Nasogastric tubes
  - CVP
  - Aortic balloon pumps

Portable X-rays

Patients cannot always go to the radiotherapy department to have their X-rays taken and may therefore require the radiographer to come to their area. In this instance protection of the patient and staff present on the unit at the time is imperative. Exposure to radiation always involves the risk of biological changes within the body. Therefore, the patient should always be exposed to the lowest amount of radiation possible and all individuals coming into contact with radiation should be protected.

Pulse oximetry

This noninvasive technique is used to measure the saturation of blood in the arterial capillaries. It is a spectrophotometric measurement of the proportion of oxygenated haemoglobin in the arteries. The absorption of light by desaturated and fully saturated haemoglobin is different. This light absorption is measured by a special light detector and appears as the percentage oxygen saturation of the haemoglobin in the arteries.

The light detector of the oximeter is attached to a tissue that is reasonably transparent to these wavelengths of light. This may be the finger, the toe or the ear lobe. As such, it is very useful in following changes in arterial oxygenation. There must be:

- a good flow of blood to the area (not effective if severe vasoconstriction is present);
- no mechanical movement of the probe, which will cause interference;
- no nail varnish, which will affect the normal haemoglobin saturation measured

If the oxygen saturation falls below 85% the pulse oximeter may become progressively less accurate. Pulse oximetry cannot be used in any form of carbon monoxide inhalation because the carboxyhaemoglobin will cause the oximeter to overread the saturation level. Pulse oximetry is used:

- to estimate arterial oxygen saturation (SpO2);
- to monitor changes in arterial oxygen saturation;
- alongside blood gas analysis to monitor the adequacy of ventilation.

End-tidal carbon dioxide monitoring

The end-tidal carbon dioxide ($P_{ET}CO_2$) monitors exhaled carbon dioxide on both intubated and nonintubated patients. The normal range for expired $P_{ET}CO_2$ is generally 4.5−5.7 kPa. This method of expiratory gas analysis can be undertaken through a nasal cannula, which simultaneously delivers supplemental oxygen. In lungs where ventilation is uniformly distributed and evenly matched to perfusion, $P_{ET}CO_2$ reasonably reflects partial pressure of arterial CO_2:

- Pulmonary embolism or decreased cardiac output is associated with a decrease in $P_{ET}CO_2$, because of decreased alveolar blood flow.
- An increase in $P_{ET}CO_2$ reflects the presence of airway narrowing or other lung disease associated with respiratory changes in the mechanical properties of the lungs.

This method of expiratory gas analysis is not commonly used in all clinical practice areas, but studies are showing its benefits and value in respiratory management. In the future it may become as normal as attaching an oxygen saturation monitor.

Lumbar puncture

In this procedure CSF is withdrawn after the insertion of a hollow needle into the lumbar subarachnoid space. The needle is usually inserted between the second and third or third and fourth lumbar vertebrae (L2 and L3, or L3 and L4). This is below the level of the spinal cord, which extends to L1 or L2, and is in the region of the cauda equina.

The fluid obtained is examined for diagnostic purposes and may be required:

● To record the pressure of the CSF using a manometer;
● In suspected meningitis or encephalitis to look for bacteria in the CSF;
● In suspected malignant tumours to look for cancer cells (cytology);
● To aid diagnosis in subarachnoid haemorrhage when there would be blood in the CSF;
● To introduce intrathecal medication such as antibiotics or cytotoxic drugs;
● To introduce contrast media for radiologic examination.

A lumbar puncture is contraindicated in the following circumstances:

● In patients with papilloedema or deteriorating neurologic symptoms, where raised ICP is suspected
● In the presence of infection, as this may lead to meningitis or abscess formation: localized skin infection around the insertion site, the presence of frontal sinusitis, middle ear discharge, congenital heart disease or prosthetic heart valves
● In patients who are unable to cooperate or who are too drowsy to give a history
● In patients who have severe degenerative spinal joint disease
● In those patients undergoing anticoagulant therapy or who have coagulopathies or thrombocytopaenia

A doctor carries out the procedure using a strict aseptic technique. The position of the patient is vitally important, and the nurse may be responsible for helping the patient to maintain this position during the procedure:

● The patient should be in the left lateral position, with maximum flexion of the spine and as near the edge of the bed as possible.
● There should be one pillow under the patient's head.
● To gain maximum stretching of the lumbar vertebrae, the client should flex his head to the chest and draw his knees to the abdomen, holding them with his hands.
● The nurse can help by supporting the client behind the knees and neck, thus ensuring the widening of the intervertebral space.

Careful positioning is necessary so that the doctor can feel the lumbar spine more easily and so insert the needle accurately. It is imperative that the lumbar puncture is performed below the first lumbar vertebra where the cord terminates.

When the needle is in position the insertion rod (stylette) of the needle is removed and a manometer attached to record the pressure of the CSF. The normal pressure of the CSF is 60—180 mm H_2O. For laboratory analysis, approximately 5—10 mL of CSF is withdrawn.

> ! If the lumbar puncture is difficult, for example in an obese client, the doctor may request that the patient sits straddled on a straight-backed chair with his or her arms folded round the back of the chair and the head resting on the hands. The patient will need support and reassurance throughout.

The nurse should note the following:

- The colour of the CSF — it should be colourless.
- The presence of blood in the CSF — the first few millilitres may be bloodstained owing to trauma after insertion of the needle but after this the fluid should run clear.
- The consistency of the CSF — it should be like water.
- The opacity of the CSF — it should be clear; cloudy CSF is typical in bacterial meningitis.

A Queckenstedt's test is performed when an obstruction to the flow of CSF in the spinal pathway is suspected. Pressure is recorded using the manometer while jugular compression is applied. Normally the pressure of the CSF would rapidly rise when jugular compression is applied and just as rapidly fall when the pressure is released. If an obstruction such as a spinal tumour or dislocated vertebra is present, the rise and fall of pressure will occur much more slowly. Pressure is applied for a maximum of 10 s and recordings taken via the manometer. Further recordings are then taken for 10 s when the pressure is released. When pressure recordings are complete, the specimens of CSF will be collected in culture bottles.

Following the completion of the procedure:

- The needle is withdrawn and the wound sealed with a plastic sealant dressing.
- The patient is asked to lie down flat in bed for 6—12 h. This should prevent the development of a headache.
- Observations for leakage from the puncture site together with neurologic observations should be continued for up to 24 h.

Radiography (X-rays)

Radiography enables film views of the internal structures of the body to be taken by the passage of X-rays (γ rays) through the body onto a specially sensitized film. Very high-energy X-rays or radioactive substances are also used in the radiotherapy department to treat some forms of cancer. This is radiation therapy. Protection from this radiation is necessary in both the abovementioned cases. The radiographer is qualified to take X-rays for interpretation by a radiologist, who is a physician who has specialized in the use of radiography to diagnose and treat disease.

X-rays are electromagnetic vibrations of short wavelength produced by passing a high voltage through a cathode ray tube. The beam crosses the patient and is partially absorbed in the process. Those energy waves (photons) that leave the patient are captured by an image receptor. The energies of the photons are decreased by differing amounts as they pass through different tissues in the body. The remnant radiation that leaves the patient produces the photographic image on the radiographic film.

An X-ray can give a variety of information about the lungs, heart, pleura, bones and mediastinal structures:

- *Radiolucent* materials allow X-rays to pass through them easily. Air is radiolucent.
- *Radiopaque* materials do not easily allow light to pass. Bone is a relatively radiopaque material.
- On a plain radiograph, gas and fat absorb few X-rays and appear dark.
- Bone and other calcified regions absorb most of the X-rays and appear white.
- Some foreign bodies such as metal and some glass are radiopaque but wood and plastic cannot be seen.

Protection from ionizing radiation

Exposure to radiation always involves the risk of biological changes within the body. The benefits of better diagnosis outweigh the risk to the patient but great care has to be taken to protect both the patient and the staff involved with taking X-rays. The patient should always be exposed to the lowest amount of radiation possible and all individuals coming into contact with radiation should be protected.

Protection occurs by:

- minimizing the time the patient is in the path of the X-ray beam;
- maximizing the distance between the radiation source and the patient;
- shielding the reproductive organs of the patient if they are within 4–5 cm of the beam. This is extremely important in children and young adults. The shields are made of lead which absorbs X-rays;
- improvement of X-ray machines so that there is less scatter of the radiation.

Time, distance and shielding are also used to protect staff:

- The time spent in the room where the radiation source is active should be as short as possible. The risk is only there when exposures are being made.

- Increasing the distance from the source of the beam greatly reduces the quantity of radiation that will reach the radiographer or nurse. This means that if the nurse has to hold the patient while he is X-rayed, there will be much greater exposure.
- If the nurse does have to support the patient, a shield should be worn. Lead aprons or gloves are used where a fixed shield is not in place.
- Any worker regularly exposed to ionizing radiation must be monitored, usually by the use of a film badge. The film inside gets darker in response to the amount of radiation exposure and it is analysed, usually monthly.
- Contact with X-rays should be *avoided in pregnancy* as exposure can lead to malformations of the foetus. There is a safe limit of 0.5 rem for a declared pregnant woman.

Contrast media

These are diagnostic agents introduced into the body by injection or via an orifice to enhance the X-ray picture in areas of the body where there is insufficient natural contrast:

- Air may be used to study the ventricles of the brain and to aid localization of tumours in the brain.
- Barium sulphate is used to study the digestive tract. It is an inert and insoluble compound that is nontoxic, cheap and readily available.
- Iodine contrast media are used to study the renal tract and vascular system.

Preparation for barium studies

- For upper gastrointestinal studies, the patient should be fasted overnight, except for water.
- Smoking should be avoided to minimize bowel gas.
- For small bowel studies, laxatives are sometimes taken the day before to empty the colon.
- For a barium enema, laxatives are given and sometimes rectal washouts so that any defects in the mucosa can be seen.

Care with contrast agents

- Barium sulphate is not used if a perforation is suspected. The body cannot remove it if it enters the peritoneum and peritonitis follows.
- Care should be taken in the elderly, especially those on steroid drugs, as there may be a danger of perforation.
- Barium sulphate should not be taken by mouth in bowel obstruction as it will solidify and can turn a partial obstruction into a complete one.

- Plenty of fluids should be taken orally following barium, as it is very constipating and can dry in the bowel, forming an obstruction.
- Any iodine-containing contrast medium may provoke an anaphylactoid action (see p. 448). It may be minor, resulting in urticaria (hives), or there may be wheezing and laryngeal oedema. Sometimes steroids and antihistamines are given as premedication to reduce these effects.
- Resuscitation equipment will always be at hand.
- Nonionic iodine contrast media with less risk of side effects have now been introduced, e.g. ioxaglate and iodixanol.
- In sickle cell trait, the injection of contrast media can cause sickling to occur.

Biliary contrast radiology

Cholecystography

- Contrast that is excreted in the bile is given orally, and it weakly opacifies the gall bladder and bile ducts.
- The gall bladder concentrates the contrast, and the films are taken 12 h after its administration.
- A fatty meal is then given, and this causes contraction of a healthy gall bladder that can be seen on the X-ray.
- If there is no contraction, this suggests damage to the gall bladder by inflammation.

Intravenous cholangiography

This is performed less frequently now as the contrast material is relatively toxic. It has been replaced by percutaneous transhepatic cholangiography (PTC or 'perc'). This is used to diagnose the cause of obstructive jaundice (see p. 349).

Angiography

- This is the opacification of the veins or arteries by the injection of appropriate contrast media.
- The femoral vessels in the groin are the favourite entry points for the catheter through which water-soluble contrast is injected and images recorded on a video recorder.
- Obstructions due to thrombosis, atheroma or embolism can be seen.
- Clotting studies should be done first to ensure there is no bleeding tendency.
- Following cannulation there is a risk of trauma to the vessel causing bleeding or thrombosis and occasionally part of the catheter has been lost into the lumen of the vessel.
- There is also a risk of allergic response to the contrast media.

Ultrasound

High-frequency sound waves are used in diagnostic medical sonography to visualize structures in the body by recording the reflections of high-frequency pulses directed into the tissue:

- Noninvasive
- Painless and almost certainly safe
- Uses a transducer, which both emits and receives the ultrasound
- Based on the emission of sound waves and the reflection of ultrasound echoes
- The ultrasound probe containing a transducer is applied to the skin over the area of interest and the image is displayed on a screen
- Jelly is used to exclude air and ensure a good connection to the skin
- The probe is moved at different angles and in different directions to display any abnormalities. 'Spot' films are also taken to record any images
- Minimal patient preparation is needed
- The bladder needs to be full of urine to examine the pelvis and the patient should be fasted to minimize gas shadows in gall bladder studies

Ultrasound is used to examine virtually all areas of the body. It:

- distinguishes solid from cystic lesions;
- assesses abdominal masses (difficult to see on X-ray);
- detects abnormal material in an organ, such as metastases;
- detects movement, as in the pulsation of an aneurysm;
- can measure physical dimensions, such as the diameter of the aorta;
- detects stones in the urinary bladder or the gall bladder;
- guides intervention procedures such as aspiration or biopsy.

Limiting factors of ultrasound

- Bone completely reflects ultrasound and obscures any tissues beyond it. This means it cannot be used to examine the brain or the spinal cord.
- Bowel gas partly reflects the ultrasound and here starving the patient or using laxatives may help.
- A thick layer of fat scatters ultrasound and so it may be better to investigate the gall bladder by other means in the very obese.

Doppler-shift ultrasound

This method is used to study blood flow. The beam is directed towards the artery and is reflected from the red cells. It can be used to generate an audible signal for detecting blood flow or may be processed to give information on the nature of the flow. Other uses include the following:

- Measuring systolic BP when low. A portable Doppler is used to detect flow beyond a sphygmomanometer cuff placed around the arm or ankle

- Detecting the foetal heart
- Studying flow dynamics, for example in carotid artery disease

Computed tomography

Computed tomography (CT) allows the visualization of the anatomy from various sectional planes by X-raying a series of thin transverse 'slices' of the patient's head or body that are then analysed by a computer. Very specialized equipment is needed and the radiographer needs extra training in this field. CT uses computerized digital imaging, as does ultrasonography and MRI. Eventually digital imaging will be used more and more in the X-ray department, reducing the use of film:

- Pathologic anatomy can be studied in great detail. Can reveal as much as an explorative operation, especially after injury to the brain. The management of serious head injuries has been transformed by the use of CT scanning. It enables appropriate surgical intervention only when necessary.
- Good images can be obtained in the obese this time! This is because fat separates the organs.
- Water-soluble contrast can be given before the scan to enhance the image.
- Very useful for areas where radiography is unsuitable: the pancreas (deep inside the body), the lungs, mediastinum, the brain and spinal cord.
- Planning radiotherapy or chemotherapy and staging tumours, e.g. lymphomas.
- Planning surgery, e.g. establishing the extent of invasion of oesophageal cancer.
- Assessing damage in abdominal or thoracic trauma.
- Guiding needles in biopsy, drainage of fluid or aspiration.

Radioisotope scanning

This is the diagnostic application of nuclear medicine to identify sites of abnormal pathology, e.g. presence of pus, extensive bone turnover, but it gives poor anatomical detail. A radioactive label is combined with a substance taken up readily by the tissue — this combination is called a tracer agent. The tracer is concentrated in a specific tissue type, e.g. the thyroid gland, and detected by a γ camera that collects and counts the level of radioactivity across the area of interest. It is used for the following:

- Liver and spleen scans to investigate unexplained abnormalities in liver function tests or suspected liver metastases.
- Bone scanning — areas of increased bone deposition and reabsorption take up the tracer. This includes secondary tumours.
- Renal scans, giving information not available from any other source.

- Labelling the patient's white blood cells.
- Lung scanning, to detect pulmonary emboli.

Magnetic resonance imaging

Strong magnetic fields and radio waves are used along with a computer in MRI to generate sectional images of the anatomy. It is a rapidly expanding diagnostic field and involves applying a powerful magnetic field to the body, which causes all the protons of all the hydrogen nuclei to become aligned. Pulses of radio waves, which emit signals that are recorded electronically, then excite these. Images are produced using sophisticated equipment that can be viewed in any plane:

- Lipids have a high hydrogen content and so are clearly seen on MRI.
- Very useful for examining the brain and spinal cord.
- Atheroma can also be demonstrated.
- Can be used to investigate blood flow and cardiac function without the use of contrast media.

Endoscopy

Any method of looking into the body uses an instrument. This can either be via an orifice, such as the nose or mouth, or via an artificial opening such as an arthroscopy. Endoscopes are now illuminated by the use of fibre optics enabling accurate diagnosis to be made:

- Gastroscopy, oesophagogastroduodenoscopy (OGD) enables the whole area to be viewed and peptic ulcers to be seen. The source of haemorrhage can often be identified.
- Duodenoscopy allows the injection of contrast into the common bile duct.
- Colonoscopy, large bowel endoscopy can be used to remove polyps and to biopsy suspicious lesions.
- Bronchoscopy — inspecting the bronchi with a narrow fibreoptic endoscope.
- Cystoscopy, cystourethroscopy — inspection of the bladder and urethra is very important in both diagnosis and treatment of diseases of the prostate, urethra and bladder.
- Ureteroscopy can now be used to remove stones from the lower half of the ureter.
- Laparoscopy is used by gynaecologists to diagnose pelvic disorders. The abdomen is inflated with carbon dioxide and a scope passed into the peritoneal cavity; can also be used to obtain liver biopsies.

Biopsy

This is the removal of a small amount of tissue for diagnostic purposes. The lesions are usually removed under local anaesthetic or at operation, e.g. lymph nodes.

Cytology

This is the study of cells by the application of special staining techniques for malignancy. A negative result may be due to sampling error. Uses include the following:

- Early detection of cancer as in cervical cytology
- Examining fluid as in a needle biopsy of the breast
- Examining ascitic fluid obtained via paracentesis or pleural effusions from chest aspiration
- Examining cells from solid masses such as the pancreas, the breast or the thyroid

3.5 NURSING CARE ISSUES

Venepuncture and cannulation

Venepuncture

This includes a puncture into a vein for the following:

- A blood sample for diagnostic purposes
- Administration of fluids and drugs
- Monitoring levels of blood components

This is a common procedure and nurses commonly are performing more, therefore ward nurses undertaking this procedure must be aware of the following:

- Relevant anatomy and physiology
- Criteria for choosing a vein and equipment to use
- Potential problems, how to prevent them and interventions
- Health and safety related to insertion and safe disposal of equipment
- Adherence to aseptic technique
- Comfort of the patient
- Adequate information regarding the procedure and complications

The veins used include the following:

- Median cubital veins
- Cephalic vein
- Basilic vein
- Metacarpal veins

Choosing a vein

Must be best for the patient. The most prominent is not always the most suitable for venepuncture, use the following:

- Visual inspection
- Palpation

Influencing factors

- Injury, disease or treatment may prevent the use of a limb for venepuncture.
- How the patient is positioned, e.g. lying on one side.
- The age and weight of the patient.
- If the patient is in shock or dehydrated, poor superficial peripheral access may be present.
- Medications can influence choice, e.g. anticoagulants, steroids, risk of bruising.
- The temperature will influence venous dilatation, e.g. if patient is cold, no veins may be visible.
- Patient anxiety about the procedure.
- Venepuncture may cause a vein to collapse.

Types of devices available will depend on local policy, as there are a number of new systems for collection now accessible commercially. To prevent occupational percutaneous injuries vacuum blood collection systems are commonly used.

Complications

- Phlebitis — acute inflammation of a vein, pain is the first indication of a potential problem
- Haematoma — bleeding into tissues
- Infiltration/extravasation — fluid leaked into tissues (oedema) due to a leakage of drug into the surrounding tissues
- Infection — sent off for microscopy, culture and sensitivity

Flushing of cannula

- Flushing guidance is often overlooked and is an essential component of good care.
- RCN (2016) note the flush volume should be equal to at least twice the volume of the catheter, usually 5—10 mL of 0.9% sodium chloride.
- An associated hazard is speed shock as a systemic reaction that occurs when a substance foreign to the body is rapidly introduced — occurs most commonly with rapid bolus injection.

It is recommended that before a nurse undertakes venepuncture she undergoes appropriate training, supervision and assessment by an experienced member of staff and keeps updated.

Cannulation

A vascular device inserted into a peripheral or central vessel to provide the following:

- Diagnostic blood sampling
- Invasive pressure monitoring
- CVP monitoring
- Pulmonary artery pressure monitoring
- Arterial pressure monitoring
- ICP monitoring
- Therapeutic administration of medications, fluids and/or blood products.
- The cannula is attached to a transducer, which converts the pressure to a waveform display.

The importance is to prevent infection; the nurse needs to pay attention to the following:

- Preparation
- Insertion
- Aftercare

Infections can cover a wide spectrum of clinical symptoms from fairly minor irritation to increased morbidity and mortality for patients. The patient may have the following:

- A fairly minor irritation at the site (local infection)
- Bacteraemia (where bacteria are present in the blood)
- Septicaemia (systemic infection), which is more serious

Infection control should be an integral part of insertion of a cannula, and all nurses involved in assisting with or undertaking cannulation have a role to play in both prevention and containment of infection. Divided into two groups:

- Exogenous — where the microorganisms originate outside the patient's body (this is usually due to cross-infection, e.g. hands of healthcare professionals and equipment).
- Endogenous — this is present owing to organisms already present on or in the patient's body.

Anaphylactic reaction to drugs

Anaphylaxis is a systemic immediate hypersensitivity reaction caused by an immunoglobulin (Ig)E-mediated immunologic release of mediators of mast cells and basophils, and with potentially life-threatening consequences (see Section 1). The focus here is on medicines:

- The increasing use of medicines and antibacterials especially, medicine-induced anaphylaxis and anaphylactoid reactions have increased.
- The scale in NHS Scotland of near patient antibiotic preparation at around 650,000 injections and a further 350,000 prepared in pharmacy, so we could anticipate 43 reported cases of anaphylaxis a year owing to anti-bacterial agents alone.
- Other causative agents: NSAIDs, anaesthetics, muscle relaxants, latex and radiocontrast media.

Anaphylaxis is often unpredictable, and the nurse needs to focus on how she can decrease risks. Strategies include the following:

- Ensure that a detailed patient history and full physical examination are done.
- Consider the route of the medicine and the rate of the medicine and/or fluid.
- Identification of patients with known causes of anaphylaxis.
- Sound knowledge of the medicine, as some cross-react and also are contraindicated if there is a known history of anaphylaxis.
- The greater number of years since the last administration of the offending agent, the less the chance of a recurrence.
- The parenteral route increases the severity and frequency of a reaction, so review the choice of the medicine and route, and if the patient still needs IV route, they remain under medical supervision for 20–30 min after medicine administration.

Recommendations for practice

Immediate actions following anaphylaxis depend on the severity of the reaction, and these can range from a mild skin reaction to cardiovascular collapse:

- Discontinue suspected medicine.
- Get help, resuscitation call (e.g. phone 2222/outreach).
- Administer oxygen, adrenaline (epinephrine), IV fluids.
- Start ABCDE/CPR if no pulse.
- Monitor patient; oxygen saturation, vital signs, ECG.
- If conscious, will be very anxious, and so the nurse's role would be to provide reassurance and adequate information and communication.
- At least 2-h observation if mild and in severe cases at least 24-h monitoring of the patient.
- Ensure prompt and appropriate reporting and recording in the patient case records and consideration of the Yellow Card Reporting scheme, which advocates the reporting of adverse medicine reactions.

- Also the patient will require advice for the future and this might include the use of a Medic-Alert (e.g. bracelet) ID system and an epinephrine kit.

Noninvasive ventilation

Artificial ventilation is invasive and creates many complications − generally confined to specialist areas (Richards & Edwards, 2014). Noninvasive ventilation (NIV) creates fewer complications. NIV is increasingly being used as an effective treatment on acute wards to provide support for patients with chronic respiratory failure. Ward nurses need the knowledge and skills to care safely for patients receiving NIV.

Physiology
Type 1 respiratory failure

- Oxygenation failure − hypoxia with normocapnia generally requires supplementary oxygen.
- Pulmonary oedema/chest infections may cause hypoxia but less likely to affect CO_2 removal as CO_2 is highly soluble.

Type 2 respiratory failure

- Ventilatory failure is hypoxic combined with hypercapnia.
- May require additional ventilatory support owing to hyperventilation.
- Inevitably leads to respiratory acidosis.

Conditions where noninvasive ventilation may be considered

- Acute respiratory failure − hypercapnic respiratory failure.
- Chronic obstructive pulmonary disease:
  - Prevent the use of mechanical ventilation.
  - Cost-effective, successful treatment.
  - Asthma − not conclusive, literature is controversial, more studies needed.
  - Acute cardiogenic pulmonary oedema − effective treatment with evidence of quick recovery.
  - Palliative care − to relieve suffering at the end of life:
    - Domiciliary NIV.
    - Prevent breathlessness in patients not admitted to hospital.
    - Enable patients with ventilatory failure a good quality of life.

Breathing involves muscular work − consumes O_2 at rest 1%−3% of total body O_2 consumption. If O_2 consumption by the respiratory muscles is increased, there is less available for heart and brain, increases to 10%−30%

aggravating tissue hypoxia. In respiratory failure management one goal is to reduce the work of breathing and improve tissue O_2 supply.

Terminology includes the following:

- Noninvasive positive pressure ventilation (NIPPV)
- Trademark names such as NIPPY and bilevel positive airway pressure (BiPAP)
- Nasal ventilation
- British Thoracic Society (2017) guidelines use NIV to describe all types of noninvasive ventilatory support including CPAP
- The guidelines refer to bilevel systems as bilevel NIV

It allows many activities to continue. Plans should include preparations for early intubation if this type of ventilation fails.

The following are the benefits:

- Reverses atelectasis
- Improves oxygenation/reduces work of breathing
- Reduces pulmonary oedema
- Improves cardiac function
- Bilevel NIV gives pressure support and CPAP combined or alone
- Relatively simple and easy to use; generally use room air with supplementary oxygen

Continuous positive airway pressure (CPAP) has been available for many years. There are some disadvantages of CPAP:

- Discomfort
- Pressure ulcers − tight-fitting masks
- Hypercapnia − arterial blood gases
- Reduced lung compliance − reduced by prolonged CPAP
- Cardiovascular instability − reduces venous return
- Gastric distension − air is swallowed
- Noise − irritating and impairs sleep
- Noncompliance − uncomfortable/stress

Assessment of patients with continuous positive airway pressure and bilevel noninvasive ventilation

- Chest wall movements
- Coordination of respiratory effort with the ventilator
- Accessory muscle recruitment
- General observations/measurements: TPR, BP and CVP
- Arterial blood gas analysis
- Samples from an arterial line
- Not safe on a general ward

- Interpretation
- FEV$_1$ (forced expiratory volume in 1 s)
- Mental state
- Patient comfort

Continued evaluation of patient's condition

- Maintenance of airway
- Suctioning forms a significant part in maintaining a patient's airway, indications: ineffective cough
- Depressed level of consciousness
- Thick, tenacious mucus
- Impaired respiratory function
- Types of suctioning:
  - Suctioning using catheter and gloves
  - Using catheter in sleeve
  - In-line closed suctioning system

Areas of contention

- The instigation of normal saline to initiate a cough reflex
- The removal of the NIV to undertake suctioning, as CPAP is immediately lost and will take a while to reinflate

Areas to consider

- Suctioning can be a frightening experience for the patient, explain the process clearly
- Size of the catheter
- Pressure used (between 80 and 120 mmHg)
- Too low will be ineffective
- Too high can cause: Atelectasis
- Hypoxaemia
- Airway collapse
- Ulceration
- Preoxygenation and duration of suctioning (no longer than 10−15 s)
- Equipment, preparation, procedure, documentation

Continuous positive airway pressure versus bilevel noninvasive ventilation

Owing to smaller starting pressures for bilevel NIV (4 cm H$_2$O), CPAP (5 cm H$_2$O), there is less reduction in cardiac output, bilevel NIV is more comfortable and quieter than CPAP. CPAP reverses pulmonary oedema more rapidly, although bilevel NIV provides better systemic perfusion. Bilevel NIV provides better long-term physiologic effects.

> ! A high proportion of hospitals in and around London offer NIV as a treatment choice. The British Thoracic Society (2017) recommends that NIV should ideally be used in high-dependency settings, where there are appropriately trained nurses and usually one nurse for every two patients. However, this is not generally the case as NIV is being used on general wards. All wards using NIV should have 24-h nurse-led support services, e.g. outreach services. The use of NIV requires ongoing investment in equipment, staff development and support.

Tracheostomy care

A tracheostomy is an opening into the anterior wall of the trachea to facilitate ventilation. It comprises the following:

- A curved tracheostomy tube, which conforms to the neck anatomy and is available in many different sizes
- An inner cannula, which should be removed and cleaned frequently to ensure patency of the tube
- A high-volume, low-pressure cuff that helps to prevent occlusion of capillary blood flow in the trachea

There are three major factors in effective pulmonary hygiene for the tracheostomy patient, as it bypasses the normal protective processes of the upper respiratory tract and inhibits the cough reflex: humidity, mobilization of secretions and suctioning.

Humidity
When a patient breathes through a tracheostomy, air is not warmed, moisturized or filtered. Therefore, additional humidity is required to keep the patient's secretions thin and mobilized as thick, crusty secretions can result in infection.

Mobilizing secretions
Regular physiotherapy aids the mobilization of secretions. Also important is frequent turning of the patient as well as encouraging deep breathing to prevent pulmonary complications. Depending on the activity level of the patient, sitting in a chair should also be encouraged.

Suctioning
Suctioning is needed when the cough becomes ineffective or secretions too thick for the patient to cough out easily. An inability to expectorate secretions

is a common problem for patients with a tracheostomy and suctioning forms a significant part in maintaining a patient's airway. If the clinical signs of the patient indicate suctioning, the correct catheter size must be at the bedside and used to minimize trauma to the tracheal mucosa. The size of the catheter should be approximately one-half the internal diameter of the tracheostomy tube.

The pressure used for suctioning is important. If the pressure is too low, suctioning will be ineffective, if too high it can cause the following:

- Atelectasis
- Hypoxaemia
- Airway collapse
- Ulceration

A higher negative pressure does not directly relate to the quantity of mucus extracted. Therefore, suctioning pressure of between 80 and 120 mmHg should be used.

In some patients it may be necessary to preoxygenate with 100% oxygen using a ventilation bag before suctioning. This procedure compensates for the oxygen removed from the trachea and bronchi during suctioning and prevents hypoxaemia. The procedure should be explained to the patient since suctioning can have a frightening effect. A clear explanation with reassurance decreases the patient's fears. The procedure is as follows:

- A sterile or nontouch technique is followed throughout using a clean or sterile glove, protective goggles and mask.
- The administration of normal saline into the tracheostomy tube is not recommended, as good humidification, in the form of nebulizers and a cold-water humidifier, eliminates the need for this practice.
- The catheter is inserted about 6 inches into the trachea. Suction is not applied during insertion but rather as the catheter is being withdrawn.
- Suctioning should be no longer than 10–15 s.
- Catheter tubing may require the following:
  - Sending to CSSD.
  - Effective disposal.
  - Cleaning with special attention to aseptic technique.
  - The patient should rest between suctioning attempts to allow for adequate reoxygenation.
  - Some patients may require manual ventilation with the ventilatory bag between attempts and after suctioning has been completed.

Suctioning of the upper airway may also be indicated if secretions or vomit are evident or suspected. Patients with a tracheostomy might find it difficult to swallow their saliva adequately or at all. Suctioning in this instance must be applied with care to avoid damage to mucosal surfaces.

Preventing complications

Complications of a tracheostomy can be prevented or minimized through meticulous nursing care and assessment.

Wound care

Attention to the tracheostomy wound can lessen the severity of infection and so it should be treated as a surgical wound. The wound may be cleaned and covered with a precut tracheostomy dressing to absorb drainage and to keep the neck plate from injuring the neck tissue. This dressing should be changed whenever it becomes soiled.

Accidental extubation

This complication can be a life-threatening situation. To lessen the chance of such an occurrence, it is essential that tracheostomy ties be secured in a knot, not a bow, at a tension allowing one finger to slip between the ties and the neck. It is recommended that a replacement tube of the same size and type and a pair of tracheal dilators be kept at the patient's bedside at all times, in case of extubation. The tracheal opening should be held open with the dilators until the replacement tube can be inserted.

Mucous plug formation

This complication can be avoided if adequate humidification is provided. A mucous plug that obstructs the airway occurs largely as a result of the following:

- Retained secretions
- Inadequate humidification
- Inadequate mobilization of secretions
- Lack of a properly fitted inner cannula

Special care considerations

Probably the greatest fear of the tracheostomy patient is the inability to speak or call for help when necessary so everything must be done to facilitate communication. Writing boards and cards should be available for the patient at the bedside and placed within easy reach. The following suggestions may be useful when communicating with tracheostomy patients:

- Allow ample time for the patient to respond since writing takes longer than speaking.
- Speak in a normal tone. Although the patient cannot talk, he can hear (often there is a tendency to speak too loudly).
- Avoid asking two questions at once. Again, allow extra time to respond in writing.

- Encourage use of the paper, writing pad or slate to ensure privacy of the communication. What is written should be destroyed or erased.

Pain

See previous sections on pain assessment and management.

Wound care

Caring for patients with wounds can be very challenging and complex, as wounds occur in people of all ages. For each individual patient it is important to identify the aim of wound care. It is not always appropriate in every case for the aim to be wound healing, as this is not always possible, as this will rely upon good vascular supply, nutritional state and any illnesses.

The structure of the skin

The skin is one of the largest organs of the body and it occupies a surface area of approximately 2 square metres. It can be divided into two main parts:

- The epidermis — composed mainly of stratified squamous epithelial tissue and four major cell types:
  - Keratinocytes
  - Melanocytes
  - Langerhans cells
  - Granstein cells
- The dermis — composed primarily of connective tissue containing collagenous and elastic fibres. Other structures found in this region include the following:
  - Blood supply
  - Lymph vessels
  - Sensory nerve endings
  - Sweat glands and ducts
  - Hair, roots and follicles
  - Sebaceous glands
  - Arrectores pilorum (involuntary muscle attached to hair follicles)

Functions of the skin

When intact, the skin essentially forms a barrier between the external and internal environments of the body. Its principal functions are as follows:

- *Protection* — against invasion by bacteria and foreign matter.
- *Perception of stimuli* enables constant monitoring of the external environment.
- *Absorption* allows certain topical compounds such as drugs to be absorbed.

- *Synthesis of vitamin D* — synthesized by the body as a result of direct exposure to ultraviolet radiation.
- *Maintenance of body temperature* — through metabolic processes the body is continuously producing heat. This is primarily dissipated through the skin, facilitated by three processes:
  - *Radiation*: the ability of the body to give off its heat to another object of a lower temperature.
  - *Conduction*: the transfer of heat from the body to a cooler object in contact with it.
  - *Convection*: the movement of warm air molecules away from the body.
  - *Water balance*: a small amount of fluid is lost each day (approximately 500 mL) through evaporation. This is termed *insensible loss.*

The healing process

The healing process includes three classifications of healing:

1. Healing by *primary intention* — the skin edges are brought together with the aid of sutures or clips (surgical wounds), butterfly plasters or Steristrips (minor trauma).
2. Healing by *secondary intention* — the skin edges are deliberately not brought together (pressure ulcer). The wound is encouraged to fill with granulation tissue from its base; common in chronic wounds.
3. Healing by *tertiary intention* — a wound has been sutured but has broken down and been resutured later.

Phases of healing

There are three phases of wound healing which are continuous, overlapping and merging with the next:

1. *The inflammatory phase* — the formation of a blood clot, loosely uniting the wound edges and stimulating the inflammatory response and leading to the characteristic appearance of a wound, e.g. swelling, heat, redness, pain, facilitating healing and repair (0–3 days).
2. *The regenerative phase* — the tissue starts to fill and granulation tissue starts the process of wound contraction. The signs of inflammation start to subside but the wound may be raised in relation to surrounding tissues (0–24 days).
3. *The maturation phase* — the process of reepithelialization begins. The scab should now slough off, as the epidermis is restored to its natural thickness (21 days–2 years).

Wound drainage

This is an opening in the skin that removes exudate or drainage (pus, blood or other fluids from the wound), which may be caused by disease, trauma or surgery (as a method of treatment, e.g. therapeutic, or to prevent complications, e.g. prophylactic). A wound drain is necessary to prevent the potential accumulation of fluid and become a focus for infection. All drainage should be accurately measured and recorded on either a wound assessment or fluid balance chart. The patient may have the drain in place for one day to weeks. The common types of wound/surgical drainage are as follows:

- Corrugated strips of rubber or plastic — used to drain fat layers and the subcutaneous tissues and occasionally the peritoneal cavity. They guide exudate onto the surface absorbent dressing, can be messy and affect normal skin.
- Tubes and catheter-type drains — most efficient type of drain and can be connected to closed drainage bags. These drains include the following:
  - Portex drains (paediatric surgery)
  - Shirley drains (liver transplants to assess/contain bleeding)
  - Jackson-pratt drain
  - Penrose drains
  - Sterimed drains (minor orthopaedic surgery)
  - Silicone drains (laparotomy or bowel resection procedures)
  - Yates' drain (hysterectomy)
- Suction drainage systems — these may involve a closed suction system, ideal for removal of blood and serous fluid. Examples include the following:
  - Drevac drain (laparotomy, cholecystectomy)
  - Portovac drains (plastic surgery)
  - Redivac drains (hip surgery)

Wound drains can either be open, closed or active:

- Open drains include corrugated rubber plastic sheets and fluid collects in a gauze pad or dressing or stoma bag.
- Closed drain tubes collect into a bag or bottle.
- Active drains are maintained under suction either low or high pressure.

Wound dressing materials

To undertake appropriate and effective management of wound, drainage and intravenous line sites, knowledge of the structure of the skin and the natural healing process is essential. In addition, the nurse should be able to recognize the various stages of wound healing and assess the wound using an assessment tool.

The best dressing

The ideal dressing product should ensure that the wound remains:

- moist with exudate but not macerated;
- free from clinical infection and excessive slough;

- free from toxic chemical particles or fibres released from the dressing;
- at an optimum temperature for healing to take place;
- undisturbed by frequent or unnecessary dressing changes;
- at an optimum pH value.

Classification of wound dressing types

Nurses are often restricted to using what is available. However, with so many similar dressings, an appropriate alternative should be available. Wound dressings are classified by their primary functions:

- Transparent or film membranes (Opsite, Tegaderm, Cutifilm, BioClusive, Opraflex).
- Are permeable to water vapour and oxygen.
- Are impermeable to water and microorganisms.
- Provide a warm, moist environment.
- Are comfortable and convenient and permit constant observation
  - Foam dressings are used for wounds of varying degree of severity and can reduce odours, and absorb exudates.
  - Collagen — used for chronic wounds and act as a scaffold for new cells to grow, aid the removal of dead tissue, aiding growth of new blood vessels and help to bring the wound edges together.
- Alginates (Kaltostat, Sorbsan, Tegagel) — used to fill cavities and sinuses. They are useful around drainage sites as they absorb exudate and serous fluid and create a gel that helps to heal the wound. These dressings require changing after 2 days, sometimes more.
- Foams (Allevyn, Cavi-Care, Lyofoam, Dermasorb, Tielle) — absorb exudate which then evaporates into the cells of the dressing and is lost as water vapour. They are nonadherent.
- Hydrogels (Geliperm, GranuGel, Second Skin, Intrasite gel) — they are used for a range of wounds that are leaking little or no fluid and are painful or necrotic wounds. Some produce a cooling gel that makes them effective at reducing pain.
- Hydrocolloids (Comfeel, Cutinova, Granuflex, Tegasorb) — take up wound fluid to form a gel that produces a moist environment on the wound surface to facilitate healing. They are self-adhesive and nonbreathable. Create moist conditions, impermeable to bacteria, long lasting and biodegradable.
- Some of these dressing types are impregnated with honey, which has been shown to have healing properties and broad-spectrum antibiotic activity.

Additional therapies

Not all wound dressing materials are suited to all types of wound, in particular, to the treatment of nonhealing or copiously draining wounds. However, an alternative method is beneficial in such situations — the vacuum-assisted wound closure (VAC) system:

- is a closed, noninvasive, active therapy system;
- uses negative pressure, which increases the effectiveness of the local circulation in the wounded area;
- actively removes excessive exudate, reducing oedema and haematoma formation;
- assists with the control of wound leakage;
- promotes angiogenesis (growth of new blood capillaries).

This method of treatment is often considered when other conventional methods of wound management have failed.

Mouth care

Mouth care (oral hygiene) is the scientific care of the teeth and mouth. The aim of oral care is to:

- keep the mucosa clean, soft, moist and intact and prevent infection;
- keep the lips clean, soft, moist and intact;
- remove food debris as well as dental plaque without damaging the gingiva;
- alleviate pain and discomfort and enhance oral intake;
- prevent halitosis and freshen the mouth.

The oral cavity harbours many varieties of bacteria, which do not normally pose any problems. Immunosuppression and systemic treatment such as cytotoxic, antifungal or radiation therapy and steroids may increase the pathogenicity of these organisms, leading to local infection. Oral complications can lead to pain, ulcers, infection, bone and dentition changes and bleeding and functional disorders affecting verbal and nonverbal communication, chewing and swallowing, taste and respiration. Therefore, mouth care is an important part of nursing practice.

Mouth care involves the following:

- Cleaning the teeth with toothpaste and toothbrush after meals
- Chlorhexidine gluconate 0.2% 5 mL, four times a day, diluted in 100 mL of water which should be retained in the mouth for at least 1 min before discarding

---

! A comfortable mouth will not only assist with appetite and food intake but will help the patient feel more sociable and confident.

Abdominal paracentesis

Abdominal paracentesis is the puncture of the abdominal wall with an abdominal trochar and cannula inserted into the peritoneal cavity. It is usually performed:

- to obtain a specimen of fluid for analysis;
- for the management/relief of symptoms, e.g. associated with ascites;
- for the administration of solutions into the peritoneal cavity, e.g. radioactive gold colloid or cytotoxic drugs (bleomycin, cisplatin);
- for abdominal ascites which is an accumulation of serous fluid within the peritoneal cavity. It can be caused by:
  - nonmalignant conditions such as advanced congestive heart failure, chronic pericarditis, cirrhosis of the liver;
  - malignant conditions such as metastatic cancer of the ovary, stomach, colon or breast.

Abdominal ascites is accompanied by symptoms of:

- breathlessness (due to pressure on the diaphragm);
- indigestion;
- alteration in bowel habits;
- fatigue;
- ankle oedema (due to reduced serum albumin);
- reduced mobility;
- nausea and vomiting, loss of appetite (leading to weight loss or anorexia);
- abdominal swelling (can cause bowel obstruction, decreased bladder capacity);
- pain (due to the increase in intraabdominal pressure and pressure on internal organs);
- change of body image.

It makes sense therefore to relieve the pressure but abdominal paracentesis is not undertaken lightly due to the risks of hypovolaemia, hypokalaemia, hyponatraemia or protein depletion.

Special care considerations

Abdominal paracentesis is an invasive procedure performed by the doctor assisted by the nurse at the patient's bedside:

- The patient should be informed about the procedure, the results that might be obtained/expected, information regarding quality of life and full knowledge of the course of the disease.
- The area of skin is prepared and draped with sterile towels and a local anaesthetic is administered.
- A specimen of 20–100 mL is obtained, then a closed drainage system is attached, a dressing applied and taped in position.

- A drainage pattern of 1 L every 4 h is recommended. If fluid is draining too fast a clamp should be applied to reduce the flow.
- Fluid drained and any other input and output should be measured and volumes recorded. A high-protein and -calorie diet may be ordered.
- Regular observations must be carried out to detect early signs of shock and infection.
- Patients may require assistance to move and gain a comfortable position.
- Appropriate pain assessment and analgesia.

Intrapleural drainage

Intrapleural drainage is a method used to remove a collection of air, fluid, pus or blood from the pleural space to restore normal lung expansion and function. The tubing used is clear, fairly rigid and may have a radiopaque strip, which enables X-ray detection.

Conditions which require intrapleural drainage include the following:

- Pneumothorax
- Pleural effusion
- Haemothorax
- Haemopneumothorax
- Empyema

In any of these conditions the pleural fluid seal is broken (e.g. by a spontaneous intrapulmonary air leak, during chest surgery or by a stab wound) and air, pus, blood or fluid will be drawn into the intrapleural space. The lung in the affected area collapses, the chest wall is no longer effective in expanding the lung and gas exchange is seriously impaired. Rapid diagnosis is essential:

- Decreased chest movement and breath sounds on the affected side of the chest on inspiration
- Difficulty in breathing (dyspnoea)
- Increased respiratory rate
- Cardiovascular changes, e.g. increasing heart rate, decreasing BP
- Sudden deterioration in condition
- Cyanosis and pleuritic chest pain
- Confirmed by chest X-ray

Treatment is aimed at restoring the lung to its original size, usually achieved by the insertion of a wide-bore intercostal catheter under sterile conditions. The positioning of the drain depends on whether it is being inserted to remove air or fluid:

- In the case of air — the drain should be placed in the second, third or fourth intercostal space in the mid-clavicular line, which is in the anterior and apical part of the chest.

- In the case of fluid — the drain should be placed in the fifth or sixth intercostal space in the mid-axillary line, which is in the posterior and basal part of the chest. This uses the principle of gravity for drainage, as fluid and blood are heavier.

Once this has been accomplished, a chest tube should be inserted and underwater seal drainage attached to draw air, fluid, pus or blood from the pleural space to prevent any further fluid build-up.

The basic principle is always to allow air and excess fluid to escape from the pleural cavity. The drainage tube from the patient is connected to a long catheter, the end of which is submerged below a few centimetres of sterile water in a calibrated drainage bottle. The decrease in pressure inside the pleural cavity during inspiration causes air to be sucked up the tube, usually to a height of about 10–20 cm (a *swing*).

It is important that:

- drainage bottles are kept below the level of the patient's chest, preferably on the floor, to prevent water being sucked into the chest;
- drains should not be clamped during movement of the patient or routinely stripped or milked;
- if suctioning is applied it is of low pressure, e.g. 10–25 cm H_2O;
- regular observation of the drain takes place, e.g. drainage, swing, suction;
- regular observation of the patient should take place and if any complaints of chest pain or difficulty in breathing or a rise in pulse rate occur immediate investigation is warranted;
- deep breathing and coughing are encouraged to promote drainage;
- the volume of fluid drained is recorded;
- precautions are in place to ensure that drainage bottles are not accidentally moved or knocked over and a spare set of equipment is available in case of emergency;
- the drainage tubes are secured or supported so that they do not pull on the chest wall or become dislodged.

! Drains shouldonly be clamped in the case of tube disconnection, bottle/system breakage, check X-ray or when the bottle and tubing need to be changed, and then the clamp should be in place for the least time possible.

A chest drain attached to a suction unit, which is turned off is considered to be a clamped drain. Turned off suction must be disconnected from the suction pump.

Urinary catheterization

This is the passage of a catheter into the bladder using aseptic technique. It is indicated for the following:

- For retention of urine — especially common in men with prostatic enlargement

- For accurate measurement of urine output in the very ill client, especially if he is unconscious
- For the relief of incontinence of urine if all other measures have failed
- To empty the bladder before surgery or certain investigations
- Occasionally to empty the bladder before childbirth
- To bypass an obstruction and thus provide a channel for micturition
- To allow irrigation of the bladder or the administration of certain drugs

There are several types of urinary catheter available and the reason for the catheterization will determine the type to be used. If a catheter is required for medium- or long-term insertion, a latex catheter should not be used as this material is likely to irritate. A Silastic or silicone catheter is less irritable to the lining of the urinary tract. A catheter that stays in the bladder is called a retention catheter and has a balloon, which is inflated following insertion. A 5- to 10-mL balloon is used for adults and 3–5 mL for children. Never inflate the balloon until some urine has drained and you are absolutely sure the catheter is in the bladder.

The smallest catheter necessary for drainage should be chosen. If the urine is clear this is likely to be a 12–14 ch for men and women. If there is sediment or blood present, a larger size may be needed. There are different lengths of catheter available for men and women.

A specimen of urine for laboratory analysis may be needed and a drainage bag may then be attached to the catheter, which is secured in position. Ensure that the patient is comfortable following the procedure.

If the bladder is very full, as in retention of urine, rapid emptying may result in haemorrhage from the bladder mucosa so 200–300 mL should be released about every 30 min. Never leave the catheter clamped for long periods, as this encourages the growth of microorganisms.

Male catheterization

Male catheterization is a procedure of inserting a catheter through the end of the male penis into the urethra into the bladder to remove urine.

There are two types:

1. Intermittent catheterization — performed for periodic relief of bladder distension, insertion every 6–8 h:
   a. Obtain a urine sample
   b. Relieve urinary retention
   c. Urologic surgery or surgery on close structures
   d. Critically ill patients requiring accurate measurement of urinary output
   e. Temporary obstruction of the bladder opening due to injury.
2. Indwelling catheters — inserted and retained in the bladder for:
   a. Continuous drainage of urine
   b. Skin ulceration caused by incontinence of urine

c. Palliative care for terminally ill patients

d. Severely impaired incontinent patients

Precautions

- A sterile technique is required – keep procedure sterile and catheter free from bacteria.
- Indwelling catheters and area should be washed with a mild soap and warm water to keep it free from accumulated debris.
- Can predispose the patient to urinary tract infection (UTI) – minimalize the amount of breaks to the enclosed one-way drainage system, avoid cross-contamination by washing hands before and after handling.
- Ensure the foreskin on the patient is drawn back after catheterization.
- Knowledge regarding male catheterization: The male urethra is longer than the female urethra.
- Has two curves in it as it passes through the penis – one can be straightened out by lifting the penis, the other curve is fixed – makes catheterization more difficult.

Complications

- Catheter obstruction
- Urinary tract infection
- Trauma to the bladder, urethra and meatus caused by incorrect insertion of the catheter or forceful removal
- Scarring, stricture, narrowing of the urethra
- Leakage around the catheter

Male catheterization is a simple procedure, but female nurses are sometimes reluctant to perform it. There should be no reason why a female nurse should not perform male catheterization following the proper training, but check:

- First with the local hospital policy, which might have made a specific statement which forbids female nurses to perform male catheterization.
- For consent with the patient, if he, or nearest relative acting on behalf of the patient, has made an express wish not to have the procedure carried out by a female nurse.
- If a more suitably qualified and competent male nurse is available it would be reasonable to assume he would undertake the procedure.

Encouraging female nurses to become competent in male catheterization has promoted improved patient care, and male patients can receive prompt attention when urinary catheterization is required.

Patient education

- Patients can be self-taught to catheterize themselves, they need to be shown how to use aseptic technique for catheter care.
- The sexuality of patients with catheters is rarely considered, however, patients who are sexually active can remove the catheter before intercourse and replace it afterwards with a new one.

Bladder lavage is the washing out of the bladder using sterile fluid to aid removal of blood clots or sediment from the bladder or to relieve an obstructed catheter. Normal saline may be used and it should be at body temperature. The procedure is aseptic and the fluid is introduced into the bladder slowly using a 50-mL syringe. The fluids are then allowed to drain from the bladder into a sterile receiver and the procedure is repeated until the prescribed amount of fluid has been used.

> ! It is important to note that the bladder is normally a sterile environment and the introduction of a catheter for urinary drainage is a potential source of microorganisms and infection. Great care is needed at all times to reduce this risk.

Oxygen therapy (see Section 4 fundamental interventions)

The unconscious patient

Consciousness is an awareness of oneself and the surrounding environment. There are three properties of consciousness, which are affected by the disease process:

1. Arousal or wakefulness (eyes open to command)
2. Alertness and awareness (orientation and communication)
3. Appropriate voluntary motor activity (obeying commands)

The causes of unconsciousness are numerous and may indicate the length of time required for recovery. The nurse should be aware of the cause of the coma and be observant for indications of deterioration in the patient's condition. The following is a list of the common causes for unconsciousness, which is, of course, not exhaustive:

- Poisons and drugs, e.g. alcohol, overdose, gases, lead
- Vascular causes, e.g. postcardiac arrest, ischaemia, haemorrhage, hypovolaemia
- Infections, e.g. septicaemia, encephalitis, HIV, meningitis
- Seizures
- Metabolic disorders, e.g. hyperglycaemia, hypoxia, renal failure, hepatic failure

- Other causes, e.g. neoplasm, trauma, cardiac failure, tetany, degenerative disorders

Complete care of the unconscious patient demands all the expert skills of the nurse, as the patient is totally dependent for his comfort and essential needs.

Special care considerations

The care of the unconscious patient is geared to the preservation of life and the avoidance of further disabilities. In addition to physiologic effects, consideration should be given to the psychologic effects of coma, e.g. isolation, sleep deprivation, sensory deprivation and overload.

The main factors of caring for the unconscious patient are as follows:

- Establish and maintain a clear airway, remove any vomit from the mouth and position in the unconscious position to prevent aspiration.
- Oxygen, suction, airway, Ambu-bag and mask, intubation by the bed or close by are essential.
- Assess the level of consciousness (use the Glasgow Coma Scale; see p. 68) and record it on the appropriate chart.
- Record and evaluate vital signs.
- Administer oxygen, prescribed drugs, IV fluids and nutrition.
- Maintain fluid and electrolyte balance.
- Carry out essential nursing care as appropriate to the patient's condition, e.g. mouth care, eye care, catheter care, turning, bed bathing, shaving, hair washing and communication.
- Positioning in the unconscious position may be required to enhance pulmonary function.
- Passive physiotherapy exercises of the limbs.
- Observe colour, temperature and pulses.

Positioning

Positioning is a fundamental and essential care element that nurses undertake on a daily basis. It is important to stress the need to correctly position and reposition patients frequently to decrease the risk of pressure sores and respiratory complications.

The semisitting or sitting position well supported with pillows, to prevent pressure sores or nerve damage, is recommended for optimizing and matching ventilation and perfusion after or during

- thoracic surgery,
- asthma,
- acute exacerbation of COPD,
- pneumonia/chest infection.

This will reduce the risk of increased breathlessness; it also reduces abdominal pressure on the diaphragm and minimizes the risk of aspiration.

The patient should be turned from side to side in the lateral or semiprone position at least every 2 h (unless contraindicated, e.g. lobectomy, pneumonectomy, chronic lung pathology) to change the distribution of ventilation and blood flow through the lungs and mobilize secretions. This has positive cardiopulmonary effects in enhancing oxygen transport by changing ventilation/perfusion of the lungs through gravitational effects.

The log role

The log role should be used when patients have to lie in the prone position and they are in danger due to their injury of further damage occurring during ordinary turning. This is a labour-intensive process and requires seven individuals: one for the head (the leader) and three either side of the bed.

Procedure

- The nurse at the head of the bed should be a qualified nurse experienced in the log-rolling procedure.
- The nurse holding the shoulders while her lower arms secure the head on either side maintains the head in position.
- The other six nurses:
  - No. 1 holds the patient from shoulder to middle waist.
  - No. 2 places arms over the middle and the upper thigh.
  - No. 3 places arms over upper thigh and knee.
  - No. 4 places arms at the thigh and knee.
  - No. 5 holds the feet.
  - No. 6 will carry out any other care required.
- When everyone is in position, the leader will decide how to indicate that all participants turn together.
- Once the signal is decided, all roll the patient with the spine in line and another nurse performs the change of sheet or necessary essential care.

Mobilization

Early and progressive mobilization is an important aspect of caring for patients. It is an extension of the physiologic principles of turning and repositioning the bedbound patient. Ambulation:

- encourages ventilation;
- increases perfusion;
- promotes secretion clearance;
- promotes oxygenation;

- decreases venous pooling, which reduces the risk of thrombus formation and pulmonary embolism;
- improves functional residual capacity (FRC);
- reduces muscle wasting;
- decreases the potential for psychologic distress, e.g. feelings of helplessness, depression and lack of control.

When and how the patient should be mobilized is decided on an individual basis in conjunction with the patient, nurse, surgeon and physiotherapist. For effective mobilization it is paramount that the nurse monitors, observes and provides optimal pain and comfort strategies and interventions during this period.

Pyrexia and hyperpyrexia

A pyrexia is a body temperature between 37.6° and 40°C and hyperpyrexia is a temperature >40°C. They are conditions in which the thermoregulatory mechanisms are intact but the body temperature is high. Infection is the most common cause of pyrexia and sepsis of hyperpyrexia but there are other causes. A number of drugs have been associated with pyrexia, e.g. diuretics, antiseizure therapy, analgesics, antiarrhythmics and antibiotics. Other causes of pyrexia include neoplasm, surgery, acute MIs, heart failure, haemolysis (seen in reactions to blood transfusions) and hyperthyroidism.

There are four stages associated with pyrexia:

1. The *chill stage* is the cold stage when the hypothalamic thermostat is reset to a higher level — the patient feels chilly, has goosebumps, and is cool to touch and pale.
2. The *plateau* is the hot stage when the body temperature has been raised to a level equal to the hypothalamic set point — the patient feels hot, warm to touch, is flushed and has raised heart and respiratory rates.
3. In the *defervescence stage* the temperature returns to normal, heat is dissipated through heat loss mechanisms, the skin remains warm to touch and flushed and eventually there is a drop in body temperature to a normal level.
4. The *crisis stage* occurs if the temperature fails to respond to treatment, the microorganism responsible cannot be eradicated and thermoregulation mechanisms can no longer control heat loss. Death may ensue.

These stages account for the discomfort experienced by patients with high temperatures. They also explain why a patient with a high temperature may initially feel cold and want to wrap up rather than be uncovered.

There are also different patterns of pyrexia, which exhibit recognizable changes in temperature over time. These patterns vary according to the time of day, which may influence decisions regarding when to monitor body temperature.

Beneficial effects of pyrexia

Pyrexia can be beneficial and is an important host defence mechanism:

- A body temperature of 40.9°C will kill some pneumococcal and gono-coccal organisms.
- The high temperature causes a reduction in serum levels of iron, zinc and copper, which inhibits the replication of certain microorganisms.
- Pyrexia as a result of viral infection increases interferon production by the infected cells, which then enters noninfected cells to inhibit infiltration by the invading virus.
- The activity of phagocytes and leucocytes is increased at temperatures between 38°C and 40°C, thus improving the infection-fighting ability of the immune system.
- A high temperature causes the breakdown of lysosomes (involved in the intracellular digestive system, which allows cells to digest and remove unwanted substances such as bacteria) in infected cells, thereby destroying cells and preventing them from initiating viral replication.

Detrimental effects of pyrexia

Pyrexia can also be detrimental to the patient:

- Basal metabolic rate will be increased, eventually leading to exhaustion.
- Glycogen stores in the liver become reduced and lead to nitrogen wastage (as protein is used for energy) and, if prolonged, may result in debility, impaired healing and delirium.
- In patients who have compromised cardiopulmonary function, the effects of increased metabolic, heart and respiratory rates can be quite dangerous. These effects can lead to an increase in carbon dioxide production and oxygen consumption.
- Dehydration may result from fluid loss during sweating and from the lungs due to increased respiratory rate, leading to hypovolaemia and electrolyte imbalance, which can be life-threatening.
- The patient feels uncomfortably hot and sweaty, with a loss of appetite, weakness and malaise, apathy and confusion.

Hyperthermia

Hyperthermia is defined as an increase in body temperature, with increased cellular metabolism, oxygen consumption and carbon dioxide production but where the body fails to activate compensatory cooling mechanisms. This condition is caused by problems of the central nervous system and does not respond to antipyretic therapy.

Hyperthermia causes cerebral metabolism to increase and the brain has great difficulty keeping up with the increase in carbon dioxide production. Cerebral vasodilatation occurs which may increase ICP and is thus dangerous in neurologically compromised patients. A temperature between 41°C and 43°C produces nerve damage, coagulation, convulsions and death. Unless effective cooling measures are initiated, irreversible brain damage and death will occur.

A hyperthermia also presents in five other conditions:

1. Heat cramps
2. Heat exhaustion
3. Heat stroke
4. Malignant hyperthermia
5. Neuroleptic malignant syndrome (NMS)

Heat cramps and exhaustion, even though they can be severe, do not generally warrant admission to hospital and those at risk can be taught ways to avoid it. However, heat stroke, malignant hyperthermia and NMS must be recognized quickly as, untreated, they may be fatal.

Tepid sponging/fanning
During a high temperature due to an infection

Treatment by cooling methods such as tepid sponging or fanning has been criticized. Cooling methods are of no use, as they result in the following:

- A compensatory response by the hypothalamus, which will activate heat-generating activities like chills and shivering.
- Compromising an unstable patient by depleting his metabolic reserve and can create a new temperature spike, which is as high or higher than the original one and may even increase the patient's temperature.
- The patient feeling weak, especially during the early stages when the temperature is still rising.

Treating a high temperature by cooling and tepid sponging can only serve to increase the temperature further and cause the patient discomfort and possible harm. The best way to treat a high temperature is by the use of antipyretic drug therapy in preference to cooling methods.

! Treating a high temperature by cooling and tepid sponging will increase the temperature further and cause the patient discomfort and possible harm.

During hyperpyrexia due to damage of the hypothalamus

In this situation the body fails to activate compensatory cooling mechanisms. This tends to increase cellular metabolism, oxygen consumption and carbon dioxide production. As cerebral metabolism increases, the brain has great difficulty keeping up with the increase in carbon dioxide production and can potentially increase ICP in already neurologically compromised patients. Unless the temperature is monitored carefully and cooling methods are instituted, irreversible brain damage and death occur.

Artificial cooling methods like tepid sponging and fanning are valuable in hyperthermia, heat stroke and malignant hyperthermias, as these generally do not respond well to antipyretic therapy. Aggressive cooling should be commenced early, as temperatures of above 41°C cause coagulation, nerve damage, convulsions, cell, tissue and organ damage and eventually death.

Hypothermia

Hypothermia is defined as a core temperature of less than 35.5°C and affects virtually all metabolic processes in the body (Richards & Edwards, 2014).

In acute hypothermia, peripheral vasoconstriction shunts blood away from the cooler skin to the core in an effort to decrease heat loss. This peripheral vasoconstriction leads to peripheral tissue ischaemia, which causes the hypothalamus to stimulate shivering in an effort to increase heat production. At 34°C, thinking becomes sluggish and coordination is impaired. Degrees of hypothermia are classified as follows:

- In mild hypothermia with a body temperature of 32–35°C, severe shivering occurs at core temperatures below 35°C and will continue until the core temperature rises or drops further to 30–32°C.
- Moderate hypothermia is between 28 and 31.9°C. At 31°C the individual becomes lethargic, heart and respiratory rates decline, cardiac output is diminished and there is confusion, hyperactivity and exaggerated tendon reflexes. CBF is decreased. Metabolic rate declines, further decreasing core temperature. This has an effect on drug metabolism as the drug half-life is increased. Sinus node depression occurs with slowing of conduction through the atrioventricular node and premature ventricular contractions (ectopics) are common. There is also an increased risk of atrial fibrillation and other dysrhythmias.
- In severe hypothermia, pulse and respiration may be undetectable and the blood coagulates more easily. Dehydration is common after a lengthy exposure to the cold. Loss of consciousness and the absence of neurologic reflexes follow.
- As the temperature falls below 20°C, the profoundly hypothermic patient becomes unable to regulate his body heat and the thermoregulatory mechanisms fail. Ice crystals form inside cells, causing them to rupture and die.

The degree and length of exposure of the patient are important. Thus, the length of time hypothermia has taken to occur is significant in that it can influence outcomes. After 12 h there will be significant fluid loss from the blood, due to shifts of fluid from extracellular to other fluid spaces and from cold-induced diuresis. In addition, there is a marked increase in mortality. It is also significant when rewarming patients as the time span of hypothermia will determine the best method of achieving this.

Accidental hypothermia

Accidental hypothermia is defined as a core body temperature below 35°C that results from sudden immersion in cold water or prolonged exposure to cold environments. It may occur in accidents involving immersion in cold water or near drowning. Older adults are at risk of accidental hypothermia, as they have poor responses to extremes of environmental temperature as a result of slowed blood circulation, structural and functional changes in the skin and overall decrease in heat-producing activities.

Therapeutic hypothermia

The term *therapeutic hypothermia* generally refers to a deliberately induced state of hypothermia, which is used to slow a patient's metabolism and thus preserve ischaemic tissue during some types of major surgery. However, hypothermia that occurs inadvertently during surgery is also termed therapeutic hypothermia because it presents during a therapeutic procedure. Both types of hypothermia can sometimes extend into the postoperative period. Therapeutic hypothermia is therefore classified into the following three categories.

Induced hypothermia

This is the intentional lowering of a patient's body temperature. It is generally used in neurosurgery and to treat hyperthermia and during cardiac surgery to decrease metabolic rate and tissue oxygen demands, protect the brain, decrease the risk of ischaemic tissue damage to the heart and thereby protect other vital organs from hypoxia.

Inadvertent, intraoperative or unintentional hypothermia

Major surgery often induces significant hypothermia (termed *inadvertent hypothermia*) because of the exposure of body cavities to the relatively cool operating room environment. In addition, procedures often involve irrigation of body cavities with room temperature solutions, infusion of room temperature intravenous solutions, inhalation of unwarmed anaesthetic agents and the use of drugs that impair thermoregulatory mechanisms. Older adults are at greater risk of suffering from this type of hypothermia.

This type of hypothermia occurs because of the following:

- Patients undergoing surgery do not adapt quickly enough to cool intraoperative environments.
- Patients are transported along cold draughty corridors before being exposed to operating theatres that have an ambient temperature of 21°C.
- Skin preparation may include the use of volatile fluids or fluids that must be allowed to dry on the skin, which leads to an increase in heat loss by evaporation.
- Medications such as muscle relaxants, narcotics and inhaled anaesthetics also contribute to decreasing body temperature as they affect the temperature regulation mechanisms and prevent body movement.
- The ability of patients to produce heat is blocked and they become dependent on the temperature of the environment.
- Once surgery begins, the use of intravenous solutions and blood at temperatures below that of the patient's body can compound the problem.

Postanaesthesia or postoperative hypothermia

This has been recognized to be an extension of induced or inadvertent hypothermia.

Rewarming methods

Passive external rewarming

Remove any wet clothing, gently dry the patient if needed and then insulate him with blankets. The patient may then be allowed to rewarm using only normal metabolic heat production. Recommended for both mild (32.2–35°C) and moderate (28–32°C) hypothermias that have an onset of less than 12 h. Movement will contribute to heat loss through convection and may reduce temperature further if not closely monitored.

If the patient's temperature fails to rise and he becomes persistently hypotensive, active external rewarming should be commenced.

Active external rewarming

The patient's skin is warmed using hot baths, hot air blowers or radiant heat. This method can also be used as an adjunct to internal active rewarming, using connective warming. It uses the principles of convection, forcing heated air directly onto the patient's skin through a disposable blanket. Used when the hypothermia has occurred slowly, e.g. over a 12-h period, and is mild or moderate in nature. However, the patient's vital signs and peripheral temperature must be closely monitored, as rewarming shock may occur in the severely hypothermic patient as a consequence of rewarming the peripheries before the core.

Active internal rewarming

These are invasive procedures, whereby the deep tissues of the body are warmed. They allow the lungs and heart to be rewarmed first. Methods include the following:

- Warm fluid for gastric and peritoneal lavage
- Mediastinal and pleural irrigation
- Continuous arteriovenous or venovenous rewarming
- Extracorporeal rewarming
- Cardiopulmonary bypass − the fastest method

These are not readily available in all hospitals and require critical care input so is not the method of choice for use in general wards. The easiest methods are as follows:

- Warmed gases to the respiratory tract − gases should be humidified as well as warmed.
- Warmed intravenous (IV) fluids − observe CVP and urine output.

If this method is used the nurse needs to be vigilant to observe for after-drop, which occurs after internal active rewarming is discontinued. A decrease in temperature of as much as 2°C may occur as blood circulates to the peripheries, recools and returns to the core. When invasive active internal rewarming methods are discontinued, attention is directed to the need for passive and active external rewarming, to prevent afterdrop in temperature.

This method is best used when the hypothermia has occurred very quickly, e.g. in less than 12 h, and is moderate or severe in nature. The treatment reduces the risk of cardiac arrest, by reducing the time the patient's core temperature is below 32.2°C.

Special care considerations

The whole process of rewarming should proceed no faster than a few degrees per hour. If a patient is rapidly rewarmed oxygen consumption, myocardial demand and vasodilatation increase faster than the heart's ability to compensate and death can occur. Hypothermia in the elderly need not be treated any differently from that in younger patients.

Heat warming processes are not the only aspects to be considered in the care of hypothermic patients. The nurse has a broader role in managing and caring for these patients and should:

- be vigilant during fluid administration;
- observe blood results and the ECG;
- document urine output;
- ensure that any drugs administered during rewarming are not toxic.

Section 4

Fundamental procedures

Section Outline

4.1 GENERAL PRINCIPLES

This section discusses how nurses can further broaden and expand their knowledge of the person as an individual.

Admission to hospital

Prior to admission to hospital the patient may have come into contact with the ambulance service or paramedic team (prehospital care), his/her GP, the primary healthcare team or the police. He/she may have referred himself/herself to the local A&E department or the minor injuries unit or be a booked admission from home.

In the A&E department, the first impressions of the hospital are formed. An A&E nurse may undertake the initial A-E assessment, the appropriate emergency interventions given and a decision may be made as to the urgency/priority of the case.

The transfer to the ward may have been a lengthy process and the patient may have been in A&E for a number of hours before being admitted. In addition, the patient may have been waiting a long time before being admitted from home. On admission to the ward, a welcoming approach, good communication, effective use of assessment tools, observation, measurement, interviewing and documentation (nursing process) skills are paramount (see Section 2).

The often-neglected psychologic and social factors need to be included. These identify the close interrelated concepts of physical, psychologic and social well-being, as disruption in any one of these aspects will have implications for the others.

A nurse's survival guide to the ward. https://doi.org/10.1016/B978-0-7020-7831-6.00004-8

Discharge planning

This is a process of developing a plan of care for a patient who is transferred from one environment to another. The significance of early discharge planning cannot be overestimated. The average length of hospital admission has been reduced dramatically owing to advances in technology, financial consider-ations and contracting requirements of purchasers. Discharge planning should be initiated as early as possible after admission and should include the following:

- Patients and their families/partners to be informed of the requirements on discharge.
- It should be designed to promote self-care or to assist with care needs when necessary.
- Involvement of the multidisciplinary team.
- The patient's physical, psychologic, social, cultural and economic needs.
- The degree of support needed at home after discharge, which should be to a safe and adequate environment.
- Planning on who will look after the patient.
- Consideration for those patients who may have specific care needs such as the following:
  - Live alone, frail and/or elderly
  - Have a limited prognosis
  - Have serious illnesses, who may be returning to hospital for further treatments
  - Have a continuing disability, learning difficulties, mental illness or dementia
  - Dependants
  - Have limited financial resources
  - Are homeless or living in poor housing
  - Do not have English as a first language
  - Require aids/equipment at home
  - Have spent an extended time in hospital
- Consideration of the need for external agencies to be involved. Assessment of needs at home may involve the:
  - Occupational therapist,
  - Social services.

Discharge should not be a matter of chance. There is the potential for patients to occupy beds unnecessarily due to late decisions regarding discharge.

Occasionally the discharge process may not proceed as planned or may be delayed. Patients may take their own discharge against medical advice and this should be documented accordingly. Some patients receiving a bad prognosis may prefer to go home and plans may need to be set up at short notice.

Transfer of a patient

Transfer of patients does not only involve moving the patient within the hospital, for example, to the imaging department, theatres, but also externally to other hospitals. This may be due to bed shortage within the admitting hospital or need for specialist care and treatment. Prior to transfer of the patient there are a number of factors to take into consideration.

Transfer should occur:

- When the staff of the referring centre feel uncomfortable with the course of the illness/injury, e.g., deterioration,
- When it is first realized that the patient requires care in a specialist centre.

Important factors of safe transfer are as follows:

- Patient should be accompanied by an experienced nurse and/or medical practitioner.
- Appropriate equipment and vehicle are sought and utilized.
- Patient fully assessed, stabilized and staff prepared prior to transfer.
- All investigations accompany patient on transfer.
- All drugs and delivery systems are readily available and prepared for immediate use.
- Monitoring systems and battery backup are familiar to accompanying staff.
- Continuous monitoring and assessment during transfer.
- Knowledge of area transferring patient to. If to another hospital, phone ahead and ensure a member of staff is waiting at the agreed point. For example, a porter waiting in the A&E department.
- Accurate and concise oral and document handover

Organizational and transfer decision-making factors

A designated consultant is responsible for the decision to transfer a patient. They should ensure the following:

- Patient transfer is appropriate.
- Patient can be transferred, risk versus benefits of transfer.
- Referring hospital is informed.
- Coordination of transfer runs smoothly.
- Appropriate staff have been allocated for transfer.
- Local policies are adhered to.
- Next of kin are informed.

Accompanying staff

- An experienced doctor, experienced in resuscitation, airway management, ventilation and organ support with previous transfer experience.

- An experienced nurse, operating department practitioner or paramedic experienced in transfer of patients.
- Current staffing levels in many hospitals mean that this level of assistance is not always available.
- Transferring hospital should provide medical indemnity, and personal medical defence cover is also recommended.

Departure checklist

- Are appropriate equipment and drugs available?
- Sufficient oxygen.
- Suction available.
- Trolley available.
- Ambulance service notified of transfer and patient's condition, nature of transfer.
- Bed confirmed at receiving hospital.
- Receiving hospital notified.
- Medical notes, X-rays and investigations available.
- Transfer letter prepared.
- Return arrangements known.
- Next of kin informed of impending transfer.

The issue that has led to a decrease in the need for interhospital transfer is the development of systems to transmit the images of a CT scan from one hospital to another. This allows the hospital to send the CT images via a phone line (telemedicine) to the specialist neurocentre where the images can be assessed. The specialist neurologist can then decide whether transport of the patient to the specialist centre is indicated.

The risks to the patient

- Lack of appropriate equipment in the transfer vehicle if an unforeseen incident occurs en route.
- Breakdown of the transfer vehicle while transferring patients – and lives have been lost.
- The vibration of the transport vehicle can cause either hypertension or cardiovascular depression.
- Acceleration forces in an ambulance can lead to transient hypertension and arrhythmias.
- The overall responsibility of the nurse during transfer is the patient's safety.

Preoperative care

This may take place in a preoperative clinic if in the hospital the nurse needs to provide safe care for patients prior to surgery. This includes ensuring a positive experience and outcome for the preoperative patient. As part of preoperative care, the nurse needs to consider patient participation and partnership as follows:

- Shared decision-making, inclusion of the patient.
- Information giving (verbal or written), including education about the forthcoming operation (preferably 10–14 days preoperatively), explanations of any drugs and pain management preferences, specific postoperative equipment or techniques that may be employed.
- Good communication skills; preoperative communication/visiting, identifying the barriers to good communication, e.g., anxiety and stress.
- Identify culture differences in interpretation and understanding. Spiritual requirements should be explored.
- Develop an effective nurse-patient relationship. Assessment of the patient's understanding and explanation of words and phrases used during information giving should be undertaken.
- The opportunity to ask questions.
- Informed consent (see p. 54). The nurse needs to ensure that the patient comprehends what is likely to happen to him/her. The nurse must act in the patient's best interests.

Screening prior to surgery

Screening prior to anaesthetic and surgery is an essential part of patient preparation. There are many specific investigations and preparations that are required for different types of surgery, e.g., of the bowel; these are detailed in Section 5. There are also standard test results that will enhance the surgeon's understanding of the patient's general condition prior to surgery as follows:

- Baseline clinical observations: blood pressure (BP), temperature, pulse, respiratory rate and urine analysis.
- Laboratory tests: full blood count, to ensure normal haemoglobin to enhance postoperative recovery, blood cross-matched for transfusion, blood urea, creatinine and electrolyte levels to check renal function.
- Further investigations, if necessary, may involve chest/abdominal X-ray, ECG, lung function tests and a CT scan.

Perioperative care

Care in the period before going to theatre may include the following:

- Ongoing physical and psychologic care.
- Skin or bowel preparations (may need to commence 48 h preoperatively).
- Nil by mouth for 4–6 h is safest because the stomach and small intestine should be empty of the last meal by this time.
- IV cannulation and infusion if relevant.

- Personal hygiene.
- Preoperative checks and premedication: this is to ensure patient safety so name bands are mandatory. A premedication may not be required and this is generally considered on an individual basis.
- Consider the removal of wigs, hairpieces, jewellery (can cause burns if diathermy is used; wedding rings can be covered with tape), dentures, glasses, contact lenses and prostheses. Removal should be delayed as long as possible to maintain body image.
- The removal of makeup and nail varnish is essential as these prevent the observation of true skin colour and the recording of oxygen saturation monitoring is affected by nail varnish.
- Preparation of the bed area for return of the patient (see the following section).
- Escorting patient to the operating theatre: ideally this should be done by the nurse caring for the patient postoperatively.
- Transportation to the operating theatre: the patient should be allowed to sit up whether travelling on a bed or trolley.
- Reception in the operating theatre complex: the patient is generally received from the ward nurse in a reception area and 'handed over' to the theatre nurse, then taken to the anaesthetic room when the anaesthetist is ready.

It is important to highlight that having to undergo surgery is one of the most stressful events in a person's life. The significance of the nurse's knowledge and skill in providing a safe and meaningful preoperative experience for the surgical patient can never be overestimated.

Postoperative care

There is a range of activities that nurses need to undertake when caring for postoperative patients. There are also specialist areas of surgery, e.g., bowel and thoracic surgery, which require more specific care, and these are covered in Section 5 as follows:

- The patient is placed in the recovery room attached to the theatre. The patient's condition is assessed and he/she is nursed in the lateral recovery position to minimize risks of aspiration until fully conscious, when he/she can be transferred back to the ward.
- The bed area has been prepared and includes the following:
  - Airways, various sizes
  - Oxygen supply, disposable mask and tubing
  - Suction equipment, selection of catheters
  - Disposable gloves, gauze swabs, bowl of water and receiver
  - Oxygen saturation monitor
  - Emergency cardiopulmonary resuscitation equipment

- A significant aspect of a surgical nurse's role is to reduce the risk of postoperative complications for patients. Surgical complications carry a potential risk to a person's recovery, as well as incurring significant financial costs. Some of the more common postoperative complications are:
  - Wound infection,
  - Deep vein thrombosis (DVT),
  - Bleeding (hypovolaemia, hypovolaemic shock),
  - Chest infection,
  - Urinary retention,
  - Urinary tract infection,
  - Paralytic ileus,
  - Nausea and vomiting,
  - Joint stiffness,
  - Pressure sores,
  - Shock,
  - Hypothermia,
  - Restlessness/confusion/hypoxia.
- It is necessary for the nurse to undertake regular monitoring of the patient and ensure the correct postoperative instructions are adhered to.

Special nursing considerations

These may include an assessment of the patient's risk of DVT formation and instigating preventive measures such as:

- ensuring patient cooperation through education,
- encouraging deep breathing and coughing at regular intervals, movement around the bed,
- early mobilization,
- antiembolic stockings,
- administration of postoperative heparin/warfarin,
- effective observation and monitoring of peripheral circulation.

Other considerations during the postoperative period can be found elsewhere in the book and include:

- dignity,
- urinary catheterization,
- nasogastric tube,
- intravenous infusion,
- nutrition,
- wound care,
- rest and sleep,
- pain assessment and management,
- discharge planning,
- patient discharge education and health promotion.

Palliative care

Palliative care is the active total care of patients whose disease is not responsive to curative treatment, encompassing both the patient and their family/carers. Issues of death and dying are often not discussed with ease. It is important that health professionals develop skills and strategies for caring for the dying patient and his/her family.

The principles of palliative care originally focused on patients with advanced cancer, but the scope has broadened and it is now offered to patients with a wide range of life-threatening illnesses such as multiple sclerosis, motor neuron disease, AIDS, chronic circulatory or respiratory disease.

Palliative care aims to:

- affirm life and regard death as a normal process,
- neither hasten nor postpone death,
- provide relief from pain and other distressing symptoms,
- integrate the psychologic and spiritual aspects of patient care,
- offer a support system to help patients live as actively as possible until death,
- offer a support system to help the family cope during the patient's illness and in his or her own bereavement.

This care takes place in specialist care hospices or in hospital and is an integral part of all clinical practice. The quality of palliative care in the hospital setting is of crucial importance despite the rapid growth of hospices and home care schemes.

The key principles underpinning palliative care comprise the following:

- Whole-person approach.
- Care, which encompasses both the patient and those who matter to them.
- Emphasis on open and sensitive communication, including adequate information about diagnosis and treatment options.
- Respect for patient autonomy and choice.
- Focus on quality of life, which includes good symptom control and nursing care.

The role of the nurse is central to the care of the dying patient and family. It requires the utmost sensitivity and attention to detail. Many dying patients wish to remain independent for as long as possible. The nurse is in a position to offer:

- skilled, supportive care to patients and families which is fully integrated with diagnosis and treatment as follows:
  - Self-help and support
  - User involvement

- Information giving
- Psychologic support
- Symptom control
- Social support
- Rehabilitation
- Complementary therapies
- Spiritual support
- End-of-life and bereavement care
- Sensitive nursing care enabling the patient to remain independent for as long as possible.
- Reporting of presenting symptoms and monitoring of symptom control.
- Coordination of care between the multiprofessional team.

www.macmillan.org.uk/home.aspx or the National Council for Palliative Care at www.ncpc.org.uk/palliative-care-explained contain some useful information in relation to health professionals and palliative care.

Nursing intervention in common symptoms

There are some aspects of symptom control that will be directly helped by skilled nursing:

- *Anorexia* — providing extra nutrition will not prolong life; liaise with the dietitian for ideas on presentation and supplements.
- *Mouth care* — assess the oral cavity; can be helped with ice cubes, boiled lemon sweets or fresh pineapple chunks.
- *Constipation* — a high-fibre diet is inappropriate; appropriate use of laxatives, privacy for defaecation and mobilization for as long as possible.
- *Dyspnoea* — involves relaxation and a range of pharmacologic interventions.
- *Fungating wounds* — sight and smell; need to eradicate smell and use a dressing that is cosmetically acceptable to the patient.

Emotional care

Emotional care relies on openness and sharing the truth about the illness. The patient will feel loss and grief for the lack of:

- independence (holidays, trips out),
- self-esteem (body image, appetite),
- recognizing signs of anxiety or depression,
- status, job and income,
- role and relationships,
- a future.

Spiritual care

Spiritual care gives the patient and family an opportunity to examine the impact of the illness on their belief systems. They need to be given the opportunity to ask the following questions:

- Why me?
- Why now?
- What have I done to deserve this?

Staying with this sort of spiritual pain and not being afraid of the questions is a helpful response. Offering the support of a relevant religious figure may not be appropriate for all but listening and being present will be appreciated.

Cultural diversity

Making nursing practice relevant to people of many cultures is a constant challenge to the nurse. Cultures differ with regard to:

- the meaning of illness,
- attitude to pain and symptoms and to medication,
- ways of coping with illness,
- attitude to place of care, physical and emotional care,
- the roles of the family,
- rituals around death, the funeral and bereavement.

Social needs

The nurse needs to ensure that patients and families have adequate information regarding the benefits to which they may be entitled. This includes the following:

- Disability Living Allowance
- Attendance allowance
- Free prescriptions
- Housing benefits
- Income support
- Council tax
- Macmillan cancer relief grants
- Power of attorney (the legal right to act on someone's behalf)
- Drawing up of a will

Complementary therapies

These are becoming increasingly popular for people who are dying and include the following:

- acupuncture
- aromatherapy

- massage
- reflexology

These are generally safe and free from the side effects of orthodox anti-cancer treatments.

Death/dying

The majority of people would prefer to die at home, but this is not always feasible and only about 25% of people in the United Kingdom do so. The following show how nurses can help to maintain comfort during the last few days of a person's life:

- Some people fear terrible pain or dying in a dramatic fashion and the nurse can do much to reassure and comfort the patient.
- A few patients find the last days intolerable and it is compassionate for the medical and nursing team to offer medication that will help relieve this.
- The majority of patients become sleepy and this merges into drowsiness and unconsciousness.
- Cheyne-Stokes breathing may occur (periods of apnoea followed by more respirations, a cycle which continues until breathing stops).

Potential organ donation

Many patients in the United Kingdom die or suffer prolonged dependency because of a lack of organs for transplantation. Therefore, if a young or middle-aged patient with a fatal condition has healthy kidneys, liver, heart or corneas, it might be relevant to discuss organ donation with the medical team. Suitable organ donors include the following:

- Victims of severe head injury.
- Severe subarachnoid or intracerebral haemorrhage.
- In the case of corneal donation, any young patient with healthy eyes or a rapidly fatal illness.

Patients who are unsuitable organ donors include the following:

- Where brain death is uncertain.
- Those generally over 60.
- Where there has been significant hypotension or hypoxia during a fatal illness.
- Where there is a history of previous disease affecting the potential donor organ (e.g., hypertension, diabetes, hepatitis B, alcohol abuse).
- Where the patient has received drugs or other treatment, which might have affected the organs to be transplanted.
- In the case of the kidneys, where there is persistent oliguria.

What to do after the patient has died?

- The family should be able to spend as much time with the deceased person as they want.
- The doctor or GP will be called to certify the death.
- Date and time of death are recorded.
- There is no need for children to be excluded from this time.
- Inform surrounding patients of the death.
- If a doctor has not seen the patient within 14 days before the death, a postmortem examination may be needed.

Last offices

This is the care given to a deceased patient, which is focused on fulfilling religious and cultural beliefs as well as health and safety and legal requirements. It should be remembered that this is the final demonstration of respectful, sensitive care given to the patient as follows:

- Screen off appropriate areas from view of other patients when the body is being removed.
- It is important that the nurse knows in advance the cultural values and religious beliefs of the family, as there are considerable cultural variations between people of different faiths, ethnic backgrounds and national origins in their approach to death and dying.
- Individual preferences should be determined and patients should be encouraged to talk about how they may wish to be treated upon dying. If in doubt, consult the family members.
- Prepare the patient according to local guidelines.
- Pack personal property in line with local policy.
- Update nursing records, transfer property and patient records to the appropriate administrative department.

A death certificate will be issued the next day from the hospital and needs to be registered within 5 days at the registrar's office in the district in which the death took place.

Bereavement

A nurse working with dying patients needs to have an understanding of bereavement. For some, death may have been sudden or unexpected, whereas for others, the result of a long illness and expected. Bereavement is an individual response and it will be different for each individual suffering loss. There have been many models and theories of grief, which help to understand and support people who have been bereaved.

Grief is not an illness, it is a pattern of reactions that take place while the person adjusts to the death of his/her loved one.

Caring for family

Caring for people whose relatives have died suddenly and unexpectedly is one of the most difficult and challenging events for healthcare professionals. The nurse is not expected to be a bereavement counsellor, but to be there for the relative before the patient has died. A well-managed death will help with the emotional health of a family. Listening and understanding imply concern and care, whereas acknowledgement of their pain and sorrow may help relatives to move forward.

The way in which families receive news of their loved ones' deaths can seriously affect how they grieve and cope. Therefore, nurses' response can play a valuable part in the recovery process, and there is a need to understand and be able to meet relatives' needs (Purves and Edwards, 2005). These include the following:

- Meeting bereaved people on their arrival.
- A separate waiting area.
- Knowing the loved one's condition − accurate information about their loved one's death.
- Notification of death by someone who uses a sympathetic tone of voice using the appropriate terms, e.g., 'dead' as others such as 'he has passed away' is open to misinterpretation.
- Helpfulness of actions − families need to know that all appropriate action has been taken to save their loved ones.
- Involving relatives.
- Viewing the body.
- Demonstrating care.
- Knowledge, education and training.
- Consistency of language.

Recognizing abnormal grief

It is important to recognize abnormal grief and to refer to specialist help. The following identifies some questions if abnormal grief is suspected:

- Are grief reactions prolonged, excessive and seeming incapable of resolution?
- Are grief reactions absent?
- Has grief been displaced or masked, e.g., by illness, drugs, alcohol or overwork?
- Was the relationship with the deceased person particularly ambivalent or dependent?
- Were the circumstances of the death unexpected or violent?

4.2 PSYCHOLOGICAL ISSUES

Promoting rest and sleep

Sleep can be defined as an altered state of consciousness from which a person can be aroused by stimuli of sufficient magnitude. The function of sleep is far from clear. It is considered as restorative and energy conserving, as protein synthesis and cell division for the renewal of tissues take place predominantly during the time devoted to rest and sleep. Sleep is needed to avoid the psychologic problems resulting from inadequate sleep, which might hinder recovery and if the function of sleep is correctly assumed, then sleep deprivation could be considered as a stressor, over and above those physical and emotional traumas already suffered.

During an average night's sleep individuals pass through four or five sleep cycles, each cycle lasting about 90–100 min. Within the sleep cycle, five successive stages have been defined by their distinctive characteristics. The first four stages of sleep are called collectively *nonrapid eye movement* (NREM) sleep and demonstrate a progressive increase in the depth of sleep. Stage five is called rapid eye movement (REM) sleep, or paradoxical sleep, and is associated with dreaming, learning and memory.

Perpetual awakening and sleep interruption have been associated with increased anxiety, irritability and disorientation, which may have a negative influence on recovery. Total sleep deprivation for 48 h can result in changes such as the following:

- behavioural irritability,
- suspiciousness,
- speech slurring,
- minor visual misperceptions,
- reduction in motivation and willingness to perform tasks which could include mobilization and other aspects of self-care,
- lethargy, irritability and disorientation and confusion,
- later, delusions and paranoia.

Recommendations for minimizing sleep interruption in patients are listed in Box 4.1.

Psychological disturbances

These can influence recovery in many ways as follows:

- Eating can be a way of finding comfort during periods of insecurity, depression, loneliness and boredom.
- Anorexia nervosa can be a way of coping with hate or anger towards a parent or fear of maturity.
- Changes in roles within a family or society can cause psychologic disturbances. Personal identity and functioning in a social setting can have an

BOX 4.1 Minimizing sleep interruptions in patients

- Turn off maximum number of lights, especially at night.
- Keep noise to a minimum (switch off suction equipment, reduce talking and whispering).
- Offer cotton wool balls for patients' ears.
- Continually reassess the need to interrupt patients' sleep to perform observations.
- Perform as many nursing observations as possible together.
- Chart amount of uninterrupted sleep per shift and evidence of sleep stages.
- Communicate the patients' need to sleep to other professionals.
- Use knowledge of patients' normal sleeping patterns and supportive family relationships to optimize environment for sleep
- Administer analgesics and sedatives according to the patients' felt need and monitor events.

influence on recovery and might involve passive or active neglect of the patient's own needs.

Social and economic status can influence recovery due to the following:

- In low-income families food concerns are often of a low priority.
- Surviving in very poor housing.
- Families may have financial problems, which compound the problem of maintaining health and recovery.

Elderly people can become anxious over issues concerning diet, or become ill, confused or forgetful. Understanding the elderly clientele means:

- Recognizing those in need of nutritional support in the community, e.g., meals on wheels or other services.
- Considering previous illness, e.g., physical disability, depression or loneliness, as this may affect recovery.
- Determining poverty, restricted access to food or shopping difficulties.
- Depression can be associated with long-term physical illness (stroke, heart failure) or symptoms (chronic pain), and the nurse needs to be alert to changes in mood or chronic fatigue.

The cost of caring to the nurse

Working closely with dying patients can cause emotional distress for the nurse and can be painful. Nurses need adequate support systems in both their professional and personal lives. The nurse needs to recognize internal signs of stress and develop strategies for coping as follows:

- Spacing of holidays and time off is important to recharge lost energy.
- Continuous training and education for stimulation.

- Take time to debrief with a colleague.
- Concise written recording can be therapeutic and help the letting go of a particularly stressful situation.
- Being honest and sharing vulnerabilities will help a team relate and work well together.

4.3 CULTURAL ISSUES

A patient's stay in hospital may be influenced by a number of factors, e.g., religious beliefs or other strongly held principles, cultural background, ethnic origins and the availability of traditional foods. Whatever a person's ethnic and cultural background, food can play a role in maintaining good health, but it will often have an important social or religious significance as well.

Some religious or cultural diets prohibit certain foods and have festivals which require strict fasting. Others require different activities following death. It is important for nurses to have knowledge and understanding of the diverse cultures currently resident in Britain and take their different practices into account.

Some religious beliefs may refuse specific treatments. Jehovah's Witnesses, Christian Scientists and members of other minority sects may refuse specific treatments such as blood transfusion. You should explain the nature of the treatment to such patients but if it is refused the doctor should be informed and the patient should sign a declaration to that effect. The patient's wishes must then dictate what treatment he/she then receives.

Knowledge of clientele

When caring for patients it is important to take account of the context in which a patient lives, as well as the situations in which the patient's health problems arise (Kozier et al., 2012). This involves being:

- Culturally sensitive − knowledge of health traditions amongst diverse cultural groups (race, gender, sexual orientation, ethnicity, socioeconomic status, educational attainment and religious affiliation). It is essential to identify a patient's beliefs, needs and values, be able to phrase questions and develop trust.
- Culturally appropriate − to give patients the best possible healthcare taking into consideration their special needs.
- Culturally competent − attend to the needs of the patient.

A nurse who knows the groups of patients they care for and their specific needs implies the following:

- Nonprejudice towards their patients despite their medical condition, his or her heritage or generalizations about groups of people.

- Nonstereotyping according to culture or ethnicity, e.g., assuming that all groups are alike.
- Nondiscrimination as all patients should be treated the same despite race, ethnicity, gender or social class.
- Consideration of their individual needs relating to their communication style — there may be cultural variations in both verbal and nonverbal communication.
- Space orientation — the body and the surrounding environment, this space between the individual and other persons varies between cultures.
- Time orientation — refers to a patient's focus on the past, the present or the future, and nurses need to be aware of the meaning of time for patients when scheduling appointments and treatments.
- Nutritional patterns — types of food eaten, the way food it is prepared, avoiding meat or milk, fasting practices, etc.

4.4 INFECTION AND ITS CONTROL

Infection control prevents the spread of infection in the community and in hospital.

Immunization

Immunization is based on exposure to the following:

- weakened or dead disease-producing microorganisms (in the form of vaccines),
- the poisons (toxins) they produce, rendered harmless by heat or chemical treatment (then called toxoids).

These will cause an individual to produce the same antibodies that would develop if the person had actually contracted the disease. Armed with the special memory that is unique to the immune system, these antibodies will 'recognize' the specific microorganisms, should they attack in the future, and destroy them.

The widely administered types of immunization are as follows:

- diphtheria, tetanus, acellular pertussis vaccine (DTP)
- polio vaccine (OPV or TOPV)
- measles, mumps and rubella
- varicella vaccine (chickenpox)
- Haemophilus b vaccine (haemophilus influenza — Hib)
- hepatitis B vaccine
- tuberculosis
- meningitis (meningococcal C)

Infection control practices

Patients who are admitted to a ward environment are immunologically vulnerable and invariably have a reduced immune response. This may be due to the individual patient's general condition, their inability to take nutrition or fasting practices in hospital. It might be due to prescribed treatments or drug therapies. Listed in Section 1 are a number of areas that nurses new to the ward environment must be made aware of, so that they may take measures in addressing the patient's potential vulnerabilities as a result of a reduced immune response. In addition, healthcare professionals must be fully cognizant of other areas that put patients at risk of obtaining a hospital-acquired infection.

To reduce the risk of infections it is necessary to understand some detail about bacteria, viruses and the sources of energy they use to replicate. Nurses can take action to remove their sources of energy and so prevent their ability to replicate and reduce the spread of infection.

Bacteria (prokaryote cells)

The prokaryote or bacterium is a single-celled organism; it consists of a nucleus, which contains the DNA, a cell wall, plasma membrane, flagella and other structures as follows:

- The cell wall is made up of carbohydrates and amino acids called peptidoglycans and determines the gram-positive or gram-negative staining properties of bacterial cells.
- The plasma membrane is a rigid external layer of material, which forms the cell wall, protects the cell against white blood cells and helps the bacterium to adhere to surfaces.
- Spores — the ability to produce spores by enclosing their cells in a resistant casing which is difficult to destroy by heat or chemicals. They are formed when the bacterium is exposed to adverse environmental conditions, e.g., no food, high/low temperature or a reduction in oxygen. When conditions improve the spores germinate and the cell starts to multiply. In this way bacteria can survive for very long periods.

Viruses

- Viruses can only replicate in living cells.
- Virus enters the nucleus of a host cell, where it instructs the cell's own mechanisms to copy the nucleic acid and translates it onto viral proteins.
- The new virus made by the host cell is released generally destroying the host cell.
- Most viruses are fragile and cannot survive outside a living cell for long, but some can survive on surfaces or on hands prior to transmission to a new

host. Viruses are fairly resistant to some disinfectants and as such outbreaks of viral gastrointestinal or respiratory infections can occur in the community and/or hospital.

Bacterial, viral growth and replication

Bacteria grow in a variety of environments, the nutrients they need vary widely, but they contain complex and molecular systems, which can use a wide variety of substances as energy sources. They can synthesize all their required organic and inorganic molecules from simple starting substances such as water, carbon dioxide, nitrogen, phosphorus, sulphur or oxygen (Table 4.1).

TABLE 4.1 The substances required for bacterial growth and replication

Energy source	Substances
Organic carbon	The Sun
Carbon	Glucose, carbon dioxide
Nitrogen	Found in cells, e.g., proteins, ammonia or nitrates, e.g., urine, atmospheric nitrogen
Inorganic ions	Sodium, potassium, magnesium, sulphate, phosphate
Environmental factors	
— Water	Gram-negative bacteria die in the absence of water, a useful infection control measure; others are more resistant to drying out, e.g., staphylococci, or are able to form spores (*Clostridium*) and can survive for months in dust particles, recommencing multiplication when a supply of water is resumed
— Oxygen	A wound with a good oxygen supply is unlikely to support anaerobic bacteria; in contrast a pressure sore with a poor blood supply is unlikely to support aerobic bacteria
— Temperature	Many bacteria die in high temperatures, and as such represent a systemic response to microorganisms
— pH (acid or alkaline)	Determined by the presence of hydrogen ions; most bacteria prefer neutrality (pH 7.35—7.45), but some microorganisms can grow in acid or alkaline environments
— Concentration of solution	Some microorganisms can stand various concentrations, e.g., very strong or dilute solutions; therefore to kill all germs in a salt bath is impossible as such enormous quantities are necessary to achieve a final concentration and as such is of no actual value

Awareness of microorganisms may show practitioners the importance of:

- thoroughly drying equipment and surface areas,
- better determine which bacteria are more likely to survive in a wet or damp environment,
- which bacteria contain spores and are able to survive when food is scarce,
- help to prevent the multiplication of bacteria by removing potential sources of nutrients, e.g., urine, blood, skin scales, etc.

Nurses/doctors/other healthcare professionals/hospital workers/relatives can reduce the risk of transmission of hospital-acquired infection in patients who might have reduced immune defences by removing the bacteria and virus source of energy. It is important to be aware that while in hospital patients may have a reduced innate response to an invasion of the body by bacteria and/or viruses, therefore, infection control practices are imperative. Continuous audit to ensure every effort is being taken to prevent the spread and multiplication of microbes is essential.

Resistance to antibiotics

Antibiotics have reduced the number of deaths since they were discovered 70 years ago. They are a vital treatment for infections such as pneumonia, meningitis and tuberculosis and essential to avoid the contraction of an infection during cancer treatments, caesarean sections and other necessary surgeries. Therefore, there is an urgency to stop the overuse and misuse of antibiotics, which is leading to many bacteria becoming resistant to these essential medicines. This is compounded by the fact that the discovery of new age antibiotics is at an all time low, even though it has been known for a long time the lack of new antibiotics will be a problem the world could face in the future.

The urgency and scale of the problem and the significance of reducing the threat from antimicrobial resistance is highlighted by the need for action as follows:

- Improving infection prevention/control practices — reduce the spread of infections
- Optimizing prescribing practices — encouraging GPs not to prescribe antibiotics for coughs or colds
- Improved education, training and public awareness — engagement of the public not to demand antibiotics

There is a need for all healthcare practitioners involved to go to: https://publichealthmatters.blog.gov.uk/2014/09/16/why-we-must-all-become-antibiotic-guardians/

Barrier nursing: the use of the single room (isolation)

When using the single room, every effort must be made to ensure that instructions are kept simple and realistic. Regular assessment and evaluation of the situation must take place to ascertain whether barrier nursing continues to remain the most appropriate form of care. There are two types of barrier nursing as follows:

- Isolation — generally used to protect staff and other patients in the ward area.
- Protective isolation — to protect the patient suffering from immuno-suppression.

Isolation

A process of care whereby infectious patients and any materials that have come into contact with or been eliminated by them are isolated from others to prevent the spread of infection. This is generally determined by the availability of facilities, the infection and how the infection is transmitted as follows:

- direct contact
- airborne
- food or bloodborne
- respiratory droplet
- skin scales or excrement

Isolation can potentially cause serious psychologic effects, such as sensory deprivation, and therefore should be kept to a minimum. The principles of isolation should be based on isolation of the organism, not the patient.

Protective isolation

A process of care, which provides a safe environment for patients who are susceptible to infection, is by isolating them from the risk of infection from all exogenous sources. It uses simple precautions which are sufficient to protect the patient, e.g., gloves and masks are not generally necessary; the most important measure is thorough handwashing.

Protective isolation is an appropriate form of care for:

- Burns
- Those who are immunosuppressed:
  - leukaemia, lymphoma, AIDS, SCID
  - drug therapies such as cytotoxics
  - radiotherapy
  - trauma
  - age
  - patients receiving bone marrow transplantation

Infection risk generally relates to the absolute level of circulating granulocytes. The frequency of infection rises as the granulocyte count drops below 0.5×10^9/L, with a dramatic increase in the risk of infection as the granulocyte count reaches zero.

Informing the patient and visitors

Giving careful explanation to the patient and visitors is essential so they understand why the barrier nursing restrictions are necessary and can cooperate fully with the procedures.

When a relative visits a patient in a single room, there is usually no reason to ask them to wear protective clothing. Visitors do not generally go from patient to patient and as such are not in contact with other patients. Visitors do not handle infectious material and an instruction to wash their hands before and after they leave the room is all that is necessary.

> **!** Staff and visitors who have an infection, such as a sore throat or cold, must not come into contact with the patient.

Handwashing

The process of handwashing is uncontroversial and is the single most important procedure for preventing the spread of nosocomial (hospital-acquired) infection. Hands have been shown to be an important route of transmission and responsible for a large proportion of cross infection.

The skin, especially the hands, is a common habitat for some bacteria such as *Staphylococcus epidermidis* (gram-positive coccus), micrococci and diphtheroids. The majority of resident organisms is harmless but may become pathogenic if allowed to penetrate through the skin via a wound, during surgery or other invasive procedures.

Other organisms, which do not generally multiply on healthy intact skin, can be acquired transiently from:

● other sites on the person's own body,
● another person,
● the external environment.

Transient organisms that can survive for several hours on the hands unless washed off include *Staphylococcus aureus*, *Escherichia coli* and *Pseudomonas*.

Thorough handwashing before attending to a patient will ensure the majority of microorganisms acquired transiently from other patients are removed. Never let the business of the ward interfere with this important procedure.

● Transient bacteria are mostly removed from the skin by washing with soap and water.

- Resident skin bacteria, e.g., *Staphylococcus aureus*, are best removed by rubbing the hands with a bactericidal alcoholic solution, e.g., chlorhexidine.
- Alcoholic hand rubs are as effective as the more time-consuming, conventional antiseptic detergent handwash methods and may be used on clean hands immediately before carrying out an aseptic procedure.

Handwashing should be carried out:

- before and after patient contact,
- before an aseptic procedure.

No-touch technique

A no-touch technique is essential to ensure that hands, even though they have been washed, do not contaminate sterile equipment or the patient. This can be achieved by the use of either forceps or sterile gloves. It must be remembered, however, that gloves can become damaged and allow the passage of bacteria. This may give a false sense of security when providing wound care, while forceps may damage tissue.

The use of gloves can encourage the rapid growth of skin flora on nurses' hands so it is essential to wash hands following removal of gloves.

Protective clothing

The transmission of microorganisms on staff clothing is theoretically possible but is unlikely to occur. This reduces the need for protective clothing. Bacteria can spread from white coats worn by doctors; if this does occur, it is more likely to arise on the front. If uniforms are in danger of becoming contaminated with body fluids, plastic aprons provide adequate protection as they are impermeable. Fabric gowns cover more of the carer's clothing but do not prevent the passage of microorganisms, especially when wet. It is recommended that if spillage is likely, e.g., in theatres or for other sterile procedures, plastic aprons should be worn underneath sterile gowns.

Disposable gloves should be worn for any activity where body fluid may contaminate the hands and for procedures involving direct contact with mucous membranes, e.g., for mouth care. Aprons and gloves must be discarded and hands washed before caring for another patient, as the hands are easily contaminated during their removal.

Nurses may leave the room when wearing protective clothing, as long as it is understood that it is contact that spreads infection and not the act of leaving the room. As long as there is no direct contact with other patients, infections are unlikely to be spread if the nurse leaves the isolation room to carry out a specific task.

Masks and eye protection

Masks are often recommended for infections that are spread by respiratory droplets. The disadvantages are as follows:

- They do not work when wet — damp masks do not filter microorganisms effectively.
- Their efficiency diminishes when worn for long periods.
- The hands easily contaminate them during repositioning or removal.

They are now recognized as unreliable against airborne infections, especially viral.

There have been reports of acquiring HIV as a result of blood splashing into the face, and masks and eye protection should be worn for any activity where there is a risk of body fluid splashing into the face.

Waste material

Waste material that is contaminated with blood or body fluids should be discarded in a yellow waste bag, in the patient's room. The outer surface of waste bags does not become significantly contaminated, and there is no reason to enclose the waste in a second bag. If leakage of body fluids is likely, a second bag or a special impervious container should be used.

> **!** All body fluids should be safely discarded directly into a bedpan washer or macerator.

Excreta (urine, faeces, vomit)

Infected excreta should be disposed of immediately down a heat-disinfected bedpan washer. Ideally a toilet should be kept solely for the patient's use. If this is not possible and disposable items are not available, a separate bedpan, urinal and commode should be left in the patient's room/anteroom. Bedpans and urinals should be bagged in the isolation room, emptied and then washed in the bedpan washer, then dried and returned immediately to the patient's room. On discharge, bedpans/urinals must be sent to the central sterile supplies department (CSSD) for disinfecting.

> **!** Staff must wear gloves when dealing with excreta.

Linen

Infected linen must be placed in a red alginate polythene bag. The bag is tied shut and then placed in a red linen bag to be sent in a safe manner to the laundry for washing. The alginate bag dissolves in the wash and allows the disinfectant to clean the linen. In this way, staff and the environment are protected from contamination.

Domestic staff and cleaning

The domestic manager must be informed as soon as barrier nursing is commenced. The ward domestic must understand clearly why barrier nursing is required and should be instructed on the correct procedure, as scrupulous daily cleaning of the barrier nursing room is essential. All furniture must be damp dusted, the floor vacuum cleaned (containing a filter) or damp mopped with hot, soapy water. Using a broom is not recommended as it disperses organisms into the air. Cleaning equipment must be kept for the patient's sole use, preferably in an anteroom.

Aseptic technique

This method is used to prevent the introduction of microorganisms into the patient's body via contamination of wounds and other susceptible sites. It can be achieved by ensuring that only sterile equipment and fluids are used during invasive medical and nursing procedures.

The following are two types of asepsis:

1. Medical or clean asepsis reduces the number of organisms and prevents their spread.
2. Surgical or sterile asepsis includes procedures to eliminate microorganisms from an area and is practised in the operating theatre and treatment areas.

An aseptic technique is used whenever there is an invasive procedure that bypasses the body's natural defences. Examples necessitating the use of an aseptic technique are as follows:

- Application of dressings to a wound, e.g., following surgery or trauma.
- Caring for any broken area of skin, e.g., pressure sores, leg ulcers.
- Invasive procedures such as catheterization and injections or the insertion of intravenous cannulae.

Guidelines for the use of an aseptic technique when carrying out nursing procedures are given very clearly in the *Royal Marsden Manual of Clinical Nursing Procedures* (Dougherty & Lister, 2015).

Staff allocation

A minimum number of staff should be involved in caring for an infectious patient. The nurse caring for an infectious patient should not attend to other susceptible patients. If barrier nursing is for an infectious disease such as chickenpox, it is preferable that only personnel who have already had the disease attend the patient. If there is doubt, then contact the occupational health department who may offer immunization.

Notification of specific infections

If a patient develops signs and symptoms of specific infection or if bacteriologic analysis identifies an organism, which necessitates barrier nursing, swift communication and action may be needed as some infections are notifiable by law. If you are unsure which infections require notification then contact the hospital microbiology department for advice. Any problems may be discussed with the infection control team.

Equipment

This includes the instruments used and any fluids or materials, which must all be sterile. Dressing packs, which have been autoclaved to ensure sterility, are obtained from the CSSD.

Any procedure should be explained to the patient beforehand and his/her understanding checked. Reassurance should be offered and on completion of the procedure the patient must be made comfortable and all equipment disposed of in a manner that will reduce any health hazard.

Patient hygiene

The patient's skin flora is an important source of infection following invasive procedures, but good patient hygiene will reduce this hazard. Washing with chlorhexidine solution has been shown to decrease bacteriuria. It can be used pre- and postoperatively to reduce the incidence of wound infections. Anaerobic organisms such as *Clostridium perfringens* colonize the skin around the thighs and buttocks, hence the need for appropriate hygiene following surgery in this area. For areas that should not get wet, e.g., indwelling intravenous central catheters, stitches should be covered with transparent film dressings as protection against wetting during showering.

4.5 ESSENTIAL INTERVENTIONS

Following an acute or chronic event, pathophysiologic changes occur to the body, some of the signs and symptoms, nurse observations and interventions have been detailed in the previous sections. However, there are some fundamental interventions that require further discussion: the administration of oxygen, fluid and electrolyte balance, pain management and nutritional support.

Administration of oxygen

Oxygen therapy

Increased oxygen content in the air used for breathing is needed when the patient is suffering from hypoxia. Hypoxia is oxygen deficiency in the body cells and may be caused by the following:

● Deficient oxygenation of the blood − due to respiratory disease or chest injuries.

- Inadequate transport of oxygen by haemoglobin — as in anaemia or haemorrhage.
- Circulatory inadequacy — as in heart disease or emergency situations, e.g., cardiac arrest.
- Inability of cells to use oxygen — rare, an example is cyanide or carbon monoxide poisoning.

Oxygen therapy is a specific medical treatment and is given as prescribed by the medical staff who will write the percentage of oxygen and the method of administration on the prescription sheet. The concentration given depends upon the condition being treated (BTS, 2017) as follows:

1. Critical illness requiring high levels of supplemental oxygen — a reservoir mask at 15 L/min, it should quickly become possible to reduce the oxygen dose while maintaining oxygen saturation between 94% and 98%
2. Serious illness requiring moderate levels of supplemental oxygen if the patient is hypoxaemic with a target range of 94%—98%:
   - Nasal cannulae 2—6 L/min
   - Simple face mask 5—10 L/min
3. Conditions for which patients should be monitored closely but oxygen therapy is not required unless the patient becomes hypoxaemic use as serious illness with a target range of 94%—98%
4. Chronic obstructive airways disease (COPD) and other conditions requiring controlled or low-dose oxygen therapy aiming for oxygen saturation of 88%—92%:
   - Use a Venturi mask at 2—3 L/min
   - 28% Venturi mask at 4 L/min
   - Nasal cannulae at 1—2 L/min

An inappropriate concentration of oxygen may have lethal effects.

Low concentrations of oxygen (24%—28%) are used to treat patients with COPD. A higher concentration in these patients may lead to a respiratory arrest as their respiratory centre is being stimulated by the low oxygen concentration in the blood.

Higher concentrations of oxygen are often prescribed in a severe asthma attack and in pneumonia, but may also be seen in shock or haemorrhage.

Oxygen toxicity may follow prolonged periods (over 24 h) of administration of high (over 50%) concentrations of oxygen. The end result of this may be pulmonary fibrosis. There are studies emerging that provide evidence from clinical studies that show conflicting data on the effects of oxygen treatment and calling for the potential harmful effects of oxygen to be considered (Shuvy et al., 2013). There is further evidence that oxygen therapy is ineffective and can be hazardous.

In hospital, oxygen is delivered from taps at the bedside in a concentration of 100%. It is then put through a variety of equipment at different rates to adjust the actual oxygen concentration the patient inspires. The inspired percentage of oxygen depends on the flow rate (0–15 L/min) set on the tap and by the delivery device. The equipment used varies and oxygen may be given by:

- Simple face mask.
- Non-rebreathing face mask (mask with oxygen reservoir and one-way valves which prevent/reduce rebreathing of expired air) – 85%–90% so not recommended for long-term oxygen administration
- Nasal cannulae/prongs – 24%–30% with a flow rate of maximum of 4 L/min for short term use
- Venturi mask – can deliver 24%–60% depending on the colour of fitting
- Tracheostomy mask

There are many kinds of oxygen masks, and the flow rate needed to achieve a certain percentage of oxygen will always be stated in the instructions that come with each mask. Some types have specific attachments that can be used to give certain percentages of oxygen and may be colour coded, e.g., Venturi masks often used in COPD.

Nasal cannulae are not suitable for all patients because they are not accurate when giving lower percentages of oxygen and if a higher percentage is needed, there is inadequate humidification. They are useful when the patient finds the conventional mask claustrophobic, as often happens in pulmonary oedema associated, for example, with acute left ventricular failure.

If high concentrations of oxygen are used, some form of humidification will be needed or the oxygen will have a very drying effect on the mucosa. If the patient's own airways have been bypassed as when oxygen is given via an endotracheal tube, humidification is essential.

The effects of oxygen administered can be monitored using pulse oximetry, which records the oxygen saturation using a noninvasive procedure. The aim is to keep the saturation above 90% if possible.

Oxygen should begin to be reduced as soon as there is indication from the patients vital signs, oxygen saturation, arterial blood gases (ABGs) that they are improving.

! Oxygen is an inflammable gas, and great care must always be taken because of this. Most hospitals are 'no smoking' zones now, but smoking must never be allowed near the oxygen.

Fluid and electrolyte balance

The constant motion of fluid and electrolytes around the body contributes to the maintenance of equilibrium. The major body electrolytes are sodium, potassium and calcium, and management of patients' fluid balance requires an understanding of fluid, sodium, potassium and calcium homoeostasis. Fluid and electrolyte balance is maintained by the renal system with some help from other organs. Fluid and electrolyte balances are closely associated, and a disturbance in one is rarely seen without some disturbance in the other.

To maintain fluid and electrolyte balance, water, sodium and potassium are in constant motion between intracellular (ICF) (about 25 L) and extracellular (ECF) compartments (divided into interstitial fluid − 12 L and plasma volume − 3 L).

Total body water

The principal component of all body fluids is water. There are complex aqueous solutions in which biochemically distinct compartments are divided by the plasma membrane (between the ICF and ECF compartments) or by specialized cell layers (between intravascular, interstitial and transcellular compartments).

Body water accounts for between 50% (females) and 60% (males) of an adult's total body weight. Men normally have less body fat than women and thus have a higher percentage of body weight as water. The percentage of body water is higher in the emaciated than the obese for the same reasons. A newborn baby is approximately 73% water. In old age the body may be only about 45% water.

The average adult has a normal fluid intake of 2−2.5 L/day obtained by drinking and from food, either as actual water in the food or by oxidation of the food during metabolism which gives rise to some 200−300 mL per day. The normal routes of fluid loss are via the kidneys, gastrointestinal tract, respiratory tract and skin. In the healthy adult:

- The kidneys excrete approximately 1500−2000 mL of fluid daily, depending on intake.
- Faecal loss amounts to some 300 mL of fluid per day.
- Losses from the skin and respiratory passages account for approximately 600−1000 mL daily.

Intake and output

In health there is near-perfect fluid balance, and the amount of fluid taken into the body daily is equal to that which is lost from the body (Table 4.2). In illness there may be excessive loss of fluid, possibly accompanied by an inability to take in fluid by the normal routes. This may necessitate the administration of fluids by intravenous infusion.

Recording fluid balance

In almost every severe illness or surgical operation, fluid balance can be disturbed, and an accurate 24-h record of all the fluid entering the patient and all

TABLE 4.2 A possible average daily intake and output

Intake (mL)		Output (mL)	
Fluids	1700	Urine	1500
Food	1000	Breathing	500
Metabolic water	300	Faeces	200
		Sweat	800
Total	3000	Total	3000

the fluid output has to be recorded. It is important this is completed accurately so that at the end of a 24-h period the difference between input [drinks, IV fluid, enteral feeding (EF)] and output (urine, diarrhoea, wound drainage, vomit) can be calculated and a negative or a positive balance documented. This score showing either a negative or positive fluid balance can provide information that can guide the nurse to investigate these findings further as follows:

- A positive balance implies the patient has more input than output and therefore the patient can be retaining fluid, which can occur in a number of situations as follows:
  - Fluid overload, left ventricular failure (LVF)/pulmonary oedema/heart failure, renal failure, urinary retention and needs to be explored looking at the cues, if the following occurs in the patient:
    - Coughing up frothy sputum (pulmonary oedema/LVF
    - Swelling of legs/abdomen (fluid overload/heart failure)
    - Check the patient's weight and compare over a number of days
  - Renal failure, go to the cues:
    - Check blood levels of urea and creatinine, potassium (will be increased) and haemoglobin (will be reduced) if renal failure is expected
    - Urinalysis protein may appear in the urine in a higher than normal concentration
    - Daily weight
  - Urinary retention:
    - Do a bladder scan
    - Pain on palpation of the bladder
    - Lower abdominal swelling
- A negative balance shows the patient has more output than input and therefore the patient can be dehydrated, suffering from hypovolaemia or hypovolaemic shock, has been over prescribed diuretic therapy and this needs to be explored:
  - Check drug charts
  - Urinalysis specific gravity can help establish whether urine is concentrated

• Blood results such as haematocrit or osmolality

The interventions for a positive balance and a negative balance are different, so careful exploration and reporting is necessary to ensure patients receive the correct treatments.

Electrolyte composition of body fluid compartments

The solute compositions of the ECF and ICF compartments are the major electrolytes, i.e., products of ionic compound dissociation in solution, and are markedly different in each compartment. *Cations* carry a positive charge and *anions* carry a negative charge. The main cations in body fluids are:

• sodium (Na^+)
• potassium (K^+)
• calcium (Ca^{2+})
• phosphorus (HPO_4)
• magnesium (Mg^{21})

The main anions in body fluids are:

• chloride (Cl^-)
• bicarbonate $(HCO_3{}^-)$

Thus, the main cation of the ECF is sodium, whereas the main cation of the ICF is potassium. The main anions of the ECF are chloride and bicarbonate, and those of the ICF are proteins (which are predominantly negatively charged) and organic phosphates. In body fluids, the total number of positive ions equals the total number of negative ions, thus maintaining electrical neutrality.

The concentration of electrolytes is measured in mmol/L milliequivalents per litre (mEq/L), which is a measure of the number of electric charges in 1 L:1 mmol/L or mEq/L = 1 mmol/L for ions carrying a single charge. Non-electrolytes are also present, i.e., molecules such as glucose or urea which are uncharged in solution.

Movement of electrolytes between compartments

Several factors contribute to and maintain the differences in solute composition between the ECF and ICF. In order to pass between the ECF and ICF, a solute must cross the plasma membrane. Some move freely across the membrane due to their concentration differences, but a majority require some form of assistance.

Measuring electrolytes

Serum electrolytes are measured in the laboratory from a sample of blood taken from the patient. This is therefore from the ECF. The levels of the various electrolytes in the blood aid diagnosis of many conditions and can also be used to monitor the progress of an ill patient.

Sodium Sodium is the main cation in the blood and is an important indication of daily fluid loss. Obligatory sodium loss via the skin, gut and kidneys is less than 10 mmol/day. The average intake of sodium in the Western world is 100–200 mmol/day. This is much more than is needed, and excess sodium intake may be linked to hypertension. Sodium excretion is controlled by the hormone aldosterone, which is produced by the adrenal cortex and causes sodium to be retained.

Sodium and water losses are linked together as are sodium and water retention. This means that the plasma sodium is dependent on the amount of ECF, and high sodium levels in the blood may be a sign of low fluid volume rather than sodium excess. The normal range for sodium in venous blood is 135–145 mmol/L.

Hyponatraemia is associated with an excess of water and develops when the serum sodium concentration decreases to below 135 mmol/L. Hyponatraemia is caused by a sodium deficit or water excess, leading to an ICF overhydration. This can occur due to fluid regimens when fluid loss is replaced with excess intravenous 5% dextrose in water. When the body is functioning normally, it is almost impossible to produce an excess of fluid by administering 5% dextrose.

Hyponatraemia is observed in conditions such as the following:

- inadequate sodium intake or diuretic therapy,
- excessive sweating stimulating thirst and intake of large amounts of water which dilutes ECF sodium,
- vomiting, diarrhoea, gastrointestinal suctioning or burns,
- congestive cardiac failure,
- hepatic cirrhosis,
- diuretic phase of acute tubular necrosis,
- adrenal insufficiency,
- compulsive water drinking,
- oversecretion of antidiuretic hormone (ADH),
- overhydration.

Hypernatraemia is defined as serum sodium greater than 145 mmol/L. Excessive serum sodium may be caused by an acute gain in sodium or a loss of water. It is always associated with hyperosmolality. The main cause of high sodium levels is inappropriate administration of saline solutions (such as sodium bicarbonate, for treatment of acidosis during cardiac arrest, or sodium chloride). This is often due to therapeutic misadventure.

Because of the high concentration of sodium, large infusions of saline solutions may increase blood osmolality, resulting in an increased load onto the circulation due to the response of compensatory mechanisms (ADH production and the renin—angiotensin—aldosterone mechanism). These processes cause movement of water to the ECF, and signs of fluid overload may be evident, weight gain, pallor, breathlessness, convulsions and pulmonary oedema being the most obvious.

Although 0.9% saline is much better than 5% dextrose (which causes water retention and dilutional hyponatraemia if infused in excess) for resuscitation/ operative purposes (i.e., correction of hypovolaemia or hypotension), it is still not ideal.

Other causes of hypernatraemia are as follows:

- Excess sodium and loss of water.
- General fever or respiratory infections which increase the respiratory rate, enhancing water loss from the lungs and sweating.
- Diabetes insipidus and mellitus.
- Polyuria.
- Severe vomiting and diarrhoea.
- Insufficient water intake can also cause hypernatraemia, particularly in individuals who are comatose, confused or immobilized.
- Oversecretion of aldosterone, as in primary hyperaldosteronism, or Cushing's syndrome caused by excess secretion of adrenocorticotrophic hormone, which also causes increased secretion of aldosterone.

Potassium Potassium is the main ICF cation. Only 2% of the body's potassium is in the ECF compartment and thus free to be measured. The healthy kidney is less able to conserve potassium than sodium, and potassium depletion can occur occasionally on a normal diet if there are increased losses from the body. The kidney controls the potassium balance in the blood. Aldosterone is released in hypovolaemia and hyperkalaemia, and aldosterone stimulates potassium excretion. The normal range for potassium in venous blood is 3.3—4.7 mmol/L.

Hyperkalaemia is a high level of potassium in the blood. The clinical features of hyperkalaemia may be very few, but if there are any symptoms there will be characteristic changes in the ECG. This will show peaking of the T waves, followed by loss of P waves and then abnormal QRS complexes.

Potassium levels are increased in the following:

- renal failure,
- the use of potassium-sparing diuretics,
- adrenal insufficiency,
- acidosis (potassium increase tends to cause acidosis).

Hyperkalaemia can kill without warning. Cardiac arrest with ventricular fibrillation may be the first sign of hyperkalaemia.

Hypokalaemia is a low level of potassium in the blood. The clinical features of hypokalaemia are decreased excitability of the nervous system and muscle weakness. In addition, there may be:

- depression
- confusion
- arrhythmias,
- ECG changes
- susceptibility to digoxin toxicity
- polyuria
- alkalosis

Blood potassium levels are decreased in:

- diarrhoea and vomiting
- other gastrointestinal losses
- excessive sweating
- use of diuretics (loop and thiazide-like diuretics)
- steroids
- salbutamol and other β_2 agonists
- nephrotic syndrome
- diabetes
- Cushing's syndrome
- excessive renin secretion
- alkalosis (potassium depletion tends to cause alkalosis)
- overhydration
- laxative abuse

> **!** Severe hypokalaemia may be asymptomatic. Muscular weakness, constipation and paralytic ileus are the most common problems.

Calcium Calcium is a necessary ion for many fundamental metabolic processes as follows:

- the structure of teeth and bones,
- muscle contractions (including the heart),
- blood coagulation,
- transmission of neural impulses,
- maintaining cell membrane stability and permeability.

The bones contain more than 99% of the body's calcium; the rest is in the serum and exists in the following two forms:

1. Ionized or free calcium (found in foods and the only type that the body can use).
2. Bound to albumin — which accounts for about half of the serum calcium.

Serum levels of free calcium are normally 4.5–5.5 mmol/L and total serum calcium, including bound and free, is usually 8.5–10 mg/dL.

Hypocalcaemia is usually associated with inadequate dietary intake of calcium or vitamin D, which is essential for optimal calcium use by the body. There are some diseases which interfere with calcium absorption from the gut as follows:

- Pancreatitis.
- Respiratory alkalosis due to hyperventilation; calcium binds to bicarbonate so less calcium is available for use.
- Renal failure on loop diuretics because of excessive calcium loss.
- Patients suffering from burns — calcium can become trapped in burned tissue.
- Blood transfusion of banked blood.
- Hypoparathyroidism — lack of parathyroid hormone leads to a drop in calcium levels.
- Low magnesium, which inhibits parathyroid function.
- A high level of phosphorus (hyperphosphataemia) as phosphorus is calcium's reciprocal.

Hypercalcaemia is defined as total serum calcium above 10 mg/dL or a free calcium level above 5.5 mmol/L. The condition is most often related to malignant tumours and prolonged immobility. Other conditions that can increase bone reabsorption include the following:

- adrenal insufficiency
- hyperparathyroidism
- hypophosphataemia
- hyperproteinaemia
- hyperthyroidism
- renal dysfunction
- thiazide diuretics
- vitamin D intoxication
- tuberculosis

Phosphorus Phosphorus is the primary anion, or negatively charged ion, in the ICF. Adults who get enough calcium usually get the daily dietary requirement for phosphorus of 800–1300 mg. This is because both electrolytes are present in many of the same foods.

Phosphorus is vital for the following:

- formation of stored energy in the cells (adenosine triphosphate, ATP),
- formation of bones and teeth,
- interacting with haemoglobin to promote oxygen release to the tissues,
- contributing to the phagocytic action of white blood cells,
- helping to metabolize proteins, carbohydrates, fats,
- normal platelet structure and function.

The serum phosphorus level is normally 2.3—4.4 mmol/L.

Hypophosphataemia is most commonly caused by diseases that raise the renal excretion of phosphorus. These include the following:

- hyperparathyroidism,
- hypokalaemia,
- administration of PN solutions do not contain enough phosphorus,
- overuse of certain antacids, e.g., those containing aluminium, calcium or magnesium inhibiting GI absorption of phosphorus,
- chronic alcohol abuse because of the associated diarrhoea, vomiting and malnutrition.

Hyperphosphataemia occurs when serum phosphorus exceeds 4.5 mmol/L. The most common cause is renal dysfunction, but it can also result from the following:

- overuse of laxatives that contain phosphorus,
- a diet too rich in phosphorus,
- increased GI absorption of phosphorus related to excess vitamin D intake,
- hypo/hyperparathyroidism,
- metabolic acidosis,
- rhabdomyolysis,
- use of cytotoxic agents,
- chemotherapy.

Magnesium A serum range of 1.5—2.5 mmol/L determines magnesium levels. It is the most abundant ICF cation. Calcium and magnesium often interact in reactions at the cellular level. Magnesium is stored around the body at the following levels:

- 53% is in the bones.
- 27% is in the muscles.
- 19% is in the soft tissues.
- 0.5% is in the erythrocytes.
- 0.3% is free in the serum.

Magnesium is vital to several body functions; it:

- is involved in enzyme reactions that result in the production of ATP or energy,

- plays a major role in maintaining and correcting electric excitability in the nerves and muscle cells, including the heart and cardiac conduction system,
- helps maintain the structural integrity of the heart.

The maintenance of normal magnesium levels is determined by dietary consumption, e.g., 280–350 mg/day.

Hypomagnesaemia is a rare condition but occurs most commonly in:

- Increased renal excretion related to the use of loop diuretics (furosemide) or some antibiotics (Garamycin, Nebcin); both types of drug speeds magnesium loss by inhibiting its reabsorption in the loop of Henle.
- Alcohol abuse, which increases renal magnesium loss.
- Renal tubular dysfunction.
- Diarrhoea and vomiting as magnesium is not absorbed properly from the lower GI tract.
- Pancreatic insufficiency.
- Pancreatitis.
- Malnutrition, malabsorption syndromes and ulcerative colitis.

The most common signs are leg and body cramps, lethargy, weakness, nausea, abdominal distension, constipation, anorexia, confusion and arrhythmias.

Hypermagnesaemia is also a rare condition, with a level above 2.5 mmol/L, and is generally unrelated to magnesium replacement as the kidney can usually excrete magnesium excesses. It is nearly always linked to renal failure. The condition can also be caused by overuse of magnesium-containing antacids and cathartics such as Milk of Magnesia and magnesium citrate.

In excess, magnesium depresses skeletal muscle contraction, nerve function and the cardiovascular system, acting like a calcium channel blocker. These patients will experience the following:

- nausea and vomiting
- drowsiness
- hypotension
- muscle weakness
- hot flushes
- reduced deep tendon reflexes
- bradycardia, complete heart block
- respiratory depression, coma and cardiac arrest

Chloride This is the major anion in the ECF and ranges between 95 and 106 mmol/L. It provides electrical neutrality, particularly in relation to sodium, and facilitates the release of carbon dioxide and oxygen from the haemoglobin (the *chloride shift*). The transport of chloride is generally passive and follows the active transport of sodium, so that increases or decreases in chloride are proportional to changes in sodium. Because bicarbonate is the other major anion in the ECF, the concentration of chloride tends to vary inversely with changes in bicarbonate concentration.

Hyperchloraemia occurs clinically when there is an excess of sodium or a deficit of bicarbonate. An increase of chloride can be expected with hypernatraemia or metabolic acidosis.

Hypochloraemia is the loss of chloride and is usually the result of hyponatraemia or elevated bicarbonate concentration, as in metabolic alkalosis. Hypochloraemia develops with:

- vomiting
- loss of hydrochloric acid from the stomach
- sodium deficit related to restricted intake
- the use of diuretics
- cystic fibrosis

Alterations in chloride levels are usually secondary to pathophysiologic processes, and treatment is usually related to management of the underlying disorder. Therefore, there are no specific symptoms associated with chloride deficit or increase.

Bicarbonate Bicarbonate forms part of one of the major buffering systems in the body, which operates in the lung and kidney: the carbonic acid–bicarbonate buffer pair. It maintains acid-base balance of the ECF; as carbon dioxide is an acid, the greater the carbon dioxide content, the more carbonic acid and conversely, the more hydrogen ions, the more carbonic acid is formed.

$$CO_2 + H_2O \leftrightharpoons H_2CO_3 \leftrightharpoons HCO_3^+ + H^-$$

The lungs can decrease the amount of carbonic acid by blowing off CO_2 and leaving water. The kidneys excrete the excess hydrogen ions, reabsorb the bicarbonate or regenerate new bicarbonate from CO_2 and water. The renal mechanism does not act as rapidly as the lungs, but the two systems are very effective together because the lungs can rapidly adjust acid concentration and bicarbonate is easily reabsorbed or regenerated by the kidneys to maintain acid-base balance.

Changes in either bicarbonate or hydrogen ion levels will change the pH. If the amount of bicarbonate is decreased, the pH will also decrease, causing a state of acidosis. The pH can be returned to normal range if the amount of carbonic acid also decreases, known as *compensation*. Conversely, if the bicarbonate increases, the pH will also increase, and compensation will include the increase of carbonic acid.

Treatment

Most of the treatment for electrolyte imbalances is to treat the underlying cause, replace any loss of electrolyte until normal values are reached or symptoms are improved, flush out the extra high concentration via increasing urine output or dilute it with carefully monitored fluid regimens or removal by dialysis.

Maintaining circulating volume and fluid balance

To maintain circulatory fluid volume, people consume liquids. However, in instances where there is a decrease in circulating fluid volume, this needs to be replaced. The main aetiologies of fluid loss are as follows:

- *Increase in temperature* — this leads to vasodilatation and may lead to symptoms of reduced circulating volume, as fluid space has increased.
- *Dehydration* — more common in the elderly but if severe, it can lead to reductions in circulating volume and hypovolaemia.
- *Loss of whole blood* — the most common cause of circulation loss; leads to decreases in the oxygen-carrying capacity of the blood and contributes to hypoxia.
- *Loss of plasma* — occurs in large partial-thickness or full-thickness burns or burns over more than 20%–25% of the total body surface area.
- *Bleeding disorders* — platelet (thrombocytopenia, thrombocytosis) and coagulation [vitamin E deficiency, liver disease, disseminated intravascular coagulation (DIC)] disorders can cause or fail to prevent an internal or external haemorrhage.
- *Third space fluid shift* — any type of trauma or cell damage (surgery, MI, pancreatitis, head injury) will automatically stimulate the inflammatory immune response. Capillaries dilate and become more permeable, causing localized swelling and lymphatic blockage, leading to loss of circulating volume.

The decline in blood volume produced by continued bleeding, plasma loss, water or fluid shifts decreases venous return and cardiac output. Replacement therapy might be required.

Colloid therapy

Colloid solutions include gelatins (human albumin solution, Gelofusine, Volplex, plasma protein fractions, salt-poor albumin, Haemaccel and Hespan) and starches (Voluven, Volulyte). They are used to restore plasma volume and improve or maintain oxygen transport, providing adequate oxygen and nutrients, which are needed for the maintenance and restoration of cellular function. Administering plasma expanders produces an improvement in oxygen availability, oxygen consumption, circulating volume, haemodynamic status and tissue perfusion.

Crystalloid therapy

Crystalloid therapy (5% dextrose, normal saline and dextrose saline) during hypovolaemic states is necessary due to sodium leaks into the surrounding cells. There needs to be a balanced use of a salt solution to restore ECF fluid volume.

Haemodilution occurs when the blood becomes so dilute that the measured blood haematocrit is reduced to 17%–21% (normal range 38%–46%). Haemodilution decreases colloid osmotic pressure, reduces haemoglobin content and coagulation factors as there is less of these elements in relation to fluid contained within blood. This increase in fluid in relation to solutes in the blood will serve to dilute body sodium, increase blood osmolarity and, via the osmoreceptors, stimulate the release of ADH. Consequently, more sodium and water will be reabsorbed from the renal tubules, causing a net increase in ECF fluid volume and total body weight.

> ! The sole use of crystalloids to avoid blood transfusions in low circulating states can lead to haemodilution.

In hypovolaemic states, it seems necessary to administer a combination of blood, colloids and crystalloids – blood to maintain clotting factors, haemoglobin levels and to prevent haemodilution; colloids to maintain the overall circulating volume; and crystalloids to maintain fluid and electrolyte balance and prevent the movement of water and sodium into the cells.

> ! It is imperative that the patient's cardiopulmonary dynamics be monitored in a way that is reliable to determine physiologic trends and responses to whichever therapy is finally chosen.

Blood transfusion therapy

The human cardiovascular system is designed to minimize the effects of blood loss, but the body can only compensate for a finite loss. Losses of 15%–30% cause pallor and weakness, whereas a loss of more than 30% of blood volume results in severe shock and can be fatal. To treat haemorrhage, whole blood is generally used as routine, especially when blood loss is substantial.

Packed red cells (whole blood from which most of the plasma has been removed) is generally only used to treat anaemia. Fresh frozen plasma is used for patients with bleeding disorders, whereby there is a deficiency in platelets or clotting factors, e.g., in DIC, warfarin overdose, trauma or thrombotic thrombocytopenia. Blood transfusions can cause serious reactions, some of which arise from the changes that occur in stored blood (Table 4.3).

TABLE 4.3 Changes that occur in stored blood

Changes that occur	Causes	End result
Acid-base changes	Stored blood is in an air-free container, and aerobic metabolism cannot take place but anaerobic metabolism does The citrate phosphate dextrose solution added to blood reduces the pH from a normal pH of 7.4 to about 7.0	This gives rise to lactic acid production. The longer the unit of blood is stored, the greater amount of acid it will contain These two processes accumulate metabolic acids and the unit of blood pH decreases to about 6.6 −6.8 after 14−21 days of storage
Alterations in electrolyte concentration	When blood is stored, the sodium and potassium undergo alteration. It can be expected that a unit of blood will contain approximately 75 mmol of sodium and 5−7 mmol of potassium There is also a progressive loss of red cell viability, and the red blood cells tend to take up water	Patients with normal cardiac and renal functions are able to handle the increase in sodium and potassium. In patients with profound trauma and shock with cardiac and renal dysfunction, the sodium and potassium content may have profound effects. This causes a leftward shift in the oxyhaemoglobin dissociation curve, and thus transfused blood cells are less capable of releasing oxygen to the tissues
The microaggregate load in stored blood	During storage there is an increased aggregation of platelets and leucocytes. To prevent these from entering the blood, it is always filtered	It is recommended that microfilters with pore sizes of 20−90 microns be used
Depletion of clotting factors	Stored blood is deficient in the factors necessary for coagulation, e.g., factors V, VIII, IX and platelets	Clotting screens and bleeding status should be closely monitored, and platelets and fresh frozen plasma administered when required
The temperature of stored blood	Blood is stored at a temperature between 1 and 6°C	Large quantities of cold blood can cause hypothermia. This compromises heart rate, blood pressure, cardiac output and coronary blood flow. Cold blood should be warmed prior to being transfused

Autotransfusion To minimize the need for blood transfusion by blood donor, during or following procedures, blood can be salvaged through an autotransfusion device. This blood can either be reinfused back into the patient during surgery if blood loss is great or saved for transfusion at a later date.

Synthetic blood products Recently artificial blood substitutes, or perfluorochemicals, have become available and are often used in cases of severe anaemia when transfusion of blood products is not an option. Oxygen is dissolved in the perfluorochemical microdroplets (which have a high solubility of oxygen) and transported to capillaries for diffusion across capillary walls.

These blood products do have side effects, which include the following:

● pulmonary oedema
● arrhythmias
● chest pain
● respiratory distress

The positive effects of perfluorochemicals do not endure beyond 24 h after infusion due to their short half-life.

These synthetic blood products may in the future:

● reduce blood recipient adverse reactions from donor blood,
● minimize the use of and improve the cost-effectiveness of blood transfusions,
● reduce the risk of spread of infections such as HIV/AIDS and hepatitis B.

Colloid versus crystalloid therapy

The use of colloid and crystalloid therapy to replace circulating volume is disputed. If crystalloids are to be used as the primary resuscitative agents in hypovolaemia, the volumes required to achieve normal haemodynamic values are 2–4 times those required with colloids. Massive crystalloid fluid resuscitation predisposes the patient to acute respiratory distress syndrome (ARDS) or pulmonary oedema.

An overuse of crystalloids to avoid blood transfusions can lead to fluid overload and haemodilution. However, once diagnosed, the excess fluid can quickly be off-loaded by a prescription of a diuretic and passed out in urine.

A use or overuse of colloids can more quickly lead to fluid overload as they contain albumin or starch, which draws fluid from the ICF compartment into the ECF compartment. However, fluid overload due to excess colloid administration is not so easily corrected by diuretics, as protein does not/should not appear in urine, allowing the overload of fluid to remain longer with the potential complication of heart failure.

Which fluid replacement therapy is preferred is generally down to the individual doctor; however, an overuse of both crystalloids and colloids are not without serious consequences if not monitored effectively.

Infusion devices

An infusion device is designed to deliver a measured amount of drug or fluid (either intravenously or subcutaneously) over a period of time with no adjustment to 'catch up'. It is set at an appropriate rate to achieve a desired therapeutic response and to avoid:

- over/underinfusion
- metabolic disturbances
- air embolism
- phlebitis
- toxic concentrations or below therapeutic doses of medications

Gravity infusion devices

Gravity flow. These depend entirely on gravity to drive the infusion. They consist of an administration set containing a drip chamber and a roller clamp to control flow, which is usually measured by counting drops. They are useful for infusing fluids which do not need absolute precision. Flow rate is calculated using a formula, which requires the following information:

- the volume to be infused,
- the number of hours the infusion is running over,
- the drop rate of the administration set (20 drops/mL crystalloid administration set, 15 drops/min blood giving sets).

The rate can be calculated from the following equation:

$$\{\text{Volume to be infused}/\text{Time in hour}\} \times \{\text{Drop rate}/60\ \text{min}\}$$
$$= \text{Drops per minute}$$

Gravity controllers. These operate by gravity and there is no pumping action.

- Drip rate controllers detect and count drops in the drip chamber and contain an automatic clamping mechanism to control the flow.
- Volumetric controllers calibrate millilitres per hour, and the accuracy of the drip flow is dependent mainly on the size of the drop formed.

Infusion pumps These pumps do not rely on gravity, and an alarm will sound if the catheter becomes occluded or displaced. There are two types.

Volumetric pumps. These are used when a large volume of infusion needs to be administered, e.g., during parenteral nutrition (PN). They work by calculating the volume delivered. All are mains or battery powered, with the rate selected in mL per hour. The accuracy is usually within 5% when measured over a period of time. These pumps:

- are able to overcome resistance to flow by increased delivery pressure and do not rely on gravity,
- are capable of accurate delivery over a wide range of flow rates,
- incorporate a wide range of features, e.g., air-in-line detectors, alarms, etc,
- are usually expensive and some are complicated to use.

Syringe pumps. These are low-volume, high-accuracy devices designed to infuse at low flow rates. The rate is controlled by the drive speed of the piston attached to the syringe driver. These devices are:

- useful where small volumes of highly concentrated drugs need to be infused,
- limited to the size of the syringe, usually a 60 mL syringe, but most will accept different sizes and brands,
- mains and/or battery powered,
- easy to operate and tend to cost less than volumetric pumps.

Specialist pumps

Patient-controlled analgesia pumps. These are syringe pumps, but the distinguishing factor is that the pump can deliver doses on demand, when the patient pushes a button. Patient-controlled analgesia (PCA) pumps are usually categorized into three types:

1. *Basal* — a baseline rate is set but can be accompanied by intermittent doses requested by the patient.
2. *Continuous* — designed for the patient who needs maximum pain relief without the option of demand doses, e.g., epidural.
3. *Demand* — drug is delivered by intermittent infusion and can be used alone or supplemented by the basal rate.

This method of delivering analgesia increases patient satisfaction as less sedation is required, anxiety is reduced and so is nursing time and stay in hospital.

Ambulatory infusion devices. These are small devices, which allow the patient more freedom to continue normal activity. These pumps are used for small volumes of a variety of drugs and fall into two categories:

- Mechanical infusion devices: Elastomeric balloons
- Spring mechanism
- Gas-powered hydrogen or carbon dioxide.
- Battery-operated infusion devices: Ambulatory volumetric infusion pump — works the same as the larger volumetric pumps but is smaller and portable

- Syringe drivers — for subcutaneous medications.

Pain management

The relief of pain is a basic human right, and human dignity and respect requires that treatable pain is relieved. Unrelieved pain has adverse physical and psychologic consequences such as masking the signs of shock, increased stress response, reduced movement and increased anxieties. The inadequate treatment of postoperative pain has been associated with poorer outcomes after surgery. Thus the quality of pain management may influence length of hospital stay and incidence of complications.

Acute pain

Acute pain is the most commonly experienced type of pain and arises from illness, injury, surgery and other medical procedures. The management of acute pain is best achieved through nonopioids and, for moderate to severe cases, a combination of nonopioids and opioids. Acute pain can feel:

- sharp
- piercing
- acute
- electric or electric shock
- needle or cut to the skin
- duration is predictable and limited
- tends to get better
- has meaning and purpose
- can be localized

Procedural pain

Procedural pain arises from medical procedures and is a form of acute pain that causes both psychologic distress and physical discomfort. Preparing patients for a medical procedure by providing accurate information about what to expect is an important component of managing procedural pain. Management of procedural pain involves the following:

- Provide age-appropriate information about the procedure and the type of pain relief planned.
- Pharmacologic interventions depend on the procedure.
- Ensure the patient is aware that something is going to hurt — people cope more effectively when prepared.
- Involve the play specialist expertise to help explain the procedure beforehand.

- Reduce adverse environmental factors, e.g., noise, cold, and cover frightening equipment.
- Limit the number of venepuncture attempts.

Chronic pain

While acute pain serves an important role of red-flagging bodily injury or disease, chronic pain when left untreated, causes significant suffering and distress. Chronic pain often results from underlying disease and can be identified by:

- burning
- aching
- always present
- throbbing
- associated with tissue destruction
- duration is unpredictable
- tends to get worse
- cannot localize

Chronic pain: Spans beyond the expected duration of an injury or disease.

- is persistent or reemergent pain without a known cause,
- results from degenerative or neurologic disease,
- results from cancer or cancer treatment.

Neuropathic pain

It is caused by a functional or anatomic abnormality of the peripheral or central nervous system. In neuropathic pain, nerves are damaged and leads to pathophysiologic changes that result in distortion or amplification of naturally generated signals. Examples include the following:

- phantom limb pain
- neuralgia
- fibromyalgia
- peripheral neuropathy

Key points to remember

- Managing pain depends upon an accurate and appropriate assessment. So assess pain regularly using a pain assessment tool (see detailed information on pain assessment tools in Section 3).
- The evaluation and management of pain should be prioritized upon admission, as failure to do so may result in delayed or inadequate diagnosis and treatment for the patient.

- Plan ahead for pain.
- Never ignore a patient's complaints of pain.
- Be aware that patients may underreport pain.
- Record the severity of pain.
- Administer adequate doses of analgesia.
- Common methods of pain management include intramuscular analgesia, intravenous opiates, patient-controlled analgesia and other nonpharmacologic interventions, e.g., music, art therapy, complementary therapies such as massage, aromatherapy and relaxation therapy.
- Use infusion pumps when available — patient-controlled analgesia/nurse-controlled analgesia.
- Monitor for adverse side effects.

Pharmacologic pain management

The experience and perception of pain are comprised of physiologic and emotional components, both of which must be considered when choosing an appropriate treatment option and route of administration. The aim is to anticipate and prevent pain whenever possible (preemptive analgesia) and to target drugs at several parts of the pain pathways at the same time (balanced analgesia). This ensures:

- lower doses of analgesics used,
- produces better analgesia with fewer side effects,
- may reduce morbidity and hospital stay.

Recommended analgesic agents

- Mild pain is best treated with paracetamol.
- Mild to moderate pain is best treated with nonsteroidal anti-inflammatory drugs (NSAIDs) or a combination of NSAIDs and opioids.
- Moderate to severe nociceptive pain, as well as neuropathic pain, is best managed with opioid analgesics.
- Pain resulting from burn, surgery, postoperative stress responses and opioid withdrawal is best treated with clonidine.
- Titrated oral opioids are commonly administered to patients with advanced stages of cancer; however, epidural or subarachnoid opioid infusions are appropriate for high-dose opioid-resistant patients (such as those with solid spinal/CNS tumours). For more information see Section 6.

Routes of administration

- Oral administration is suitable for mild pain.
- Intramuscular injections are painful so other routes may be preferred.

- Local anaesthetics by subcutaneous or topical administration should be used for short-term relief of painful procedures.
- Regional techniques should be used to provide epidural anaesthesia and peripheral nerve blocks.
- A continuous or patient-controlled intravenous drip which has already been established is a suitable method of administration for moderate to severe pain.
- Patients can easily learn how to use a PCA device in order to provide pain relief without serious toxicity or side effects.

Patient-controlled analgesia.

- The PCA pump uses an intravenous or subcutaneous line and a syringe with ordered medication, which is locked inside the pump.
- The pump is programmed so that when the patient pushes a button, an analgesic dose is administered.
- If it is too soon, the pump will not deliver the dose because a lockout interval is programmed into the pump by the nurse.
- The level of pain needs to be carefully assessed so that the programmed pump dose alleviates the pain effectively.
- The advantage of the PCA is that it allows some measure of control over his/her pain relief.
- The pump can also be set to administer an analgesic dose at designated time intervals without the patient needing to push the button.

Nutritional support

Recording and monitoring this area of nursing care can affect the patient's recovery and as such it is an essential part of the nurse's survival on the ward.

Nutrition

Food contains nutrients, which are digested by enzymes, which are controlled and regulated by hormones. There are six principal classes of nutrients as follows:

- minerals
- vitamins
- carbohydrates
- fats
- proteins
- water

The essential function of minerals and vitamins (*micronutrients*) is the regulation of physiologic processes. The energy-yielding nutrients are carbohydrates, fats and protein or *macronutrients*. These provide primary and alternative sources of energy. Water is the overall vital nutrient sustaining all life processes. Nutrients produce and maintain the human body, build and rebuild tissue, provide energy and regulate metabolic processes.

Guidance on the adequacy of nutrition is required and standards have been devised against which measured intakes can be compared. These standards are known as Recommended Daily Amounts. In 1991 the Department of Health, in the COMA Report, updated the dietary reference values (DRVs). These are not intended to be used in evaluating the adequacy of an individual's daily diet, as we do not need to eat the DRV of every nutrient every day, but to establish the wide variety of foods that patients can eat as part of a healthy diet.

Malnutrition

The maintenance of health depends upon the consumption and absorption of appropriate amounts of energy and all the necessary macro- and micro-nutrients. Too little of some over a period of months may lead to malnutrition. Malnutrition is defined as a state which occurs when there is an imbalance between nutritional intake and nutritional requirements. When nutrition ceases during periods of fasting, there is a loss of energy stores and malnutrition will ensue.

Malnutrition can be obtained in the community

Nutritional reserves fortify the patient for the demands of hospitalization, and where there is malnutrition, poor outcomes may often result. A patient admitted to hospital from the community may already be suffering from the effects of malnutrition, either due to their psychologic, social situation or due to a reduction in physiologic state.

Psychologic disturbances Eating for some people can be a way of finding comfort during periods of insecurity, depression, loneliness or boredom. Anorexia nervosa can affect an individual's mood state and motivation to maintain a satisfactory nutritional status. These people can become vulnerable, which may impair their nutritional needs in favour of their psychologic and social needs.

The recently bereaved who is alone may not wish to bother to cook for just one, so does not bother; nutrition may suffer as a result.

Reactions to a stressful situation can lead to a decrease in nutritional requirements, such as a depressed mother at home who eats convenience foods due to lack of time or a busy secretary who does not have time to eat.

Social and economic status

- Low-income families' food concerns are often a low priority.
- Surviving poor housing conditions in deprived areas and on a very low income tends to take greater precedence over nutrition.

Nutrition related to religion and social customs

- Eating patterns may be influenced by religious beliefs or other strongly held principles.
- Some religious or cultural diets inhibit certain foods and have festivals, which require strict fasting.
- Some religious beliefs and eating practices may, over a period of time, affect an individual's nutritional requirements and may lead to undernutrition.
- Vegetarians are also at risk from malnutrition if they do not pay attention to a well-balanced diet. It is the more restrictive vegetarians where the likelihood of nutritional deficiency is higher.
- It is important for nurses to have a knowledge and understanding of the diverse cultures currently residing in Britain and take their different nutritional practices into account.
- Nurses need to acquire sound knowledge of religious beliefs, cultural habits, lifestyle and attitudes of their patients.
- This will assess and ensure that the dietary instruction of different religious and social groups while in hospital fits in with their own traditional customs and eating habits.

Elderly people

- Malnutrition is revealed as a common problem amongst elderly people receiving hospital treatment.
- The elderly group can become anxious over issues concerning diet, become ill or disinterested in food, confused or forgetful and commence completely inappropriate diets.
- Illness, long-term diseases or disabilities of elderly people often occur. These are generally the most common cause of a reduced nutritional intake, causing lack of eating competence, the ability to transfer food from the plate to the stomach through the mouth, due to physical disability, depression or loneliness.
- Poverty, problems with shopping for food and preparation of meals, as well as with chewing and swallowing are all difficulties that also need to be considered.
- Nurses admitting an elderly patient to hospital need to be observant and aware of these issues to prevent further malnutrition and its complications from occurring.

Physical dysfunction

- Many patients are at risk of malnutrition due to a disease state — debilitating chronic illnesses, such as heart failure, chronic obstructive airways disease, emphysema, find eating a chore as they struggle for breath during each mouthful and may have been consuming only small amounts of food for some time.

- Patients with malignant disease are at risk of malnutrition due to either the disease causing mechanical interference with food ingestion or treatments such as radiotherapy or chemotherapy. In patients with cancer, malnutrition is the most common secondary diagnosis.
- Other patients with illnesses such as inflammatory bowel disease or ulcerative colitis may experience malabsorption, weight loss and infections, as well as the disease itself.
- Patients who have been ill at home for a period of time prior to being admitted to hospital are at risk of malnutrition.

Malnutrition obtained in hospital

In hospital they continue to be at risk of developing malnutrition.

The malnutrition observed can be due to a lack of education and interest in nutrition, not only by nurses but also by other members of the multidisciplinary team. However, the malnutrition observed can often be as a direct result of some hospital practices.

Feeding not a high priority

- Early starvation begins after several hours without any food, and glycogen stores are very small and may last only 24–48 h.
- The need for feeding or nutritional supplement is only identified when the patient has been stabilized. This has generally been suggested at about 48–72 h following admission.
- During this period, fat stores may have become depleted, and a third of the brain's energy may now be derived from ketones.
- Nutrition must be seen as a priority in a patient's treatment, as the success of all other treatments may depend upon the nutritional status of the individual.
- Nurses need to consider patient feeding as one of their priorities. This might help to ensure that an essential component of patient care is not neglected.

Nil by mouth

- For a surgical patient or a patient undergoing medical investigations, the current processes involve a period of prolonged starvation.
- Withholding of meals for diagnostic tests may compound nutritional depletion, cause anxiety, fear, discomfort, which may further reduce food consumption.

- Fasting times for surgery or investigations are necessary to reduce the risk of aspiration during procedures, but prolonged fasting does not guarantee an empty stomach, as different foods empty from the stomach at different rates.
- Many patients are deprived of food and fluid beyond the accepted maximum fasting time of 12 h.
- If theatre is cancelled, there is no way to get the patient some food until the evening meal, and this can go on for several days until surgery/procedure is finally undertaken.
- In the ward environment, it should be noted that a patient who is 'nil by mouth' from midnight, in reality, may have been fasting since the previous evening meal.
- It is suggested that regard should be given, by nurses, to the possibility that a patient received from surgery or following investigations, may have been fasting for as long as 24 h.
- If nurses are in any doubt about fasting practices, they should consult their local nil-by-mouth policies within their own trust.

The use of 5% dextrose

- Patients who have been without food for a number of days might be placed on an intravenous infusion.
- The practice of maintaining nutritional status on intravenous 5% dextrose solution promotes malnutrition. One litre of 5% dextrose solution contains 170 kcal; thus, a patient receiving 3 L per day is expected to survive on 600 kcal/day.
- Fluid requirements may be overprescribed as adults should only require between 1800 and 2000 mL of fluid each day, but even with 3 L per day, there will still be a gross shortfall in nutritional requirement.
- Clearly, the use of 5% dextrose to maintain nutritional balance is inadequate.
- The common practice of replacing 5% dextrose with a 50% dextrose solution is also inadequate as this increases the production of carbon dioxide from excess glucose oxidation, which elevates the respiratory workload and serves to promote respiratory acidosis.
- Such results emphasize the essential need to commence adequate and effective nutritional support rapidly and early in a patient's stay in hospital.

The physiologic effects of malnutrition

Carbohydrates are the first source of energy utilized by the body (*glycolysis*) and are needed to maintain a normal blood glucose level.

- During starvation carbohydrates are not available directly from the gut, but the body can utilize carbohydrates stored as glycogen in the liver and skeletal muscles as a source of energy.
- During approximately the first day of fasting, low glucose levels stimulate glucagon secretion by the pancreas. As a result, glycogen is converted to glucose (*glycogenolysis*) and released from the liver. This restores blood glucose levels to normal. Glycogen can be lost without any physiologic consequences.
- These mechanisms supply blood glucose but cannot maintain blood glucose levels for very long.
- Fat stores may be used for energy. This requires a major body adjustment, as all other body tissues must reduce their oxidation of glucose and switch over to fat as their energy source.
- As the liver metabolizes fat, ketone bodies are produced in large quantities, which are oxidized by the body into carbon dioxide, water and ATP. As a result of fat utilization as a source of energy, an individual can fast for several weeks, provided water is consumed.

If fasting continues, the brain, having become deprived of glycogen stores, has to gradually adapt to the use of ketone bodies as the major source of energy. When this occurs, depression of the central nervous system may ensue, leading to coma. As other body cells are also limited in the amount of ketone bodies they can metabolize, excess ketone bodies appear in the blood, resulting in ketosis, which, if food intake is not initiated, can lead to a metabolic acidosis.

When fat reserves are completely depleted, the body will break down large quantities of muscle protein as a source of energy to maintain cellular functions. Large amounts of amino acids can be released and converted to glucose in the liver by *gluconeogenesis* or the amino acids may be oxidized directly. It is estimated that once protein stores are depleted to about one-half of their normal level, death results. During fasting, amino acids contribute to blood glucose only after liver glycogen and fat stores are depleted.

Improving dietary intake

The success of nutrition is largely dependent on the nurse's interest, knowledge and understanding. Improving dietary intake may prevent further invasive treatments, e.g., PN or nasogastric feeding, to improve nutritional intake.

To improve dietary intake, a thorough nutritional assessment needs to take place. Then an individual personal food plan must be decided, in partnership with the patient, to cover the following factors:

- It should fulfil basic nutritional needs, in increased amounts, to meet additional metabolic demands.

- It should encompass 'comfort foods' or familiar ethnic dishes and well-liked foods.
- The patient's cultural and religious beliefs, likes and dislikes, appetite and motivation should be considered.
- Variety in food texture, colour and flavour.
- Build-up foods may be negotiated with the patient and added in between meals.
- Timing and frequency of food and drink.

A strict record of all food, offered and eaten must be kept. Evaluation of the personal food plan must be implemented to determine whether there is a need for further changes or adjustments to the diet or knowledge base of the patient.

Nurses may have to discuss changing eating habits and attitudes to food due to surgery or illness. This may be very complex and difficult to accomplish due to issues such as culture, religion, socioeconomic status, age, physical disability or psychologic problems. Nurses should try to discuss dietary matters with patients and how they may be able to maintain an adequate diet following discharge from hospital.

Parenteral nutrition

PN is 'the provision of all nutritional requirements via the intravenous route'. Instead of food being fed into and absorbed from the gastrointestinal tract, nutrients are infused directly into the venous circulation, thus bypassing the gut. PN contains essential nutrients in quantities to meet all the daily needs of patients. It is administered using an aseptic technique into a central line, which is situated usually in the subclavian or internal jugular vein.

PN is indicated for patients with:

- prolonged ileus
- uncontrolled vomiting
- chronic diarrhoea or malabsorptive states
- severe radiation enteritis
- short bowel syndrome
- gastrointestinal obstruction
- severe pancreatitis with fistula
- hypercatabolic states
- critical illnesses
- multiple trauma or burns
- hepatic or renal failure
- inflammatory bowel disease

The types of patients selected for PN are as follows:

- patients who are unable to eat or absorb orally for a period >5 days,
- patients who are malnourished and unable to eat or absorb food,

- unconscious patients who may aspirate if fed orally,
- patients who are hypercatabolic or have multisystem failure and are unable to maintain adequate nutritional intake,
- bowel rest for patients with fistulae, pancreatitis or inflammatory bowel disease.

There are generally two routes of administration as follows:

1. Central venous line, usually subclavian vein: this may lead to problems with infection.
2. Skin-tunnelled catheter for long-term nutrition or a peripherally inserted central catheter.

The PN solution contains the following:

- Amino acids — both essential and nonessential, 1—2 g/kg/day.
- Glucose — carbohydrate energy source, provides 3.75 kcal/g. Use 25%—50% dextrose and increases the insulin to prevent liver complications.
- Fat emulsion — fat energy source, generates 9 kcal/g. Use 10%—20% solution plus increased insulin to prevent liver complications.
- Electrolytes, e.g., sodium, potassium, magnesium, calcium and phosphorus.
- Vitamins, minerals and trace elements are required.

There are many choices of PN regimen as follows:

- Premixed.
- Either prepared by hospital pharmacy or purchased.
- A regimen for a particular patient formulated to the patient's needs for energy and nutrition.

Standardized PN regimens are available and depend on body weight. They are ordered daily as the patient's requirements change. They can last up to 7 days but must be kept in the fridge. Some require mixing prior to administration.

The nurse's role in delivery

- Administration sets need to be changed every 24 h.
- Feeding line should never be used for the administration of additional medicines — PN is incompatible with numerous other medicines.
- A completely separate line should be used for medications, blood products' If a CVP reading is required the transducer needs to be attached to a separate lumen of the CVP line.
- Volumetric infusion pumps should be used.
- Never attempt to 'catch up' if the infusion is running slowly.
- Incomplete bags should be discarded.

The nurse's role in management

- Aseptic conditions:
  - tubing,
  - dressings,
  - connections of feeding solution,
  - site of the subclavian catheter observed for inflammation/infection,
  - no blood products should be infused through the line.
- Monitoring of PN:
  - Regular measure of vital signs such as temperature, pulse, respiration and blood pressure
    - Body weight – increases
    - Fluid balance – positive balance
    - Urine testing – sugar and ketones
    - Blood testing – urea, nitrogen, creatinine, urea, glucose, sodium, potassium.
- Mouth care due to nil-by-mouth state.

Complications

These are many and should be detected by appropriate monitoring.

Central line complications

- pneumothorax
- arterial puncture
- air embolism
- sepsis
- vein thrombosis
- catheter blockage and accidental removal

Metabolic complications

- fluid overload,
- hyperglycaemia,
- hypoglycaemia,
- translocation of bacteria/sepsis,
- a reduction in trace elements and vitamins,
- metabolic acidosis – chloride/CO_2,
- refeeding syndrome,
- electrolyte disturbances:hyperammonaemia,
- hyponatraemia,
- hypernatraemia,
- hypokalaemia,
- hypocalcaemia,

- hypophosphataemia,
- hypomagnesaemia.

Some of these may require a review of the PN solution, rate of administration, additional fluids, blood products and drugs. PN should not be terminated until oral or EF is well established.

Enteral feeding

EF includes any method of delivering nutrients for absorption by the gastrointestinal tract. This generally includes feeding via the nasogastric route, even though this type of feeding can be achieved through the nasoenteric route (i.e., placed in the duodenum or jejunum).

There is clear evidence that long periods of time without enteral nutrition can produce detrimental gastrointestinal responses and serious complications. It is advocated that the use of EF be initiated early, when oral diet is insufficient. Early EF immediately following any type of surgery is possible (i.e., within 6 h of insult) and is only generally to be contraindicated in complete gut failure, which is apparently very rare.

Types of tube

Nasogastric/nasoduodenal tubes are the most commonly used and are suitable for short-term use such as postoperatively or during radiotherapy. The wide-bore tube is used initially to allow easy assessment of gastric contents, e.g., aspiration of the nasogastric tube 4 hourly to determine gastric content and pH. When feeding is commenced, aspiration is continued until it is evident the patient is successfully absorbing. The narrow-bore tube should replace the wide-bore one for long-term feeding needs and should be used whenever possible as it is more comfortable for the patient and less likely to interfere with swallowing or cause oesophageal irritation. It collapses when aspirated and is not suitable during the initial assessment stage, but has many benefits following effective assessment.

A *gastrostomy* tube may be more appropriate than a nasogastric tube when:

- long-term feeding is anticipated, as it avoids delays in feeding and discomfort associated with tube displacement and is cosmetically more acceptable,
- there is upper gastrointestinal obstruction.

The tube of choice is the percutaneous endoscopically guided gastrostomy. These are made from polyurethane or silicone and are held in place with an inflatable balloon. The one disadvantage of this method is that it requires some form of sedation and radiologic support to ensure that it is in place and may need an anaesthetic for insertion.

A *jejunostomy* tube is placed into the jejunum and is the preferable method if a patient has undergone upper gastrointestinal surgery or severe delayed gastric emptying.

Methods of administration

1. Bolus feeding — indicated in situations when the patient is restless or confused, as the tube may become displaced and the patient is at risk of pulmonary aspiration.
2. Intermittent continuous feeding — feeding needs to be interrupted to allow gastric emptying prior to positioning and intense physiotherapy due to the risk of pulmonary aspiration, reducing the nutrition that the patient receives. It is not suited for restless or confused patients.
3. Gravity drip — whereby it is just allowed to flow through over a given period of time.
4. Pump-assisted feeding — connected to a pump for the majority of the day. The pump can be set at various flow rates per hour from 1 to 300 mL.

The complications of enteral feeding

These complications can be easily recognized and prevented if the nurse understands and anticipates the following potential problems:

- pulmonary aspiration
- nausea and vomiting
- diarrhoea
- blockage of tube
- trauma to the nose
- overfeeding

It is important to ensure that patients are able to meet their nutritional requirements orally before terminating EF. It may be useful to maintain an overnight feed while the patient is establishing oral intake.

Overfeeding Excess carbohydrate and lipid intake can cause hepatic steatosis and abnormal liver function. Lipid may also be deposited in the lung and impair diffusion of gases and produce infusional hyperlipidaemia. Overfeeding with excess carbohydrate can lead to excess carbon dioxide production, which can precipitate respiratory failure.

The energy requirements of disease have often been overestimated. The recommendation that more energy should be provided to counter the effects of pyrexia (13% of basal metabolic rate per degree centigrade rise in temperature) is inappropriate. It is also recommended not to account doubly for the energy cost of breathing; for patients with ARDS, their resting energy expenditure may represent only 20%—30%, rather than 50%, and a normal subject with no respiratory problems will only be 2%—3%.

The energy requirements of patients who are unwell are usually similar to, or less than, those of healthy subjects; the reason being that the basal hyper-metabolism often seen in inpatients is offset by the decrease in physical activity. The normal daily energy expenditure in adults is generally 1700—2500 kcal (30—35 kcal/kg) (1 kcal is 4.184 J). It is recommended that hypocaloric feeding be the current practice in hospital feeding regimens, especially in the early stages of injury (e.g., 1500 kcal/day for up to 1 week). This would reduce the risk of liver and lung complications and metabolic instability and their consequences.

An increase in calorie intake should take place in the recovery phase, when nutrition level is normal and the patient is no longer at risk. This regimen, to reduce prescribed energy intake initially in patients with acute illnesses and/or malnutrition, should be followed irrespective of whether the patients are preoperative or postoperative, receiving parenteral or enteral nutrition or are in intensive care units.

Section 5

A systems approach

Section Outline

In this section, some common medical and surgical conditions that you will meet on the wards are considered and care and management of the patient is discussed. In some areas a problem-solving approach has been used and the care is planned in a little more detail following the activities of living. Using these examples as a guide, you will be able to plan the care for other patients using this section.

5.1 THE CARDIOVASCULAR SYSTEM

More than a quarter of all deaths in the UK are caused by cardiovascular disease (CVD). There are nearly 160,000 deaths each year and an average of 435 people a day or one death every minute. However, death rates from CVD have fallen by more than three quarters since 1961 when more than half the deaths in the UK were caused by CVD (BHF, 2017).

CVD includes the following conditions:

- Hypertension
- Angina
- Myocardial infarction
- Cardiac arrhythmias
- Heart failure

Ischaemic heart disease (IHD) or coronary heart disease (CHD) is caused by an inadequate blood flow via the coronary arteries to the heart muscle. This leads to angina and possibly a myocardial infarction. There are approximately 2.3 million people living with CHD in the UK, and more than 60% of these are male (BHF, 2017).

CHD is usually due to a narrowing caused by deposits of atheroma (fatty plaques) in the coronary arteries. These plaques may rupture and cause complete occlusion to a coronary artery, resulting in death of the myocardial muscle and a myocardial infarction.

Hypertension

Hypertension is raised blood pressure and is present in about one in three of the UK population above 55 years of age. Many of the patients you nurse are likely to be on medication to reduce their blood pressure. A blood pressure of 120/80 mmHg is regarded as normal by the World Health Organization (WHO, 2015) and a blood pressure of 140 mmHg as systolic or 90 mmHg as diastolic or above is considered to be raised.

Hypertension is a most important risk factor for diseases of the cardio-vascular system, including stroke, CHD, and peripheral vascular disease (PVD). Diseases of the cardiovascular system kill more people in Britain than all other causes of death combined, and hypertension is sometimes called the 'silent killer'.

Patients have raised blood pressures and feel well. They may have no symptoms, but the raised blood pressure may be slowly damaging their bodies. The risk to the person rises progressively as the blood pressure rises. The patients who you nurse with CVD may have had raised blood pressure for many years.

The control of hypertension can lead to the prevention of its cardiovascular complications. A raised systolic blood pressure is now regarded as being more significant than a raised diastolic pressure as a risk factor for CVD, and iso-lated systolic hypertension (systolic blood pressure of 160 mmHg or more) is associated with a two to three times greater death rate from heart disease (Table 5.1).

In the vast majority of cases there is no definite cause of hypertension and the term essential or primary hypertension is used.

There are risk factors associated with essential hypertension, and these include the following:

● Genetic factors (high blood pressure tends to run in families)
● Low birthweight
● Obesity
● Smoking
● High salt intake
● High alcohol intake
● Stress

Only in less than 10% of patients can a definite cause be found for the raised blood pressure. This is called secondary hypertension.

TABLE 5.1 British Hypertension Society (BHS) classification of blood pressure (BP) levels

Category	Systolic BP (mmHg)	Diastolic BP (mmHg)
Optimal BP	<120	<80
Normal BP	<130	<85
High normal BP	130−139	85−89
Grade 1 hypertension (mild)	140−159	90−99
Grade 2 hypertension (moderate)	160−179	100−109
Grade 3 hypertension (severe)	>180	>110
Isolated systolic hypertension (grade 1)	140−159	<90
Isolated systolic hypertension (grade 2)	>160	<90

These levels will be at least 5 mmHg lower if ambulatory monitoring of blood pressure is used or home monitoring of blood pressure. The reader is referred to the full NICE guidelines on hypertension.

The most common cause is kidney disease, especially diabetic nephropathy. Other causes are mostly endocrine and include the following:

- Phaeochromocytoma (tumour of the adrenal medulla)
- Conn's syndrome (hyperaldosteronism)
- Cushing's disease (overactivity of the adrenal cortex or due to administration of long-term steroids)
- Hyperthyroidism
- Acromegaly (excessive growth hormone in adulthood)
- Hyperparathyroidism

Malignant hypertension is **a** dangerous form of accelerated hypertension where the blood pressure rises rapidly and diastolic blood pressure is >120 mmHg. This may lead to progressive kidney failure, retinal haemorrhages, heart failure, cerebral oedema and stroke. If no treatment is given, less than 20% of these patients survive for 1 year.

Diagnosis

All adults should have their blood pressure checked at least every 5 years. In mild hypertension, lifestyle changes alone may be recommended at first, and these may include weight loss, reduction in salt intake, safe exercise, stopping smoking, and stress reduction. National Institute for Health and Clinical

Excellence (NICE) guidelines (updated 2017) recommend the use of ambulatory blood pressure monitoring when diagnosing hypertension:

- A blood pressure in the doctor's surgery of 140/90 mmHg or more is followed by ambulatory blood pressure monitoring (ABPM) at home. If this is higher than 135/85 mmHg this is classed as Stage 1 hypertension.
- Stage 2 hypertension is a clinic reading of 160/100 mmHg or higher followed by ABPM average of 150/95 mmHg.
- In severe hypertension the clinic systolic BP is 180 mmHg or higher or the clinic diastolic BP is 110 mmHg or higher.

Medication

The British Hypertension Society (BHS) and the NICE have together issued guidelines on the pharmacologic management of hypertension (www.nice.org.uk).

Step 1

- For those younger than 55 years of age, *angiotensin-converting enzyme (ACE) inhibitors*, e.g., ***ramipril*** or an angiotensin receptor blocker (ARB) such as ***losartan*** (used if intolerance such as a cough with ACE inhibitors), are the first-line treatment.
- For those above 55 years of age or black patients of any age, *calcium channel blockers*, e.g., ***diltiazem,*** are the first-line therapy. If these are not suitable because of the presence of oedema or intolerance or heart failure, then a thiazide diuretic, e.g., ***chlortalidone*** or ***indapamide***, should be given rather than the conventional bendroflumethiazide.

Step 2

- A CCB in combination with either an ACE inhibitor or an ARB.

Step 3

- If the hypertension is not controlled, further drugs are added to the regimen and a patient may be taking an ACE inhibitor or an ARB, a diuretic and a calcium channel blocker for hypertension.

Step 4

- If still not controlled then a further diuretic, e.g., spironalactone, in a low dose may be added to the therapy. If this is not tolerated or insufficient, then an *alpha-blocker* such as ***doxazosin*** or a *beta-blocker* such as ***atenolol*** is added to the drugs already being taken.

ACE inhibitors − These drugs block the formation of angiotensin II from angiotensin I that is manufactured from renin, produced by the kidney. As these drugs may cause a sudden drop in blood pressure, the first dose is given before going to bed at night. If the patient cannot tolerate an ACE inhibitor (usually due to the side effect of a dry cough) then an angiotensin-II receptor blocker (antagonist) (ARB) such as losartan should be prescribed.

Calcium antagonists − Amlodipine is an example. These drugs cause vasodilatation and are also useful in clients with angina. Side effects include headache and flushing.

Diuretics − Bendroflumethiazide was the most common and a small dose of 2.5 mg daily is usually prescribed. This drug has some vasodilatory action. The current guidelines replace bendroflumethiazide with chlortalidone or indapamide.

Beta-blockers should not be given to patients with airway obstruction. The most common drug used is atenolol which is a cardioselective beta-blocker and often used in the treatment of angina.

Patients admitted with a very high blood pressure will usually have this controlled slowly rather than giving drugs to act quickly by the intravenous route. The aim is to reduce the diastolic blood pressure to <110 mmHg over approximately 24 h.

Low blood pressure

Often a fall in blood pressure is more significant than the absolute value, and monitoring of blood pressure is an activity that as a nurse you will be performing daily.

A systolic blood pressure of less than 90 mmHg is considered low. A systolic BP less than 70 mmHg will:

- lead to reduced tissue perfusion throughout the body and a state of shock,
- reduce the blood supply to the heart,
- reduce renal blood flow and thus reduce urine output − leading to renal tubular necrosis,
- reduce blood flow to the brain and eventually lead to unconsciousness. It may result in permanent brain damage.

Causes of hypotension

- Depletion in blood volume, e.g.:
  - Blood loss as a result of trauma
  - A leaking aneurysm
  - Bleeding from the gastrointestinal tract or postoperatively
- Dehydration from any cause such as diabetic ketoacidosis and diarrhoea or vomiting
- Loss of serous fluid from severe burns
- Pump failure:
  - Myocardial infarction

- Pulmonary embolism (if very large)
- Depression of the myocardium due to acidosis or septicaemia
- Drugs that depress the contractility of the heart, e.g., beta-blockers
- Large fall in peripheral resistance:
  - Sepsis
  - Peritonitis
  - Pancreatitis
  - Anaphylactic shock
  - Neurogenic shock

Management

- This will depend on the cause of the hypotension.
- Record observations of blood pressure, pulse and respirations as prescribed.
- When the blood pressure is low, the pulse rate will usually be increased (*tachycardia*).
- The respiratory rate may also be increased, as in acidosis or haemorrhage, but in severe instances the rate may be reduced and respirations may be shallow.
- Fluid replacement may be commenced by intravenous infusion and a plasma expander may be given.
- If blood has been lost the doctor will group and crossmatch the patient and order a transfusion.
- The urine output has to be closely monitored as hypotension can lead to impaired renal function. It may be necessary to catheterize the patient if the urine output falls and it should remain above 30 mL/h.
- Oxygen may be prescribed.
- The patient may be anxious and will need reassurance.
- Investigations such as an electrocardiogram (ECG), chest X-ray and blood cultures to identify infection may be ordered.

Postural (orthostatic) hypotension

This is a drop in systolic blood pressure of at least 20 mmHg on standing from sitting or lying down positions.

Normally, reflex actions compensate for changes in gravity on standing which could cause venous pooling. If the autonomic nervous system is not functioning so well, especially in the elderly, the sympathetic response may not occur. Postural hypotension may also occur for other reasons such as venous pooling in pregnancy, vasodilator drug action, prolonged immobility or a low blood volume may occur with diuretic use.

Postural hypotension is often accompanied by dizziness, blurring or loss of vision and fainting.

Coronary artery disease

This is due to coronary atherosclerosis and presents as stable angina or acute coronary syndrome (ACS). ACS includes unstable angina, ST elevation myocardial infarction (STEMI) and non–ST elevation myocardial infarction (NSTEMI). The latter two are differentiated by the ECG tracing.

Fatty atheromatous plaques are laid down on the endothelium of the arteries. They start as 'fatty streaks' and progress to cause narrowing of the vessel. The plaque may eventually leak and rupture, attracting platelets and forming a thrombus, resulting in a myocardial infarction.

The focus now is on primary prevention as we know that certain risk factors are associated with the development of atheroma. We are not able to change some of these such as:

- Age
- Male sex
- Family history

Others we may be able to change with treatment. These include the following:

- Raised blood cholesterol and lipids (hyperlipidaemia)
- Hypertension
- Diabetes mellitus
- Lack of exercise
- Smoking
- Obesity
- Diet high in saturated (animal) fats

Moderate alcohol consumption (one or two drinks per day) is associated with a reduced risk of CAD but if intake is high the risk of CAD increases.

CVD risk level is now assessed using prediction charts that take into account the above risk factors. These charts are printed in the back of the British National Formulary (BNF) and are used to determine whether medication such as drugs to reduce cholesterol should be prescribed to those free of symptoms.

Those with symptoms of angina or previous heart attacks are at high risk and should be treated intensively to reduce further risk.

Angina

This is pain, usually in the chest, felt as a result of lack of blood supply (*ischaemia*) to the heart. There is a narrowing of the coronary vessels, usually due to deposits of atheroma but sometimes due to spasm. Coronary blood vessels usually need to be narrowed by at least 70% for the pain of angina to be felt.

Types of angina

- Stable angina — 'angina of effort' — the most common form.
- Variant (Prinzmetal's) angina — may occur at rest — usually due to spasm of a coronary artery.
- Nocturnal angina — wakes the patient up — may occur with vivid dreams.
- Unstable angina (see acute coronary syndrome) — rapidly worsening angina of recent onset or occurring at rest.

Clinical features of stable angina

- The pain is usually in the central chest but may extend down the left arm or both arms or into the neck and jaw.
- Some patients may experience pain just in the arm, the neck, the jaw or the back.
- It is usually described as a tightness or squeezing pain, gripping or a heavy discomfort.
- The pain is brought on by exertion (angina of effort), excitement or extreme cold, all of which increase the oxygen demand of the myocardium.
- The pain fades fairly rapidly on rest.
- A glyceryl trinitrate (GTN) tablet sublingually or GTN spray buccally usually gets rid of the pain.
- The pain will always occur after a similar amount of physical exertion.
- The distribution of the pain will be the same each time, but in more severe attacks it may extend further.
- Sometimes the pain of angina is mild and the patient confuses it with heartburn or ignores it.

Management of stable angina

This patient is likely to be treated in the community, and their condition will be explained to them. Stable angina has an annual mortality of less than 2%, so the patient will be informed of the good prognosis.

General advice will aim to restore normal exercise capacity and will include the following:

- Cessation of smoking
- Weight loss if necessary
- Treatment of hypertension if present
- Treatment of raised cholesterol levels if necessary
- Dietary advice on how to achieve a low saturated fat intake and a low salt intake.

Pharmacologic management

Nitrates

- These may be given in several forms and relieve the pain of angina by causing vasodilatation. They are coronary vasodilators but also reduce the work of the left ventricle by reducing venous return due to venodilatation. All nitrates may produce a troublesome headache.
- GTN may be given as a tablet sublingually or as an aerosol spray. Its onset of action is very rapid, 1–2 min, and its duration of action is under 30 min. The spray has a longer storage life.
- GTN may also be given in the form of a sustained-release transdermal patch where the GTN is absorbed through the skin.
- *Isosorbide dinitrate* is a longer-acting nitrate that may be given once or twice daily.
- *Tolerance* and reduced therapeutic effects may occur with prolonged use of long-acting nitrates, including transdermal patches. The patches should be removed for several consecutive hours in each 24-h period to prevent this from happening.

Beta-blockers

- Contraindicated in asthma, beta-blockers reduce the heart's demand for oxygen and also reduce pulse rate and blood pressure.
- An example of a general beta-blocker is *propranolol*, but cardioselective beta-blockers such as *atenolol* are usually used. These block the beta-1 receptors in the heart in preference to the beta-2 receptors found in other parts of the body, e.g., the bronchi, but are still not regarded as safe in those with asthma.

Calcium antagonists

These vasodilate and may be used in angina or hypertension. An example is *amlodipine.*

Aspirin

- Used as an antiplatelet drug, aspirin prevents platelets sticking together and so reduces the chance of a thrombus (blood clot) and a coronary event.
- Patients with angina may take *aspirin* 75 mg daily unless contraindicated.

Lipid-lowering drugs

- As a raised low-density lipoprotein (LDL) cholesterol is a risk factor for CHD, and statins such as atorvastatin are often prescribed. These drugs reduce the total cholesterol by inhibiting an enzyme in the liver that allows the manufa*cture of cho*lesterol from saturated fats.

Coronary angioplasty and stenting

Percutaneous transluminal coronary angioplasty (PTCA) is a procedure in which a segment of atheromatous artery is dilated by a balloon that has been introduced on the tip of a very thin catheter using X-ray fluoroscopy. *Intracoronary stents* are usually inserted into the artery to prevent restenosis. These are thin wire mesh structures that act as permanent linings to keep the coronary artery patent. Sometimes drug-eluting stents are used in a further attempt to prevent restenosis at the site of the stent. NICE has issued guidance on the use of stents in CAD, and this is available on their website.

Surgical treatment of angina

Coronary artery bypass grafting

The narrowed coronary artery that is causing the angina is replaced by a graft usually taken from the internal mammary artery (less likely to narrow over time) or saphenous leg vein. Patients with severe three-vessel CAD can also be grafted. The number of CABG procedures annually in England is around 20,000 (NHS, 2015).

Acute coronary syndromes

This term is used to describe STEMI, NSTEMI and unstable angina. The plaque is now rupturing or has eroded and platelet adhesion has occurred. Sometimes it is difficult to differentiate between unstable angina and a myocardial infarction – the term ACS is therefore used to describe both.

Cocaine is a powerful coronary vasoconstrictor and raises blood pressure and pulse rate. Cocaine users may present with chest pain, and a minority may go on to ischaemia and infarction.

- Unstable angina.
- More ominous symptoms than stable angina.
- The episodes of pain are more frequent.
- They may occur without obvious cause and at rest.
- Some patients present atypically with pleuritic pain, indigestion or dyspnoea.
- 12-lead ECG may be normal in ACS but there may be ST depression and T-wave inversion.
- The patient is admitted to hospital.
- Urgent angiography is required for diagnosis and treatment in those in danger of progressing to myocardial infarction or death.

- Antiplatelet drugs are vitally important. **Aspirin** is given but other *antiplatelet drugs* such as **clopidogrel** are additionally used.
- *Low-molecular-weight heparins* (LMWHs) such as **enoxaparin** are used as anticoagulants.
- Beta-blockers may be given to reduce the demand of the heart for oxygen and nutrients.
- Statins and ACE inhibitors are also routinely given in ACS and appear to stabilize the plaque.
- Coronary revascularization is recommended.

Myocardial infarction (MI) occurs when the muscle cells in the myocardium die due to ischaemia. MI is diagnosed by the clinical history, a 12-lead ECG and biochemical markers such as troponin and creatinine-kinase-MB that are raised. Troponin is a protein released from the heart during a heart attack, and sensitive test measuring its level results in improved diagnosis.

ST elevation myocardial infarction

This is a heart attack or coronary thrombosis that presents with an ECG showing ST elevation. A blood clot (thrombus) occurs in one of the coronary arteries supplying the heart muscle with oxygen and nutrients. The lack of blood supply leads to death of the area supplied by that artery. The word 'infarct' means death.

In the UK, someone has a heart attack approximately every 3 min and about 66,000 people die each year from heart attacks. Today at least 7 out of 10 people survive (BHF, 2018). Death is usually due to cardiac arrhythmias, and in hospital the patient will usually be nursed in a coronary care unit where members of staff are experienced and equipment is available. If an arrhythmia occurs, it can be treated immediately and DC countershock administered in ventricular fibrillation (VF) if needed.

Clinical features

- Chest pain which is tight or crushing in nature; 80% of patients have this.
- The pain may be similar to that of angina but more severe.
- The pain lasts longer than angina — usually more than 20 min.
- Pain may radiate to the arms, throat and jaw.
- The pain may not respond to sublingual GTN, and morphine is usually needed.
- Nausea and vomiting may occur.
- Sweating.
- Pallor.
- Hypotension.
- Tachycardia.
- Anxiety.

Always ask patients about the type of pain they have — their vocabulary may help to confirm the diagnosis.

> The elderly or diabetic patient may sometimes have a 'silent' MI where no chest pain is experienced and the symptoms are atypical — dyspnoea, fatigue and syncope may be present.

Early medical management

The patient is likely to be very frightened; so the nurse will need to offer reassurance, using a calm and confident manner.

The main aim is revascularization:

- A 12-lead ECG should be done as soon as the patient is admitted. If this baseline ECG is normal (rare), it should be repeated every 15 min for as long as the patient is still in pain.
- The patient will be connected to a cardiac monitor for immediate detection of cardiac arrhythmias. These are common following a STEMI.
- An intravenous cannula will be inserted to allow drugs to be given easily and immediately.
- Blood samples will be taken for cardiac markers (see below), full blood count (FBC), biochemistry, lipids and glucose.
- Analgesia will be given as needed to try to keep the patient pain free.
- The patient will be made comfortable using the headrest and pillows.
- Oxygen may be prescribed.
- Observations of blood pressure and pulse will be monitored half hourly at first.

It is important that the blocked coronary artery be made patent again as soon as possible and blood flow reestablished to the cardiac muscle. The first choice is primary PCI (percutaneous coronary intervention) by angioplasty if available, but if angioplasty is not available a fibrinolytic drug ('clotbuster') will be commenced as soon as possible unless there are any contraindications.

The first thrombolytic drug was streptokinase, derived from bacteria. This means the drug can only be used once as the body makes antibodies that render it ineffective when administered a second time.

Other genetically engineered alternatives, e.g., alteplase or tenecteplase, are now more frequently used. Tenecteplase has the advantage of only needing one bolus dose.

Contraindications for the use of fibrinolytics include recent haemorrhage, trauma or surgery, history of cerebrovascular disease, severe hypertension, history of peptic ulceration and pregnancy.

It is important to observe for any signs of bleeding when the patient is on thrombolytics.

Cardiac markers of myocardial necrosis

- These are substances that are released into the bloodstream by the damaged myocardium and may be measured by biochemical assays.
- Examples are cardiac troponin and creatinine kinase (CK).
- They rise following cardiac damage, and this may confirm the diagnosis of myocardial infarction.
- CK is a relatively nonspecific marker as it is also released by damaged skeletal muscle. It peaks within 24 h of MI and falls back to baseline in 48 h. Total CK is no longer used, but a calculation of the myocardial fraction of CK is used.
- Cardiac troponin levels are used to diagnose an acute myocardial infarction. This is a more sensitive and accurate test than other markers such as CK.
- Troponins are highly specific to damaged cardiac muscle. They are released into the circulation about 6—8 h after injury to the myocardium and peak at 12—24 h, remaining elevated for 7—10 days. This may make it difficult to diagnose a recurrent MI.

If troponin is within normal limits 18 h after the onset of the chest pain, an acute myocardial infarction (either STEMI or NSTEMI) can be discounted.

Aspirin

Aspirin, 75 mg daily, has been shown to reduce mortality following an MI and also to work in an additive manner with thrombolytics in the prevention of a second MI.

Clopidogrel is another antiplatelet drug that is administered alongside low-dose aspirin in ACS. The drug is continued for up to 1 year.

Heparin

Heparin is an anticoagulant that works rapidly but has a short duration. It is used in the treatment of pulmonary embolism and deep venous thrombosis, but it may also be used in ACS.

LMWHs are usually used, and they are administered once daily by sub-cutaneous injection. Examples include dalteparin (Fragmin) and enoxaparin (Clexane).

Cardiac arrhythmias

Cardiac arrhythmia is the most common and most lethal complication of an MI. The most dangerous irregularity is VF, which constitutes a cardiac arrest. This is shown in Fig. 5.1. Immediate treatment of VF using defibrillation (DC shock) may be lifesaving.

Drugs used to treat cardiac arrhythmias include the following:

- *Amiodarone* − It is used in atrial fibrillation (AF) and other supraventricular arrhythmias but also ventricular arrhythmias including nonresponsive ventricular tachycardia (VT). Amiodarone should be given by a central line if possible when given intravenously.
- *Adenosine* − It is an extremely short-acting drug useful in paroxysmal supraventricular tachycardia but often used as an aid to the diagnosis of broad or narrow complex supraventricular tachycardias.
- *Verapamil* − A calcium antagonist that is occasionally used in narrow-complex tachycardias. It must not be given to a patient who is being treated with a beta-blocker, as both drugs reduce the force of cardiac contractions.
- *Beta-blockers* − Beta-blockers act mainly by decreasing the effects of the sympathetic nervous system on the heart. They may be used with digoxin to control the ventricular response in AF and are also useful in some forms of supraventricular tachycardia. *Esmolol* and *sotalol* are examples.
- *Atropine* − It is used to treat bradyarrhythmias (slow rate), although a pacemaker may sometimes be needed.

There are many different cardiac arrhythmias which may follow an MI. When you work in CCU, collect the rhythm strips from several patients, label them correctly and point out their identifying features. Note the treatment of the arrhythmia.

Acute MI is commonly associated with fatal dysrhythmias, and the detection and treatment of these was the primary reason for the creation of

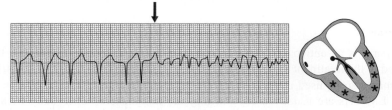

FIGURE 5.1   Ventricular fibrillation. *From Hampton, 2003. The ECG Made Easy. Elsevier, reproduced with permission.*

CCUs. Dysrhythmias may occur because of abnormal impulse formation, abnormal conduction or ectopic activity.

Following an MI, patients invariably show overactivity of the autonomic nervous system. Parasympathetic overactivity is common after an inferior or posterior MI. Sympathetic overactivity (tachycardia and transient hypertension) may be present in nearly half of all patients (especially with anterior MI) and lowers the threshold for VF.

Different cardiac arrhythmias and their causes are shown in Table 5.2.

Consequences of cardiac dysrhythmias

- Impairment of circulation or myocardial oxygenation has consequences that are extremely variable but are more pronounced in the presence of cardiac disease.
- The healthy heart can withstand many abnormal rhythms. The diseased heart cannot, and sustained tachycardias may lead to circulatory collapse or ischaemic pain.

TABLE 5.2 Causes of different cardiac arrhythmias

Abnormal impulse formation and ectopic beats	Conduction disturbances
At the sinus node Sinus arrhythmia Sinus bradycardia Sinus tachycardia Sinus arrest	In the sinus node SA block
In the atria Atrial ectopic beats Atrial tachycardia Atrial fibrillation Atrial flutter Wandering atrial pacemaker	In the AV node First-, second-, and third-degree AV block
In the AV node Nodal ectopic beats Junctional rhythm Junctional tachycardia	In the bundle of His Left bundle branch block Right bundle branch block Left anterior and posterior hemiblocks
In the ventricles Ventricular ectopic beats Idioventricular rhythm Ventricular tachycardia Ventricular fibrillation	Others Intra-atrial block Ventricular pre-excitation Atrioventricular dissociation

AV, atrioventricular; *SA*, sinoatrial.

- Management of acute dysrhythmias aims:
  - to restore normal sinus rhythm and
  - to prevent recurrence of the dysrhythmia.
- Establishment of sinus rhythm is not always possible (e.g., in AF), and treatment is then designed to slow the ventricular rate and improve cardiac output.

Sinus bradycardia

- Sinus rhythm slower than 60 beats per minute during the day or 50 beats per minute in the night.
- Bradycardia occurs in about 30% of patients following MI.
- Normally indicates parasympathetic overactivity, with release of acetylcholine from autonomic fibres in the atria and AV node.
- Afferent vagal fibres are more common on the inferior surface of the heart, and inferior MI is complicated more by this. Slowing of the heart is useful and protective in that it limits myocardial work but may result in hypotension secondary to a reduced output. Coronary perfusion may also be reduced.
- Usually symptomless, sudden onset of bradycardia may result in hypotension with dizziness or syncope.
- Causes include the following:
  - Hypothermia, hypothyroidism, raised intracranial pressure.
  - Drug therapy with beta-blockers, digitalis or other antiarrhythmics.
  - Acute ischaemia and infarction.
  - Chronic degenerative causes.

Junctional bradycardia

- If the sinus node fails to initiate an impulse and there are no other focuses in the atria, the AV junction takes over the pacemaker function.
- Most commonly occurs after acute MI, particularly if the patient is hypoxic or acidotic.
- Relatively slow (40−60 beats per minute) but sometimes may speed up, and junctional tachycardia (>100) may occur.

Heart block

This is a block to the conduction of impulses and may occur at any point in the conducting system of the heart.

Atrioventricular block is a block either in the atrioventricular (AV) node or the bundle of His (AV bundle).

A block lower down in the conducting system is *bundle branch block*, and this occurs in the bundle of His either in the right or left bundle branches.

Various conduction disturbances can occur and are usually asymptomatic, but some patients may present with syncope.

There are three forms of AV block:

- First-degree AV block, where there is prolongation of the PR interval to no more than 0.22 s and every atrial depolarization is followed by delayed conduction to the ventricles.
- Second-degree heart block, where some P waves conduct and some do not. There are several forms — Mobitz I block (Wenckebach block), Mobitz II block and 2:1 or 3:1 (advanced) block where every second or third P wave conducts to the ventricles. The reader is referred to one of the more advanced medical texts in the Further Reading for more details.
- Third-degree (complete) AV block, where all atrial activities fail to conduct to the ventricles. The electrical activity from the atria and ventricles is completely unrelated.

Ventricular standstill and asystole

- Occurs when impulses fail to reach the ventricles or impulse formation ceases.
- If the problem is in the conduction system, atrial P waves may continue to occur.
- There will be no ventricular activity unless a ventricular pacemaker takes over.
- The ventricles are left without electrical stimulation, and ventricular standstill occurs.
- No cardiac output and cardiac arrest results.
- More often, no electrical activity (either atrial or ventricular) is seen, and the term *asystole* is used.

This form of arrest has a poor prognosis and has the following causes:

- Metabolic acidosis
- Electrolyte imbalance
- Hypoxia and drugs
- Acute MI

About 25% of arrests in hospital and 10% out of hospital are of this type.

Tachycardias

- An increase in rate is the normal response of the heart to increased work. This occurs so that cardiac output will increase.
- However, abnormal tachycardias are frequently associated with a diminished cardiac output.

- Increase in heart rate is at the expense of diastole, and the heart has less time to fill.
- If ventricular filling is reduced, cardiac output will be reduced.
- Coronary blood flow takes place in diastole and therefore ischaemia may result.
- Symptoms provoked by tachycardia may include angina, dyspnoea, palpitations or syncope.
- Most tachycardias are produced by reentry or enhanced automaticity.
- Narrow complex tachycardias include junctional tachycardias (SVTs), atrial flutter and AF.
- Each may present as sustained or paroxysmal tachycardia.

Atrial flutter

- Rate 220–350/min (usually about 300).
- ECG shows flutter waves which have a saw-tooth appearance in the inferior leads.
- There may be some AV blockade resulting in a ventricular rate of about 150 (i.e., 2:1 block).
- Atrial flutter is always unstable and should be converted to sinus rhythm.

Atrial fibrillation

- One of the most common cardiac arrhythmias.
- Affects approximately 1 in 20 of those above the age of 65 years in the UK.
- Complicates 10%–15% of MIs and is associated with a poor prognosis.
- Normal atrial contraction is replaced by a series of irregular fibrillation waves (350–600/min) caused by multiple and changing micro reentry circuits.
- Myocardial contraction is ineffective for atrial emptying, and the atria remain functionally in diastole.
- Reduces cardiac output by 10%–20%.
- Although AF makes the heart less efficient, the most important consequence is thromboembolism, especially *stroke*.
- Patients with chronic AF are usually prescribed anticoagulants in an attempt to prevent embolism and stroke.

Sinus tachycardia

- Sinus rhythm greater than 100 and commonly between 100 and 150.
- P waves are normal and have a 1:1 relationship with the QRS.
- Found in one-third of patients with MI – an attempt to maintain cardiac output when there is reduced stroke volume.
- May be worsened by fear, pain or anxiety.

- Adequate analgesia will often settle this post-MI.
- Mortality for those with MI is higher in sinus tachycardia than for those with sinus bradycardia.

Atrial ectopic beats

- Common in health and disease.
- Seen as premature P waves on ECG.
- Very common after an MI. May indicate sympathetic overactivity, hypoxia or anxiety.
- Usually asymptomatic and cause no haemodynamic upset.

Ventricular dysrhythmias

- These include ventricular ectopics, VT, ventricular flutter and VF.
- Myocardial ischaemia predisposes to ventricular dysrhythmias as normal electrical conduction pathways may be disturbed.
- Myocardial irritability following an MI is the most common cause of ventricular arrhythmias.
- Necrotic myocardial tissue is a focus for this ectopic activity.
- Predisposing factors following an MI include potassium imbalances or drugs.

Ventricular ectopics

- These are premature ventricular complexes which can occur at any time in diastole.
- The QRS complex is premature and widened. Danger is progression to VT.
- Beta-blockers post-MI seem to reduce serious dysrhythmias as well as limiting infarct size.

Ventricular tachycardia

This is a life-threatening reentry dysrhythmia. QRS complexes are wide and regular at a rate of 100–220 beats per minute. The atria continue to beat and dissociated P waves may be seen. The atrial rate is usually slower as it arises from the SA node.

There are four types of VT:

- The most common is *monomorphic VT* and the complexes are of uniform appearance (monomorphic). Each episode of VT continues for a variable time and usually terminates in a long pause before sinus rhythm returns.
- *Polymorphic VT (torsades de pointes)* is a dangerous dysrhythmia. The QRS undulates around the isoelectric line, with a marked change in

amplitude every 5–30 beats. Episodes may be precipitated by drugs that prolong the QT interval or by electrolyte imbalances. Usually terminates spontaneously but may lead to VF.

- *Ventricular flutter* is characterized by a rapid ventricular rate of about 180–250 beats. The ECG has been likened to a row of hairpins. It often precedes VF.
- *Accelerated idioventricular tachycardia* is an escape rhythm which is slow, usually about 60 and not exceeding 120. After about 30 beats, sinus rhythm usually returns but may occasionally be replaced by sustained VT or VF.

Ventricular fibrillation

- Electrically and mechanically, the heart is completely disorganized and cardiac arrest ensues.
- The ECG shows fine and coarse waves of irregular size, shape and rhythm.
- Fine VF may mimic asystole and produce an apparently flat line on the ECG.
- About 90% of deaths following acute MI are due to VF. Nearly half occur in the first half hour.
- Primary VF occurs in the first 12 h after MI. Usually associated with a good prognosis as the heart is usually still functioning well.
- Reperfusional VF may occur following thrombolysis, but this probably reflects a good prognosis as the infarct-related artery has been reopened.
- Secondary or late VF occurs when function has been severely compromised by the infarct and prognosis is poor.

The Resuscitation Council (UK) has produced guidelines for the management of peri-arrest arrhythmias, and these can be obtained from their website (www.resus.org.uk). They have been designed to allow the advanced life support provider to treat the patient effectively and safely in an emergency.

Sudden cardiac death

This is defined as death due to cardiac causes within 6 h of the onset of symptoms. About 80% of cases in the UK are probably due to coronary artery disease, and about 40% of deaths due to coronary artery disease occur this way. Most cases are due to fatal ventricular arrhythmias with myocardial ischaemia.

Cardiac failure

Heart failure occurs when the heart is no longer acting as an efficient pump and thus cannot respond to the demands made upon it.

The heart is really two pumps in series — the right side of the heart and the left side — and either side may fail independently. There may, however, be a failure of both sides together, or left heart failure may lead to right.

The term *congestive cardiac failure* is usually taken to mean right-sided failure following left heart failure but may be used differently by some practitioners. Due to this confusion, this term is best avoided, although you will certainly still meet it on the wards. Biventricular failure is a failure of both ventricles and is the most common form of heart failure. Although we do divide heart failure for clinical purposes into left and right cardiac failures, it is rare for one part of the heart to fail totally in isolation.

Chronic heart failure can be *compensated* with stable symptoms and no obvious fluid retention or *decompensated* if acute or showing deterioration. In decompensated heart failure, there are obvious clinical features present.

Left heart failure

Commonly known as left ventricular failure (LVF), this results from damage to, or overload of, the left ventricle. This could be due to an increased load on the left side of the heart or reduced muscular power.

Causes for LVF include the following:

- IHD (the most common cause)
- Systemic hypertension
- Mitral and aortic valve disease
- Cardiomyopathies
- Overtransfusion

Fig. 5.2 shows that if the left ventricle is not pumping adequately, there will be a buildup of blood in the left side of the heart. This will cause a backlog in the left atrium and then the pulmonary veins and also in the blood vessels within the lungs themselves. The raised pressure in the vessels will cause fluid to leave the blood vessels and enter the lung tissue, causing *pulmonary oedema*.

Symptoms depend on the severity of the failure. There may be fatigue, pulmonary congestion and breathlessness on exertion, orthopnoea and paroxysmal nocturnal dyspnoea. It is commonplace in an accident unit for patients to come in as an emergency with severe dyspnoea due to LVF. This most commonly occurs during the night and in the early hours of the morning when the patient has been lying in bed.

The patient on the ward can also suddenly develop a worsening LVF and need rapid treatment.

Clinical features and physical signs of acute pulmonary oedema due to LVF include the following:

- Severe breathlessness
- Moist, wheezy breathing

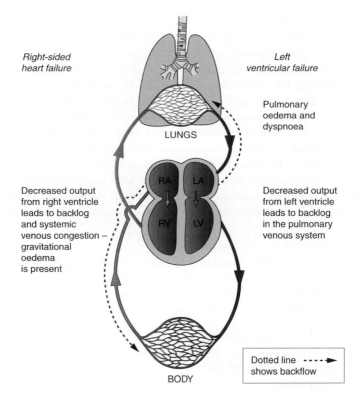

FIGURE 5.2   Congestion in left- and right-sided heart failure.

- Basal lung crackles
- Anxiety — feeling of suffocation
- Tachycardia
- Cold, clammy skin
- White, frothy sputum — may be pink in terminal stages

Care and management

- Aid the patient to sit up in bed and thus allow maximum lung expansion.
- Reassure him that this terrible suffocating feeling will be relieved.
- Administer oxygen if prescribed by nasal cannula.
- A portable chest X-ray may be performed.
- Urgent diuretics are needed to relieve the pulmonary oedema. It is likely that the doctor will administer furosemide intravenously. This will start to work rapidly as it also has a vasodilatory effect as well as a diuretic effect. In about 30 min or less the patient should start to feel better.

> Do warn the patient that he will need to pass urine more than once and that this is just what we want him to do. If he is not aware of this he will worry about his constant need to urinate.

- Nitrates are also administered as venodilatation reduces the preload on the heart.
- A small dose of diamorphine (2.5 mg) is often administered intravenously. This relieves the panic and anxiety but also helps to reduce the strain on the heart.
- In a milder and more chronic form LVF will cause shortness of breath on exertion and perhaps some breathlessness in the night with a cough that occurs on lying down. The patient will be treated with oral diuretics such as furosemide and may be prescribed an ACE inhibitor such as ramipril.

Right heart failure

Failure of the right side of the heart occurs secondary to lung disease but also secondary to left-sided heart failure. It may also occur following a large pulmonary embolus or in those with right-sided valvular disease.

You will nurse many clients with right-sided heart failure because of the high incidence of chronic respiratory problems in Britain.

Clinical features and physical signs

When the right ventricle cannot pump adequately the backlog of blood occurs in the right atrium and then the venae cavae. This causes the venous system to become congested. Physical signs may be common than actual symptoms:

- Due to the raised pressure in the veins, fluid leaves the capillaries and enters the tissues, giving rise to gravitational oedema.
- This means that the earliest sign of right-sided heart failure is pitting oedema. This will occur in the feet and legs of those who are ambulant (gravitational) and in the sacrum if the patient is in bed and may spread to the groin.
- Jugular venous distension.
- The fall in cardiac output results in salt and water retention by the kidneys, which causes a raised blood volume and more oedema.
- Ascites (fluid accumulated in the peritoneal cavity) may occur.
- Pleural effusion (fluid in the pleural space) may add to the breathlessness.
- All the abdominal organs are engorged with blood, and the liver may be tender and enlarged.

- Loss of appetite.
- Lethargy and fatigue.

Management and care

Breathlessness. The patient will usually be more comfortable to sit upright in bed or in a chair. Some clients prefer to even sleep sitting in a chair.

Oxygen should be administered if it has been prescribed. This is usually at a low concentration because the patient is likely to have chronic lung disease.
Oedema.

- An accurate record of fluid intake and output is kept.
- To assess the oedema, daily weighing may be done.
- Diuretics such as *furosemide* will be prescribed.
- Reduced salt intake will help to prevent further accumulation of fluid in the tissues.
- Fluid restriction may become necessary if diuretics fail.

Fatigue. The patient will feel tired as the heart cannot respond to any increased demands made upon it. Rest is important to reduce the strain on the heart and also to promote a diuresis as this allows more cardiac output to flow to the kidneys.

! This client is very susceptible to deep venous thrombosis while resting and active leg movements must be encouraged.

Abdominal discomfort

- Venous congestion can cause problems throughout the gastrointestinal tract.
- Loss of appetite and constipation are common.
- Straining to go to the toilet should be avoided and so a laxative may be ordered.
- Congestion of the liver may lead to slight jaundice.

Skin care. Poor circulation, oedema and rest in bed all increase the risk of pressure sores developing.

Orientation. If circulation is very poor, cerebral hypoxia may occur and the patient may become confused and disorientated. Conscious level may deteriorate.

Administration of medication

Diuretics help to reduce the oedema. *Furosemide* is the most potent diuretic and is often used in heart failure. Potassium is lost with this diuretic but the patient is likely to be prescribed potassium-sparing drugs such as spironalactone or ACE inhibitors, which retain potassium and help to counteract the loss.

Digoxin may be prescribed but its role is unsure. It does increase the force of the cardiac contractions but benefit is now not thought to be via this route. It may be prescribed if the patient has AF as well as heart failure as digoxin also reduces conductivity within the AV node, thus helping to control ventricular response in AF. Digoxin does appear to benefit some patients with advanced heart failure but it has a narrow therapeutic range. The toxic level of digoxin in the blood is close to the therapeutic level, and the nurse should be aware of the signs of digoxin toxicity. These include the following:

- Slow pulse rate — below 60 beats per minute (bpm)
- Anorexia
- Nausea and vomiting
- Diarrhoea
- Blurred vision
- Arrhythmias

! The pulse rate is checked before digoxin is administered and the dose is usually omitted if the pulse rate is below 60 bpm.

ACE inhibitors such as **ramipril** are prescribed in heart failure. They help to take the strain off the heart by causing vasodilatation and also have a slight diuretic action. They do cause some retention of potassium, and when they are prescribed, care should be taken to monitor electrolytes if another potassium-sparing diuretic is also being given.

Spironolactone is an aldosterone antagonist and has been found to improve long-term clinical outcome in heart failure. Aldosterone is a hormone produced by the adrenal cortex. Its secretion leads to sodium retention and therefore water retention by the body and potassium loss. When aldosterone is antagonized by spironolactone the reverse occurs and there is sodium and water loss from the body with some potassium retention. Hyperkalaemia may occur, especially if ACE inhibitors are also prescribed.

Ivabradine is now recommended by NICE in certain cases of chronic heart failure. It is only initiated by a heart specialist. It reduces heart rate by its action on ion currents in the sinoatrial node which is a different mechanism from other drugs used (e.g., beta-blockers).

! A reduced potassium level leads to increased cardiotoxicity of digoxin.

Anticoagulants, e.g., **heparin**, may be ordered for some clients if the risk of thromboembolism is assessed as severe.

NICE has produced guidelines for the treatment of chronic heart failure due to left ventricular systolic dysfunction, and these can be found on their website (www.nice.org.uk).

Principles of nursing management

Communicating. The patient needs constant reassurance, clear explanations regarding care and a calm atmosphere.

Breathing. The patient may be very breathless and should be sat up in bed or in a chair, well supported with pillows, and given a bedtable to rest his arms upon. Oxygen may be given but only if prescribed.

Maintaining a safe environment. Hypoxia may lead to confusion. The nurse needs to be with the patient should this occur.

Eating and drinking. There may be reduced appetite, and small attractive meals should be offered. Dietary advice should be followed.

Eliminating. Urine output must be measured accurately because of the diuretic therapy and the oedema. Constipation may be present and a laxative may be needed.

Personal cleansing and dressing. The patient may have a dry mouth and ice cubes may be appreciated. Mouth care may also be needed.

Mobilizing. Initially the patient will need to rest but beware of the risk of deep vein thrombosis (DVT) and the need for passive or active leg movements.

Sleeping. The breathlessness may appear worse at night. Ensure that the patient is comfortable. He may need to sleep in a chair. Sedation should be avoided if at all possible. An open window may help if the ward is rather airless.

Biventricular heart failure is a chronic condition and the patient will need to be on medication for the rest of his life. He will need a varying degree of support to live in the community.

Stroke

A stroke is an acute event, in which a neurologic deficit appears more than a few minutes or hours, sometimes in a stepwise fashion, persists for more than 24 h and is presumed to be due to impairment of the blood supply to one part of the brain. A stroke is sometimes referred to as a cerebrovascular accident (CVA).

The interruption of blood flow to the brain may be due to an embolus or thrombus (80% of cases) or a haemorrhage into the brain (20% of cases) from a weakened intracranial arterial wall. Motor and sensory loss or disturbance will ensue. Recovery is variable but in many cases can be complete.

Stroke is the fourth single most common cause of death in Britain and the largest single cause of severe disability. Each year approximately 100,000 people in the UK will have a stroke. There is around one stroke every 5 min (State of the Nation Stroke Statistics, 2017).

The Government first published a 'Stroke Strategy' in 2007. The F.A.S.T. (face, arm, speech, time) campaign began in 2009 and educated the public on the recognition of features of stroke and the need for early treatment and hospitalization. Between 2009 and 2013 this resulted in a 54% increase in stroke-related 999 calls, leaving thousands of people left disabled by stroke with more rapid intervention and treatment. Thousands more are recovering from their strokes, helped by specialist stroke units. However, one in five stroke patients are still treated on general medical wards (The Stroke Association, 2015).

Rehabilitation following a stroke is an absolutely vital part of the care and there are regional stroke rehabilitation centres to fill this need.

Transient ischaemic attack

This is an episode of acute neurologic deficit, of presumed vascular origin, which resolves completely in 24 h. The patient may present with the features of a stroke but these resolve over this short period. There may be a small infarction and this will show up on magnetic resonance imaging (MRI). The condition is an emergency, and high-risk patients need urgent diagnosis (within 24 h) and treatment to prevent possible further development into a stroke. The phrase often used is 'time is brain'.

There should be facilities available for imaging of the carotid arteries and intervention where needed. At present this is not the case in all areas.

Aspirin as an antiplatelet should be started immediately if not being taken already.

Predisposing factors (stroke and transient ischaemic attack)

- Incidence increases with age.
- Higher in men at all ages (male:female is 1.5:1).
- Hypertension is the major predisposing factor, the aim is a systolic BP of less than 140 mmHg.
- Atheroma of part of the cerebral circulation, causing narrowing of the blood vessels.
- Disease of the heart valves and AF may instigate the formation of emboli in the heart which may then break off and travel to the brain. Warfarin should be prescribed if possible in AF to prevent the formation of emboli.
- Other factors include diabetes mellitus, smoking and hyperlipidaemia.
- Lack of physical activity.
- Regular high consumption of alcohol.

Speed is vital in the recognition and treatment of stroke, but stroke is often preventable and primary prevention with health education and lifestyle changes is essential.

Adopting a healthy lifestyle with a Mediterranean diet and exercise should decrease the incidence of stroke.

Control of hypertension is also essential. Every 10 mmHg reduction in systolic blood pressure reduces the risk of major cardiac events by 20% according to the BHF.

The wider use of statins to reduce LDL cholesterol levels should also reduce the incidence of stroke.

Black and minority ethnic groups have a higher incidence of stroke and so should be targeted with preventative measures.

Clinical features of stroke

- Depend on the position and extent of ischaemia or haemorrhage.
- Abrupt onset.
- Vary enormously in severity and symptoms and signs.
- Slow worsening over hours, or a stepwise deterioration over days, may occur (evolving stroke).
- Loss of consciousness may occur.
- Headache, dizziness.
- Fitting.
- Vomiting.
- Motor disorders (hemiplegia or hemiparesis).
- Aphasia (difficulty in speech) may be partial or complete loss of the ability to communicate. If the stroke affects the dominant hemisphere of the brain where the speech centre is located (left side in right-handed people), aphasia is likely to occur.
- Sensory disorders — visual impairment, loss of sensation (hemianaesthesia).
- Consciousness may deteriorate as cerebral oedema increases.
- Affected muscles are flaccid at first (the limbs on the affected side feel floppy; if the arm is lifted and released, it falls back onto the bed). After about 48 h, the muscles become spastic — rigid and difficult to move.

! A stroke affecting the right side of the body has originated in the left side of the brain and vice versa.

Initial management

All patients with a suspected stroke should be taken immediately by ambulance to a stroke unit where a diagnosis can be made and thrombolysis is offered throughout the day or night. Thrombolysis should be given within 3 h of the onset of symptoms but only after the exclusion of haemorrhagic stroke.

Some patients may be eligible for thrombectomy. This is a procedure that removes the clot from the brain, but there are only a few specialist centres in the UK at present that offer this treatment.

Admission to specialist stroke units has been shown to decrease mortality and improve the long-term outcome for stroke patients. Most hospitals do now have a stroke unit but standards of care vary over the country.

Aspects of care

High-dependency care is often needed for the first 24 h. Most stroke progression occurs within this period, and so assessment and rapid recognition are vital.

- Refer to Section 3 on assessment of the unconscious patient.
- An urgent brain scan (CT or MRI) will be done to differentiate between a blood clot or a bleed.
- Neurologic function and the patient's level of consciousness need monitoring.
- Respiratory function and oxygen saturation should be monitored.
- Regular recordings of pulse, blood pressure and respirations are made.
- Note any irregularity of the pulse − cardiac rhythm is monitored.
- Investigations include an ECG and chest X-ray.
- Thrombolysis is used to treat patients whose stroke is due to a clot.

Communicating

- Provide continuous reassurance to the patient, even if he appears unconscious.
- Provide accurate information for relatives.

Where possible, both the patient and carers should be involved in formulating a plan of care.

Eating and drinking

- The patient must not be given anything by mouth until the swallowing reflex has been assessed and is present.
- If the patient cannot drink, a nasogastric tube may be passed or an intravenous infusion commenced.

Eliminating

- A catheter may be inserted if the patient is unconscious.
- This will prevent retention or incontinence and allow the urine output to be measured accurately.

Personal cleansing and dressing

- Carry out frequent mouth care, especially if the patient is breathing through his mouth, receiving oxygen or not drinking.
- Keep the skin clean and dry.

Mobilizing

- Physiotherapy is essential here.
- If immobile, the patient will need to be turned frequently and carefully to prevent pressure sores developing.
- Carry out gentle passive exercises to flaccid limbs, under the guidance of the physiotherapist.
- Correctly position the limbs after turning the patient.

Continuing care and rehabilitation

In the convalescent and rehabilitative phase the goals are to prevent complications, to aid maximum independence and to provide support for the family.

Rehabilitation should be supported by a multidisciplinary team (MDT), and access to speech therapy and physiotherapy is essential. More than a third of patients in the UK are discharged to a community rehabilitation team or to an Early Support Discharge team, but these are still not available in around 20% of hospitals.

Maintaining a safe environment

- Keep the surrounding floor area free from obstructions.
- Ensure the patient wears shoes rather than slippers for walking practice.
- Keep the bed at a suitable height for the patient.

Communication

- Offer encouragement to both the patient and the relatives and ensure they make a positive contribution to the plan of care.
- Check that any information given has been understood and repeat as necessary to ensure understanding.
- The patient may not be able to respond and the nurse will need to liaise with the speech therapist and use picture boards or the alphabet where appropriate.

- Observe for emotional lability (weeping outbursts are common with stroke patients). One-third of patients develop depression following a stroke.
- Breathing.
- Ensure the patient is positioned carefully in the bed or chair to permit maximum lung expansion.
- Encourage breathing exercises as taught by the physiotherapist.
- Observe for signs of a chest infection.

Eating and drinking

- Avoid foods that could cause choking (e.g., crumbs).
- Remember that food may lodge in the mouth on the paralysed side.
- Help to make mealtimes interesting and a time to look forward to. Involve relatives or carers where possible.

Eliminating

- Help the patient to achieve continence without the aid of a catheter.
- Avoid constipation by providing high-fibre foods if appropriate and the use of a gentle laxative if necessary.

Personal cleansing and dressing

- Frequent mouth care and washes, watching again for any food debris in the mouth.
- Assist with washing and dressing as necessary.
- Do not leave the patient unattended in the bath.
- Use appropriate lifts and hoists.
- Try out adaptations to clothing, e.g., Velcro instead of buttons.
- Seek the advice of the occupational therapist regarding dressing and suitable clothes and aids.
- Appreciate that progress may be by very small steps and give the patient praise for any advances he makes in self-care.

Mobilizing

- With the physiotherapist, make achievable short-term goals for the patient to work towards.
- Carry out exercises in the physiotherapist's absence, using aids and equipment provided and as taught by her.
- Maintain the limbs in a straight position when the patient is at rest.

Working and playing

- A positive attitude demonstrated by all caring professionals will encourage the patient to believe that progress can be made.
- If the patient cannot communicate, do ask the relatives if he usually likes to listen to the radio and do provide such distractions some of the time.
- Occupational therapy workshops may be available to practise therapeutic activities.
- The social worker may be able to give advice concerning possible employment changes.

Sleeping

- Keep the limbs carefully positioned at night.
- Observe for an increase in depression or anxiety at night.
- Provide company when possible if the patient is awake.

End of life care

- Stroke carries a mortality of about 20% within the first month. Many patients are unable to communicate effectively, and providing high-quality care in these circumstances can prove difficult and requires a team of specialist nurses.
- The management of any pain is important, as is emotional and psychological support.
- Provide accurate information, in a sensitive manner, to both the patient and his relatives, to enable them to plan for the future.
- Listen to the worries of both the patient and his relatives and to any anger and bitterness they may feel.
- Arrange a visit from the hospital chaplain where this is appropriate.

Peripheral vascular disease

This is narrowing of the arteries supplying the legs and feet. Peripheral vascular disease (PVD) usually presents as a chronic ischaemia of the legs due to atheromatous disease involving the aorta, iliac, or femoral arteries. It is more common in men above 50 years who are smokers.

Clinical features

- Ischaemia — a cramp-like pain in the calves during exercise and relieved by rest (intermittent claudication).
- Rest pain.
- The limb will be cold to the touch, lack hair, and the skin will be dry.

- Nonhealing ulcers or gangrene may occur.
- Absent pulses in severely diseased areas.

  Both limbs are usually affected but one may be worse than the other.

Investigations

- X-rays may show calcification.
- Doppler ultrasound may help to define the severity.
- Arteriogram using contrast media to show the narrowing.

Management

- Reduce risk factors such as smoking, treat hypertension and control diabetes if present, lose weight if obese.
- Lipid-lowering therapy (usually statins) if total cholesterol is above 3.5 mmol/L.
- Antiplatelet therapy with low-dose aspirin.
- Keep limbs warm but do not apply heat.
- Avoid infection and trauma to the feet.
- Regular exercise encourages new vessel formation and improves walking capacity.
- Cilostazil or naftidofuryl may be prescribed. These drugs have vasodilatory effects and improve walking distance in intermittent claudication in those who do not have pain at rest.
- Bypass surgery is not usually needed in intermittent claudication. Sometimes angioplasty and arterial stenting may be required.

Acute ischaemia of the legs

- May be due to an embolism.
- Extremely painful, pale, pulseless limb.
- Treatment is removal of the clot.
- If gangrene develops, amputation may be necessary.

Aortic aneurysms

An aneurysm is a bulge in the vessel wall usually due to atheroma. It is a weak point and the danger is that it will leak or rupture. It may be asymptomatic and found as a pulsatile mass on examination or as calcification on an X-ray. An ultrasound will show how large the aneurysm is and if a leak has occurred. It is most common in the abdominal aorta (AAA or 'triple A').

Surgery is usually carried out when the aneurysm is increasing in size or has reached a diameter of more than 5.5 cm. A family history of ruptured aneurysm also increases the likelihood of a surgery.

Rupture is life-threatening and causes intense pain in the back and the patient is shocked due to blood loss.

A dissecting (splitting) aortic aneurysm usually starts in the ascending aorta, and pain is severe and central, often radiating to the back. It may feel similar to a myocardial infarction.

Emergency surgery may be necessary, but grafting is much more successful when carried out on an unruptured aneurysm.

Deep vein thrombosis

- Venous thromboembolism (VTE) often occurs in normal vessels.
- Important causes are stasis and hypercoagulability.
- The majority occurs in the deep veins of the leg.
- A thrombus forms in the vein, and inflammation of the venous wall follows.
- Can occur in any vein in the leg but most often in the calf.

Risk factors

All patients admitted to hospital should undergo a risk assessment for VTE when they are admitted. Risk factors include the following:

- Trauma or surgery, especially of the pelvis, hip or lower limb. Surgery lasts for more than 90 min or 60 min if pelvis or lower limb is involved.
- Immobility, especially for 3 days or over.
- Varicose veins with phlebitis.
- Obesity.
- Previous deep vein thrombosis (DVT) or family history of DVT.
- Pregnancy.
- High doses of oestrogens (slight increased risk with oral contraception).
- Polycythaemia, sickle cell anaemia, thrombocytopenia, nephrotic syndrome, cardiac failure, recent myocardial infarction and malignancy are all conditions that increase the risk of a DVT.
- Active cancer or cancer treatment.
- Dehydration may increase the risk.

NICE (clinical guideline 92) have produced guidance: Thromboembolism – reducing the risk. This is available on their website at www.nice.org.uk.

Clinical features

- May be asymptomatic and the features of a pulmonary embolism may be the first sign.
- Pain in the calf – may be swelling, redness and engorged superficial veins.

- Affected calf may be warmer.
- Ankle oedema may be present.

Management

- Diagnosis is by ultrasound or Doppler ultrasound.
- Venography will detect practically any thrombosis but is not usually necessary.
- Main aim of treatment is to prevent pulmonary embolism.
- All patients with thrombi above the knee should be anticoagulated as these are the ones that usually cause a pulmonary embolism.
- Anticoagulation of below-knee thrombi is recommended for 6 weeks to prevent extension of the clot.
- Bedrest is advised until fully anticoagulated and then mobilization with an elastic stocking.
- *Heparin* is usually given for 48 h. LMWHs have replaced unfractionated heparin as they do not require monitoring and are more effective as well as being safer. They enable patients to be treated in the community.
- Oral anticoagulants, e.g., rivaroxaban, digabatrin or warfarin may be given for at least 3 months but may be longer depending on whether the cause of the DVT is known.
- If warfarin is used, the international normalized ratio is usually maintained between 2.0 and 3.0.
- Anticoagulants do not affect the thrombus that is already present.

Prevention

- Prophylaxis depends on the risk and the type of surgery, if applicable. Those with risk factors for bleeding will only receive anticoagulation when the risk for bleeding does not outweigh the risk of thromboembolism.
- Antiembolism stockings are given when appropriate.
- Choice of prophylactic measures will depend on both the type of surgery and other risk factors.
- LMWH is given to those at specific risk, e.g., surgery to the leg or pelvis or immobility and cardiac failure. If there is renal failure, then heparin (unfractionated) is usually used.
- Following hip and knee surgery, oral anticoagulants such as dabigatran are used.
- Early mobilization is important after surgery as most cases of DVT occur in the first 72 h postoperatively.
- Leg exercises should be encouraged.
- Patient should not sit on a chair with his legs immobilized on a stool.
- Full guidance is in the NICE guidelines mentioned above.

5.2 THE RESPIRATORY SYSTEM

There are some clinical features that are common to many disorders of the respiratory tract. These include the following:

- Cough
- Dyspnoea — a subjective sensation of shortage of breath
- Orthopnoea — breathlessness when lying flat
- Wheeze
- Sputum
- Haemoptysis — coughing up blood

Asthma

Asthma is a common and chronic inflammatory condition of the airways. As a result of the inflammation the airways are hyper-reactive and narrow easily in response to a wide range of stimuli. While initially reversible the inflammation may lead to an irreversible obstruction of airflow.

The bronchoconstriction that occurs is an abnormal narrowing of the airways caused by bronchospasm, mucosal oedema and increased secretion of sticky mucus. Alveoli can become blocked with plugs of mucus. Expiration becomes an active rather than a passive process.

Precipitating factors may include exercise, housedust mites, pollens and spores, pets, smoke, chemicals, certain foods, drugs (especially beta-blockers and nonsteroidal antiinflammatories) and emotional factors.

Extrinsic asthma

- Commonly develops during childhood.
- Identifiable factors provoke wheezing.
- Often associated with other features of atopy such as hay fever and eczema.
- Sometimes nocturnal cough may be the only symptom.

Intrinsic asthma

- Begins in adult life.
- Airflow obstruction is more persistent.
- Most exacerbations have no obvious stimuli other than a respiratory tract infection.

In an asthma attack there is:

- Dyspnoea
- Cough
- Wheezing
- Sense of tightness in the chest

It may be precipitated by exposure to one or more of a wide range of allergens.

> ! Asthma can produce symptoms of all grades varying from very mild to life-threatening. Its danger should never be underestimated, and several hundred people die each year from asthma.

Recording airflow obstruction

- Mini peak flow meters are a cheap and reliable way of doing this.
- They are used in hospital, and patients will use them at home to assess the control of asthma and the response to treatment.
- Peak flow recordings in a diary allow patients to see a deterioration in airflow, although they may be asymptomatic.
- Peak flow recordings are taken in hospital before salbutamol is administered and repeated about 20 min after administration to assess improvement. An increase of 15% is considered to be significant.
- In hospital when the patient is very breathless, it may not always be appropriate to immediately measure the peak flow rate.

Medication in asthma

The British Thoracic Society (BTS) published revised guidelines in 2016. The BTS Asthma Guideline Quick Reference Guide is now available as an app to download onto an i-phone or Android.

The guidelines go through the diagnosis and nonpharmacologic measures that may be used in asthma as well as the pharmacologic treatment of both chronic asthma and acute severe asthma.

The BTS recommend a pharmacologic approach that starts with inhaled corticosteroids. If these are not working, then adherence and inhaler technique should be checked, together with eliminating any trigger factors present.

Other drugs that may be added are long-acting beta-2 agonists.

High dose beta-2 agonists such as salbutamol are used as first line in patients with an acute asthma attack.

Aerosols

The duration of action of an aerosol inhaler depends on the dose administered and the drug it contains. Salbutamol usually lasts 3–5 h and salmeterol around 12 h.

Short-acting bronchodilators are used to treat an attack, long-acting are taken regularly to prevent an attack.

Steroid inhalers are widely used to prevent attacks of asthma and decrease the inflammatory process within the lungs. Oral candida is a common complication, and the risk may be minimized by using mouthwashes after administration and using a spacer.

Combination inhalers are now more widely used with an inhaled cortico-steroid and a long-acting beta2 agonist. Their use improves inhaler adherence.

Advantages of aerosols

- Provide more rapid relief
- Administered directly to the bronchioles, therefore smaller doses required
- Fewer side effects

The dose needs to be stated explicitly — the number of inhalations at one time, the frequency and the maximum number of inhalations allowed in 24 h.

If the patient is using his aerosol excessively, this is usually due to undertreatment of his asthma.

Nebulized salbutamol is used frequently in the treatment of acute asthma both in hospital and in general practice.

Acute asthma

- Acute asthma is divided for assessment purposes into a moderate exacer-bation, an acute severe asthma attack and life-threatening asthma.
- A moderate exacerbation means that there are increasing symptoms with a peak flow of 50%—75% of the best or predicted peak flow and no symp-toms of severe asthma present.
- Acute severe asthma has a peak flow of 33%—50% of that predicted or of the best, a respiratory rate of 25 rpm or more, a heart rate of 110 bpm or above and an inability to complete sentences in one breath.
- Life-threatening asthma is said to occur in acute severe asthma if ONE of the following is present:
  - PEF <33% of best or predicted
  - Cyanosis
  - Silent chest
  - Poor respiratory effort
  - Arrhythmia
  - Poor respiratory effort
  - Oxygen saturation of haemoglobin less than 92%
  - Blood gases show a normal $PaCO_2$ (4.6—6 kPa) but $PaO_2 > 8$ kPa
- In near-fatal asthma the $PaCO_2$ is raised or mechanical ventilation is needed
- Speed of onset varies — some attacks come on over minutes, in some deterioration occurs slowly over days

Management of an asthma attack

- A calm and reassuring atmosphere will help the patient.
- Sit the patient up.

- Administer oxygen as prescribed — the aim being to maintain oxygen saturation between 94% and 98%.
- Administer *salbutamol* nebulizer driven by oxygen as soon as possible.
- *Ipratropium bromide (Atrovent)* nebulizer may sometimes be used, especially if there is a poor response to salbutamol or the asthma is acute severe.
- *Hydrocortisone* intravenously or oral *prednisolone* may be given.
- Occasionally a single dose of intravenous *magnesium sulphate* may be administered if the patient is not responding to treatment.
- Antibiotics are not given routinely in asthma but if there is a chest infection they may be intravenously administered.
- Chest X-ray in acute severe asthma.
- Blood pressure measurement — if hypotensive, this is a sign of deteriorating condition.
- Pulse and respiratory measurements — bradycardia is a very severe sign. Usually there is a rapid pulse rate.
- Pulse oximetry measurement (see p. 134).
- If oximetry is poor, blood gases may be measured (see p. 118).
- Occasionally, artificial ventilation is needed, depending on the blood gas analysis and if the patient is exhausted.

Chronic obstructive pulmonary disease

This term is recommended to describe pathologic airflow limitation that is not fully reversible. Chronic airflow limitation (CAL) and chronic obstructive airway disease (COAD) were the terms previously used. About 1.2 million people in the UK suffer from diagnosed chronic obstructive pulmonary disease (COPD).

In the UK the most common causes of COPD are chronic bronchitis and emphysema, which often occur together. They are linked closely to cigarette smoking, and patients are usually diagnosed as having both chronic bronchitis and emphysema. COPD is the preferred term to describe chronic bronchitis and/or emphysema.

> **!** *Chronic bronchitis* is said to be present when there is a *productive cough* for most days of three consecutive months for more than 1 year. The disorder is characterized by excessive mucus production.
>
> *Emphysema* is characterized by *permanent enlargement of the air sacs* within the lung tissue. There is destruction of pulmonary tissue and a loss of elastic recoil.

The breathlessness is caused by the limitation of expiratory airflow that causes the residual volume to be increased. The thorax is overinflated, and inspiratory capacity is now impaired.

Inflammation within the lungs leads to destruction of the alveoli in emphysema and decreased delivery of oxygen to the alveoli with decreased removal of carbon dioxide.

Predisposing factors

- The dominant cause of this condition is cigarette smoking.
- Atmospheric pollution and occupational dust exposure are other factors in Britain.

Clinical features

- Chronic bronchitis and emphysema develop over many years and patients are rarely symptomatic before middle age.
- Minor symptoms at first — morning cough and a little sputum.
- Breathlessness initially occurs on exertion but gradually increases so that eventually dyspnoea will occur even at rest.
- If bronchitis predominates, periodic chest infections often occur.
- Cyanosis may be present — 'blue bloater'.
- If emphysema predominates there is extreme breathlessness but the patient is often not cyanosed — 'pink puffer'.
- Respiratory wheeze.
- Use of accessory muscles of respiration.
- 'Pursed lips' during expiration. This increases intrathoracic pressure.
- Often dyspnoea at night, causing wakefulness and leading to exhaustion.
- Extreme anxiety during very breathless periods.

Routine prescribing of supplemental oxygen is not advised in stable COPD patients without resting hypoxaemia, but correction of hypoxaemia to achieve an arterial oxygen tension of at least 7.3—8.0 kPa is the immediate priority of management in acute exacerbations of COPD.

Often low-flow oxygen administered by nasal prongs (1—2 L/min) or Venturi-type facial masks (28%) is sufficient.

Administration of oxygen and arterial blood gases are carefully monitored over time as in a few patients, arterial PCO_2 may increase (CO_2 retention) and acute respiratory acidosis may occur. It is not understood why this happens. In many sufferers of COPD, the respiratory centre has become tolerant to increased carbon dioxide levels and relies upon hypoxia and a decreased oxygen level in the blood to drive respirations.

In most patients with COPD, the aim is for a saturation of 88%—92% compared with 94%—98% in most other patients not at risk of hypercapnoeic respiratory failure.

! It is essential always to check the percentage of oxygen prescribed for these patients and never exceed it.

Management

- Reduce mucosal irritants and encourage the patient to stop smoking.
- If very breathless, complete rest may be needed.
- Provide oxygen as prescribed, usually at 24%–28%.
- Ensure the patient is sat up in bed, well supported with pillows, with his arms resting on a bedtable to allow maximum lung expansion.
- Administer the prescribed bronchodilators via nebulizer.
- Obtain sputum specimen for culture and sensitivity.
- Administer antibiotics if prescribed.
- Refer for chest physiotherapy to loosen and help to expectorate sputum.
- Observe the patient for increased breathlessness and cyanosis or any changes in mental state.
- Provide reassurance as needed when breathlessness is extreme.
- Carry out the prescribed pulmonary function tests – this may include measurements taken with a peak flow meter.

! Try to demonstrate empathy with this very frightened, breathless patient. Stay with him and offer reassurance during his worst periods.

Drug therapy

Restoration of normal function is not possible. The aim of therapy is to reduce the disability.

Bronchodilators

- Selective β-2 agonists such as **salbutamol** and **terbutaline** are the most useful. They are best given by inhalation and a nebulizer may be used.
- Muscarinic antagonists such as **ipratropium bromide (Atrovent)** may be helpful, given by inhaler or nebulizer.
- Long-acting β-2 agonists (LABAs) such as **salmeterol** may be prescribed as may long-acting muscarinic antagonists (LAMA), e.g., **tiotropium.**
- Some patients find mucolytic drugs helpful.

Corticosteroids

- These are not recommended as monotherapy in COPD.
- They are usually administered via inhaler, often combined with a LABA, when the FEV_1 is less than 50% of normal.
- The potential for side effects with inhaled corticosteroids is discussed with the patient.
- Oral corticosteroids are not normally recommended.

Antibiotics

- Antibiotics given promptly in an acute attack may shorten the exacerbation, but are not given for prophylaxis in COPD.
- Patients may be given a supply of antibiotics to keep at home and to take when their sputum turns green.
- Some bacteria are resistant to ampicillin, and a cephalosporin, such as cefaclor, may be used more.

Diuretics

If oedema is present (lung disease may cause right-sided heart failure), diuretics may be prescribed.

Advice for healthy living

- Stop smoking.
- Influenza vaccine each autumn.
- Keep warm and dry during the winter months.
- Advice on the effective use of an inhaler.
- Antibiotics available if needed in an exacerbation.
- Exercise when possible.

In 2010, NICE updated the clinical guidelines for the management of COPD. This is available on their website (www.nice.org.uk).

Bronchiectasis

> **!** Bronchiectasis is a dilatation of the bronchi, which may be localized in one tree or generalized.

The dilatation leads to impaired clearance of bronchial secretions and these become infected.

Causes

- Most cases used to arise in childhood and were inflammatory following pneumonia or whooping cough.
- Obstruction of an airway due to inhalation of a foreign body or enlarged lymph nodes.
- Cystic fibrosis.

Clinical features

- Cough.
- Sputum production — the sputum may be copious and thick, green and foul-smelling.
- Wheeze and breathlessness.
- Haemoptysis.

Management

- Physiotherapy and postural drainage are very important. These must be done on a daily basis and the patient or family is taught to do this at home.
- Antibiotics when there is an acute exacerbation.
- Bronchodilators if necessary.

Respiratory failure

- Respiratory failure occurs when pulmonary gas exchange is sufficiently impaired to cause reduced oxygenation of the blood (hypoxaemia) or reduced carbon dioxide elimination leading to hypercapnia: Type 1 respiratory failure is defined by a PaO_2 of <8 kPa and a normal or low $PaCO_2$.
- Type 2 respiratory failure is defined by a $PaCO_2$ of >6.5 kPa and often hypoxaemia as well.

Causes of respiratory failure are shown in Table 5.3.

Pneumonia (Fig. 5.3)

> ! Pneumonia is an inflammation of the substance of the lungs.

It is usually due to bacteria but may also result from chemical causes, aspiration of vomit, radiotherapy or an allergic mechanism.

Pneumonia is an acute illness characterized by:

- a cough — may be dry at first,
- purulent sputum — haemoptysis sometimes,
- fever,
- raised respiratory rate,
- pleuritic pain,
- confusion may occur in the elderly and may be the only sign.

There will be changes on the chest X-ray to show consolidation of the lung.

TABLE 5.3 Classification of causes of respiratory failure

Mechanism	Acute causes	Chronic causes
Restrictive neuromuscular diseases (failure of respiratory muscles)	Tetanus, botulism, poliomyelitis, polyneuritis, spinal cord injury	Muscular dystrophy Myasthenia gravis
Chest wall diseases (failure of chest expansion)	Pneumothorax Flail chest (trauma)	Kyphoscoliosis Obesity Pleural effusion Mesothelioma Ankylosing spondylitis
Lung diseases	Radiation pneumonitis	Interstitial fibrosis Sarcoidosis
Obstructive	Foreign bodies Angio-oedema Bronchiolitis Asthma	Chronic obstructive pulmonary disease Bronchiectasis Epiglottitis
Abnormal perfusion	Pulmonary embolism Fat embolism	Recurrent emboli Vasculitis
Impaired diffusion	Shock	Sarcoidosis Pneumoconiosis Interstitial pneumonitis Interstitial fibrosis
Interstitial disease	Interstitial pneumonitis	
Pulmonary oedema	Acute left ventricular failure Toxic gases Mitral stenosis	Chronic left ventricular failure

---

! Pneumonia may be localized and affect one lobe – *lobar pneumonia*.
It may be diffuse and affect the lobules of the lung and the bronchioles – this is *bronchopneumonia*.

Some bacteria causing pneumonia:

- *Streptococcus pneumoniae*
- *Mycoplasma pneumoniae*
- *Haemophilus influenzae*
- *Staphylococcus aureus*
- *Legionella pneumophila*
- *Myobacterium tuberculosis*

There are viral, fungal and protozoal pneumonias as well.

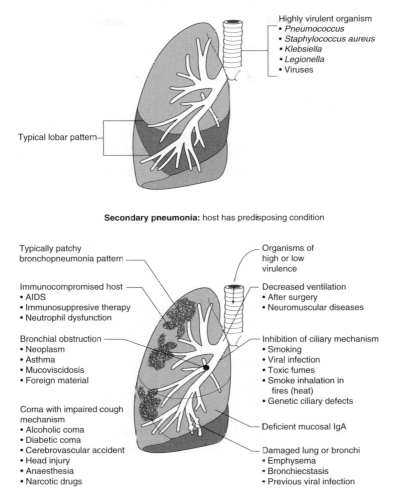

Primary pneumonia: previously healthy host

Highly virulent organism
• *Pneumococcus*
• *Staphylococcus aureus*
• *Klebsiella*
• *Legionella*
• Viruses

Typical lobar pattern

Secondary pneumonia: host has predisposing condition

Typically patchy
bronchopneumonia pattern

Immunocompromised host
• AIDS
• Immunosuppresive therapy
• Neutrophil dysfunction

Bronchial obstruction
• Neoplasm
• Asthma
• Mucoviscidosis
• Foreign material

Coma with impaired cough
mechanism
• Alcoholic coma
• Diabetic coma
• Cerebrovascular accident
• Head injury
• Anaesthesia
• Narcotic drugs

Organisms of
high or low
virulence

Decreased ventilation
• After surgery
• Neuromuscular diseases

Inhibition of ciliary mechanism
• Smoking
• Viral infection
• Toxic fumes
• Smoke inhalation in
  fires (heat)
• Genetic ciliary defects

Deficient mucosal IgA

Damaged lung or bronchi
• Emphysema
• Bronchiectasis
• Previous viral infection

FIGURE 5.3 Primary and secondary pneumonia. *From Chandrasoma, 1995. Taylor/Concise Pathology, second ed. McGraw-Hill, New York. Reproduced with permission of The McGraw-Hill Companies.*

Aspiration pneumonia

• Aspiration of gastric contents into the lungs can cause severe illness, which may be fatal. Gastric acid in the stomach contents is very destructive.
• Aspiration material enters the right lung more readily than the left due to the wider right bronchus.
• Infection is usually with an anaerobic organism derived from the upper respiratory tract.

Factors predisposing to aspiration pneumonia include the following:

- Altered consciousness — drug overdose, anaesthesia, epilepsy, CVA, alcoholism.
- Dysphagia and oesophageal disease — stricture, fistula, hiatus hernia, reflux.
- Neurologic disorders — myasthenia gravis, motor neuron disease.
- Nasogastric tubes.
- Terminal illness.

Community-acquired pneumonia

This is a pneumonia that develops in the community or within 48 h of admission into hospital.

Pneumonia in the immunocompromised patient

- With the use of immunosuppressive drugs and the emergence of HIV infection, these types of pneumonia have become much more common.
- These are the so-called 'opportunistic' infections.
- These may be rapid pneumonias that are extensive and life threatening.
- They may be viral, fungal, protozoal or bacterial in origin.
- *Pneumocystis carinii* is the most common opportunistic infection.

Management of pneumonia

- Mild cases will not be admitted to hospital.
- Sputum should always be sent for culture.
- Chest X-ray will be performed.
- Antibiotics will be prescribed — these will depend on the type of pneumonia. **Cefuroxime** and **clindamycin** are examples.
- Fluids should be encouraged to avoid dehydration — in the very ill, intravenous fluids may be necessary.
- Physiotherapy may be needed to help expectoration.
- Pleuritic pain may need analgesia.
- Oxygen may be prescribed.
- Temperature and respirations will be monitored.

Pneumonia in the elderly can be a serious illness and may go undiagnosed. Early diagnosis and treatment increase the likelihood of recovery. Vaccination against pneumococcal pneumonia is recommended together with an influenza vaccination.

Lung abscess

A localized suppurative infection in the lung where a cavity forms and fills with pus.

Causes

- May follow a severe pneumonia — especially, aspiration pneumonia.
- More likely to occur with TB, *Staphylococcus aureus, Klebsiella*, aspiration pneumonia or septic emboli.
- Anaerobic bacteria are involved in most cases.

Clinical features

- Pneumonia that is persistent or worsening.
- Foul-smelling sputum in large amounts.
- Breathlessness.

Management

- Antibiotics usually given intravenously for 2–3 weeks.
- Sometimes surgery is necessary.

Pulmonary tuberculosis

- An infection due to Myobacterium tuberculosis (TB).
- The primary infection is usually symptomless, most commonly involves the lungs and heals leaving dormant tubercle bacilli in about 20% of old calcified lesions.
- When the host's immune system is at an ebb the tubercle bacilli may be reactivated and spread to all organs of the body including the lungs, the kidneys and bones.
- There is a high incidence in patients infected with HIV.
- Pulmonary TB is the most common form of TB.
- In 2016, there were 5664 cases of TB in England (Public Health England, 2017). This is part of a sustained annual decline.

Clinical features

- Gradual onset of symptoms over weeks or months.
- Tiredness, malaise, anorexia and weight loss.
- Fever.
- Cough.
- Sputum may be mucoid, purulent or bloodstained.

- May be a dull ache in the chest.
- There may be a pleural effusion (fluid in the pleural cavity).
- Chest X-ray will show shadows and perhaps fibrosis.

Management

Some severely ill patients may require admission to hospital for a short period.

Sputum is sent for culture of acid-fast bacilli. The growth in culture is slow. The nursing management depends on the severity of the illness.

! The most important factor in the treatment of tuberculosis is compliance with a drug regimen for 6 months.

Drug therapy

This is in two phases: an initial phase using four drugs and a continuation phase using two drugs in fully sensitive cases. Full details can be found in the BNF and NICE produces clinical guidelines for the management of TB (www. nice.org.uk). There are two regimens recommended in the UK but variations occur in other countries:

- *Rifampicin* and *isoniazid* are given daily as a combination tablet 30 min before breakfast for 6 months.
- For the first 2 months *pyrazinamide* and *ethambutol* are also given.
- The four-tablet regimen is used initially in an attempt to eliminate bacteria rapidly and control resistance.
- Streptomycin is not usually used in the UK but may be if there is resistance to isoniazid or if standard drugs are not tolerated.
- Fixed-dose combination tablets are recommended.
- Drug resistance after initial drug sensitivity tends to develop in those who do not comply with regimens.

Pulmonary embolism

This is the obstruction of one of the pulmonary arteries by an embolism, which is usually in the form of a blood clot originating from a DVT in the leg. There is often a history of DVT or of tenderness in the calf.

Pulmonary embolism should be suspected in a patient who collapses suddenly 1–2 weeks after surgery.

Massive PE is second only to sudden cardiac death as a cause of sudden death.

! A large pulmonary embolus is a medical emergency and can result in death.

Clinical features

These depend on the size of the embolus but include:

- Sharp, knife-like pain in the chest, usually well localized in a small embolus.
- If the embolus is large the pain may be more central.
- Shortness of breath.
- Anxiety and distress.
- Haemoptysis.
- Hypotension.
- Tachycardia.
- Pallor or cyanosis — cyanosis suggests a large embolus.
- Collapse.
- Massive PE may present as a cardiac arrest or shock.

Others present with nonspecific signs and symptoms and the diagnosis may be missed.

Management

Again, this will depend on the severity of the episode and may include the following:

- Reassurance of the patient.
- Monitoring of vital signs — blood pressure, pulse and respirations.
- Cardiac monitor.
- Continuous pulse oximetry.
- Administration of oxygen as prescribed.
- Pain relief — opioids may be needed.
- Investigations — chest X-ray, ECG, CT angiography, arterial blood gases.
- Anticoagulation — LMWHs may be used or unfractionated *heparin* may be administered as an intravenous loading dose followed by continuous intravenous infusion via an infusion pump. An oral anticoagulant such as rivaroaban is started.
- Analgesia — nonsteroidal antiinflammatory drugs may work well. *Diamorphine* may be given, but there is sometimes a reluctance to give opiates in a large embolus as these may lower the blood pressure more.
- Thrombolytic therapy may be *used* in a large embolism.

Lung cancer

This is the most common cancer in the world and the most common cause of cancer death in the UK. There has been an improvement in 5-year survival in the past 15 years, and it was 9.5% in 2011 (Cancer Research UK, 2016).

The public need to be more aware of the symptoms of lung cancer as early diagnosis is needed.

Lung cancer is the second most common cancer in women, breast cancer being the most common. It is also the second most common cancer in men, after prostate cancer.

The vast majority of lung cancers are caused by smoking. The risk increases with the number of cigarettes smoked each day.

There are two main types of lung cancer:

- Small cell lung cancer (SCLC) − about 20%−25% of cases.
- Non-small cell lung cancer (NSCLC) − other cases. Included in this category are squamous cell carcinoma, large cell lung cancer and adenocarcinoma (the most common type in nonsmokers).

Clinical features

- May be unspecific
- Cough
- Haemoptysis
- Dyspnoea
- Chest pain (may be mild)
- Wheeze
- Malaise
- Weight loss
- Hoarseness
- Anaemia
- Clubbing of the fingers
- Enlarged supraclavicular lymph nodes
- Direct spread may involve the pleura and there may be a pleural effusion

Metastatic complications

- The growth frequently metastasizes to bone, giving severe pain and sometimes pathologic fractures.
- The liver is frequently involved.
- Secondary deposits in the brain may lead to personality changes or epilepsy.
- May metastasize to the adrenal glands.

Investigations

These should be chosen to give the most information about diagnosis and staging with the least risk to the patient. The type of investigation depends on whether staging is also necessary and whether treatment with curative intent may be possible. For full details the NICE guidelines should be referred to:

- Diagnosis is usually by chest X-ray, and 90% of tumours will show on presentation. At this point, the tumour has sometimes been present for many years and there have been no symptoms until recently. CT scan will detect smaller tumours and is evaluated for screening.
- An abnormal chest X-ray leads to referral to the lung cancer MDT.
- A CT scan of thorax, upper abdomen and lower neck is done to look for lymphatic spread.
- Further diagnostic tests are then used to stage the disease. These may include:
  - Endobronchial or endoscopic ultrasound
  - Fine needle aspiration
  - A bronchoscopy and biopsy
  - A specimen of sputum will be sent for cytology if unable to tolerate bronchoscopy
  - Bone scintigraphy or MRI

The NICE guidelines for the diagnosis and treatment of lung cancer include an algorithm showing the diagnostic and staging clinical pathway for lung cancer. This is available on their website.

Management

The prognosis in lung cancer is very poor and a lung cancer clinical nurse specialist should be available at all stages of care to support both the patient and their carers:

- In the early stages of NSCLC, surgery may benefit the patient and excision may be attempted. This usually consists of removal of a lobe of a lung (lobectomy) and may be followed by chemotherapy or radiotherapy. More extensive surgery (e.g., pneumonectomy) is only attempted when absolutely necessary to clear the margins of the tumour. Sometimes smaller amounts of lung (segmentectomy or wedge resection) are attempted for smaller tumours where there is limited fitness of the patient.
- Radical radiotherapy may be indicated where there is curative intent.
- In SCLC, surgery may be possible in the early stages.
- *Cisplatin*-based combination chemotherapy is used in SCLC and prolongs survival.
- *Newer drugs that target the immune system are now being used with some success.*
- For many patients the aim is symptom relief.
- Palliative radiotherapy is offered when curative treatment cannot be offered. It will help to relieve any bronchial obstruction or haemoptysis and may also be given to relieve bone pain.

- Stenting may be used in pending bronchial obstruction.
- Pleural effusion may need draining if it is troublesome.
- Effective assessment and relief of pain are essential.
- Opioids such as morphine will probably be used for pain relief and to relieve the cough. Morphine may be administered in slow-release tablet form or elixirs. A syringe pump may be used to administer continuous morphine.
- Opioids are constipating, and laxatives should be prescribed.
- Relief of other symptoms such as nausea or confusion.
- Palliative radiotherapy and/or dexamethasone may be offered in brain metastases.
- The patient and carers will need much emotional support during this distressing time.

The pleura

Dry pleurisy

- Pleurisy is inflammation of the pleura that leads to pain on inspiration or coughing.
- In dry pleurisy there is no pleural effusion.
- There is a sharp pain, worse on inspiration or coughing.
- Causes include pneumonia and lung cancer.

Pleural effusion

This is an excessive collection of fluid in the pleural space (Fig. 5.4). The fluid may be serous fluid, blood, pus or lymph.

! A collection of blood in the pleural space is a *haemothorax*.
  A collection of pus in the pleural space is an *empyema*.

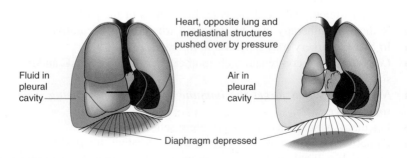

FIGURE 5.4   Pressure collapse of the lung. *From Govan et al., 1993. Pathology Illustrated. Elsevier, reproduced with permission.*

Causes

- Heart failure
- Hypoproteinaemia
- Pneumonia
- Lung cancer
- Tuberculosis

Clinical features

- Dyspnoea which is variable dependent upon the size of the effusion
- Dull chest pain
- Symptoms due to the underlying cause, e.g., carcinoma of the lung

The effusion will be seen on a chest X-ray as a water-dense shadow with a concave-upwards upper border.

If the effusion is causing dyspnoea it should be drained. The fluid is best removed slowly and an indwelling chest drain may be inserted.

Pneumothorax

A pneumothorax is an accumulation of air in the pleural space (see Fig. 5.4).

Causes

It may occur spontaneously, most often in young thin men. Other causes include:

- Trauma
- Asthma
- COPD
- Tuberculosis
- Pneumonia
- Lung cancer
- Cystic fibrosis and any diffuse lung disease

Clinical features

- There may be no symptoms if small and in a young fit man.
- Dyspnoea dependent on the size of the pneumothorax. Varies from mild to very severe.
- Pleuritic pain, sometimes transient.
- The pain usually begins abruptly, and the patient may have felt 'something snap' before the onset of the pain and the dyspnoea.

The pneumothorax will show on the chest X-ray as an area devoid of lung markings.

Management

- Analgesia.
- Oxygen if prescribed (care if COPD).
- A small pneumothorax will resolve without treatment and analgesia and rest may be the only prescribed care with a repeat chest X-ray the next day.
- A larger pneumothorax may be aspirated or a sealed underwater chest drain inserted.

> ! Tension pneumothorax is a life-threatening condition.

A breach in the lung surface acts as a valve, admitting air into the pleural cavity when the patient breathes in but preventing its escape when he breathes out. This may displace mediastinal structures and compromise cardiopulmonary function. Unless the air is rapidly removed, cardiopulmonary arrest will occur.

5.3 THE BLOOD

Blood consists of red cells, white cells, platelets and plasma. Plasma is the liquid component and contains clotting factors and proteins as well as carrying nutrients and waste products.

The red cell

Anaemia

Anaemia is present when there is a decrease in the level of haemoglobin (Hb) in the blood below the reference range for the age and sex of the individual. Usually, there is also a decrease in the red cell count (RCC) and packed cell volume (PCV). Normal values for the cells in blood are shown in Table 5.4.

TABLE 5.4 Normal values for adult peripheral blood

	Men	Women
Haemoglobin (g/dL)	14–17	11–16
Red cell count ($\times 10^{12}$/L)	4.5–6.0	3.9–5.1
White cell count ($\times 10^{9}$/L)	4.0–11.0	4.0–11.0
Platelets ($\times 10^{9}$/L)	150–400	150–400

Clinical features

- May have an insidious onset.
- Lethargy.
- Faintness.
- Breathlessness.
- Tachycardia.
- Angina if atherosclerosis is present.
- Pallor of skin and mucous membranes.
- Cardiac failure may occur in the elderly or those with compromised cardiac function.
- Confusion in the elderly.

Classification of anaemias

Terms that refer to cell size end with 'cytic', whereas terms that describe the red cell colour end with 'chromic'. The classification of anaemias is shown in Table 5.5. In microcytic anaemia the red blood cell is smaller and paler than usual.

Iron deficiency anaemia

Iron is needed for the formation of the red oxygen-carrying pigment in the erythrocyte. It is present in the diet and is absorbed from the small intestine. Green vegetables, red meat, eggs and milk contain iron.

Deficiency is common in premenopausal women as they have an additional loss of iron in the menstrual flow.

Causes

- Blood loss from menstruation.
- Chronic blood loss, usually from gastrointestinal tract. May be the only clue in cancer of the colon.
- Inadequate intake in the diet.
- Increased demands in pregnancy or growth.
- Decreased absorption with small bowel disease or following gastrectomy.

TABLE 5.5 Classification of anaemia

Microcytic	Macrocytic	Normocytic
Iron deficiency	Vitamin B_{12} deficiency	Aplastic anaemia
Anaemia of chronic disease	Folate deficiency	Haemolytic anaemia

Additional symptoms include brittle hair and nails due to decreased epithelial cell iron, a red smooth tongue (atrophic glossitis), spoon-shaped nails (koilonychia) and, rarely, pharyngeal webs at the back of the throat which cause difficulty in swallowing (dysphagia).

Treatment

- Treat the underlying cause. It is important to exclude any serious underlying cause such as cancer of the gastrointestinal tract or peptic ulceration.
- Oral iron, e.g., *ferrous sulphate*, 200 mg three times daily for about 6 months.
- Side effects include gastrointestinal disturbance — usually constipation but may be diarrhoea. This can be reduced by changing to a different iron preparation, e.g., *ferrous gluconate.*
- Some patients may need iron injections if absorption is so poor.

Anaemia of chronic disease

This starts as a normochromic (erythrocytes are normal colour), normocytic (cells are normal size) anaemia and occurs in a variety of chronic diseases, e.g., rheumatoid arthritis (RA), chronic infections, renal and liver failures, neoplasia (malignancies) and inflammatory disease, e.g., Crohn's disease. There is a slightly reduced survival of the red cell (normal survival about 120 days) and a low level of erythropoietin release (hormone produced by the kidney that stimulates the production of red cells). Iron stores tend to be normal or increased.

Treatment

- This type of anaemia only responds to treatment of the underlying disease and not to the administration of iron.
- Erythropoietin may improve some patients. Erythropoietin is a hormone produced by the kidney that stimulates the formation of new red blood cells in the bone marrow.

Macrocytic anaemia

Here the red cells are large and immature. They have defective DNA synthesis. The most common causes are deficiencies in either vitamin B_{12} or folate, both of which are needed to synthesize DNA.

Vitamin B_{12} deficiency

This vitamin is obtained from animal sources (meat, fish, eggs and milk). To be absorbed in the gastrointestinal tract it has to bind to the intrinsic factor, which is secreted by the gastric parietal cells in the stomach.

Vitamin B_{12} is stored in the liver, where there is sufficient supply for 2 years or more.

Causes

- Low dietary intake – usually vegans
- Impaired absorption
- Intrinsic factor deficiency
- Pernicious anaemia
- Following gastrectomy
- Small bowel malabsorption:
  - Ileal disease or resection
  - Tropical sprue
  - Coeliac disease
- Pancreatic disease
- Chronic pancreatitis

Pernicious anaemia

This is an autoimmune disorder in which there is atrophy of the gastric mucosa and a failure of intrinsic factor and gastric acid production that leads to a decreased absorption of B_{12}. It is the most common cause of vitamin B_{12} deficiency in Western countries:

- Common in late adult life and the elderly.
- In Britain, women are affected more commonly than men.
- Common in those with blue eyes and fair hair.
- Associated with other autoimmune disorders, e.g., hypothyroidism.

Clinical features

- Onset insidious with increasing symptoms of anaemia.
- Usually quite severe by the time it is diagnosed.
- Lethargy, tiredness and weight loss.
- Pallor and sometimes slight jaundice due to the increased breakdown of the immature red cells.
- Glossitis may occur.
- Neurologic features include subacute combined degeneration of the cord with peripheral neuropathy and symmetrical paraesthesia of the hands and feet. Ataxia may follow and eventually paraplegia. Higher cerebral function may be affected, leading to dementia.

Investigations

- Blood count and film.
- Measurement of serum vitamin B_{12}.

- Serum bilirubin may be raised.
- Parietal cell antibodies are present in 90% of cases.
- The Schilling test differentiates pernicious anaemia from malabsorption as the cause of vitamin B_{12} deficiency.

Treatment

- Intramuscular hydroxycobalamin (B_{12}).
- Injections are needed because the vitamin cannot be absorbed orally; 1 mg is given twice weekly for 3 weeks to replenish body stores and then 3 months for life.
- Treatment can reverse early neurologic signs and stop the progress of later changes.

Folate deficiency

Folic acid is a B vitamin, and its role is interdependent with B_{12} as both are needed by rapidly dividing cells. It is found in liver, yeast extract and green vegetables. There is an increased requirement in pregnancy and supplements should be given to prevent neural tube defects (e.g., spina bifida).

Causes

Decreased intake:

- Elderly
- Alcoholism
- Milk-fed premature infants

    Malabsorption:

- Coeliac disease
- Tropical sprue
- Gastrectomy
- Crohn's disease

    Drugs:

- Phenytoin

    There is an increased requirement in pregnancy, lactation, prematurity, growth in childhood.

Clinical features

They are those of anaemia.

Treatment

- Underlying cause must be treated.
- Deficiency corrected by oral administration of folic acid 5 mg daily.
- If the cause of the macrocytic anaemia is not known, folate must not be given on its own as it may aggravate the neuropathy of B_{12} deficiency.

Aplastic anaemia

This is very rare and is due to suppression of the bone marrow leading to failure in production of all blood cells. This means there is a shortage of white blood cells and platelets as well as erythrocytes. It may be inherited but is more commonly acquired.

Many drugs have been associated with aplastic anaemia. Some anticancer drugs cause this in a dose-related manner but with some drugs it may be an idiosyncratic reaction, e.g., chloramphenicol.

A blood count shows pancytopenia (low count of all blood cells).

Treatment

- Elimination of the cause if possible.
- Supportive care with transfusions and antibiotics.
- Bone marrow transplant may be possible in some patients — the young or those older with a very severe form of the disease.
- Immunosuppressive therapy may be used for older patients with a less severe form of the disease.

Haemolytic anaemia

- This is due to the rapid breakdown of red cells before the natural end of their normal lifespan.
- There is evidence of both increased red cell production (*reticulocytosis*) and increased red cell destruction.
- Causes of haemolytic anaemia are shown in Box 5.1.

Clinical features of increased haemolysis

- Pallor
- Jaundice
- Splenomegaly (enlarged spleen)

Red cell membrane defects

- Most common in this country is **hereditary spherocytosis.** This is inherited in an autosomal dominant manner. Found in 1–2 per 10,000 of the population.

BOX 5.1 Causes of haemolytic anaemia

Inherited	Acquired
Red cell membrane defect	*Immune*
Hereditary spherocytosis	Autoimmune haemolytic anaemia
Hereditary elliptocytosis	Haemolytic transfusion reactions
Haemoglobin abnormalities	*Nonimmune*
Thalassaemia	Rare cases of nocturnal
Sickle cell disease	Haemoglobinuria
	Mechanical haemolytic anaemia
Metabolic defects	*Miscellaneous*
Glucose-6-phosphate dehydrogenase deficiency	Infections (e.g., malaria)
	Drugs/chemicals
	Hypersplenism

- There is a defect in the production of the protein spectrin which results in the production of spherical red cells, which are more rapidly destroyed.
- Most patients can live a normal life, although being slightly anaemic.
- An acute haemolytic crisis may occur at certain times (e.g., an acute infection) and require a blood transfusion.
- There is an increased need for folic acid as more red cells are being manufactured.
- Diagnosis is by the blood film.

Treatment

- The treatment of choice is a splenectomy. This is usually delayed until after childhood to minimize the risk of overwhelming pneumococcal infection.
- Following splenectomy, all patients should receive pneumococcal vaccine and long-term prophylactic penicillin.

Haemoglobin abnormalities

Normal adult haemoglobin is made up of two polypeptide globin chains (alpha and beta) and an iron-containing pigment (haem). The haemoglobinopathies are abnormalities of the polypeptide chains.

Thalassaemia

- These are a group of disorders arising from one or more gene defects and resulting in reduced production of one or more of the globin chains.
- This leads to precipitation of the globin chains in the red cells and ineffective erythropoiesis (red cell manufacture) and haemolysis (red cell breakdown).
- There are two main types:
  - alpha-thalassaemia: reduced alpha-chain synthesis
  - beta-thalassaemia: reduced beta-chain synthesis.

In both types there are several clinical forms of the disease varying from asymptomatic and mild to severe with presentation in the first year of life. In the most severe form of thalassaemia, there is complete absence of alpha-globin and infants may be stillborn (*hydrops fetalis*).

Thalassaemia trait (thalassaemia minor)

- The most common abnormality
- Heterozygous form of the disease
- Very mild defects of the red cells
- Common in certain parts of the world and affects 20% of people from certain areas of Africa, Asia and the Mediterranean.
- No treatment is required but need to check for any anaemia.

Treatment of thalassaemias

- Detection of severe forms in the fetus means that termination can be offered. This would be tested for if the mother was found to have thalassaemia trait.
- Blood transfusion is the mainstay of treatment.
- Iron overload may result from repeated transfusions. This may lead to damage to endocrine glands, liver, pancreas and heart, with death in the second decade from cardiac failure.
- Treatment with desferrioxamine (an iron-chelating agent) may prevent iron loading.

Sickle cell syndromes

- This results from the production of an abnormal haemoglobin — haemoglobin S.
- It is a hereditary defect due to the substitution of the amino acid valine for glutamic acid in the beta-chain.

- It is found most commonly in those of African origin (25% carry the gene). It may confer a biological advantage against infection with malaria and so natural selection has increased the incidence of the HbS gene in this group.
- When deoxygenated, HbS molecules link together and this causes increased rigidity of the red cells and the characteristic sickle shape.
- The sickled cell has a shortened survival and is unable to pass through the very small capillaries (microcirculation). This may cause a chronic anaemia and chronic organ damage from vascular occlusion. Sickling may be precipitated by infection, dehydration, cold or hypoxia.

Clinical features

Sickle cell trait

- Those heterozygous for HbS (one gene HbS and one normal Hb gene) have sickle cell trait and are asymptomatic unless the oxygen tension is reduced (at high altitude, in an aircraft or under general anaesthesia).
- Still get renal microinfarcts due to obstruction of small capillaries and may complain of haematuria. May develop renal impairment.

Sickle cell disease

- Homozygous patients (both genes are HbS) suffer from chronic haemolysis, but this is usually compensated. Hb ranges usually between 5 and 10 g/dL.
- Usually mild jaundice.
- Acute haemolytic crises are precipitated by infections, pregnancy, drugs, surgery and anaesthesia.
- This may precipitate microvascular occlusion and tissue death.

Sickle cell crisis

- Associated with fever, malaise and severe pain.
- Can occur in most parts of the body.
- Organs affected include eyes, brain, bone, muscle, lung, spleen, liver, kidney and skin.
- May have pleuritic chest pain.
- Cerebral infarction leading to fits and hemiparesis.
- Priapism (prolonged erections).
- Carries a high mortality in young children, and death is usually from renal failure or overwhelming infection.
- Management is aimed at prevention of infections and other situations leading to a crisis.

Treatment of an acute crisis

- Oxygen
- Rehydration
- Antibiotics
- Adequate pain relief — opioid analgesia often required
- Anaemia can be treated by blood transfusion

Metabolic defects

- The most common is glucose-6-phosphate dehydrogenase deficiency (G6PD).
- G6PD is a vital enzyme to combat oxidative stress in the red cell.
- Deficiency is a heterozygous X-linked trait (carried on the female chromosome).
- Found predominantly in African, Mediterranean and Middle Eastern populations.
- Red cell breakdown occurs. precipitated by some oxidizing drugs (e.g., sulphonamides), oxidants in foods and infection.
- Usually presents with haemolysis and anaemia.
- Large number of foods and drugs may be implicated and should be avoided.
- To diagnose, the enzyme activity can be measured.

Acquired haemolytic anaemias

- Most common type is due to the presence of autoantibodies (against self). These attach to the red cells and reduce their survival time.
- Diagnosed by a positive Coombs' test.

Polycythaemia

- A group of disorders in which there is an increased Hb concentration in the blood. There is a raised RCC and PCV.
- In true polycythaemia there is an absolute increase in the red cell mass. In apparent polycythaemia the red cell mass is normal and the rise in PCV is secondary to a decrease in plasma volume.
- Stimulus for increased red cell production is hypoxia, and polycythaemia may occur secondary to oxygen lack, as at altitude or in chronic lung diseases.
- Associated with thrombotic (blood clot) disorders such as myocardial infarction, stroke, PVD and DVT.
- There is increased viscosity (thickness) of the blood which results in reduced flow.

Polycythaemia rubra vera (primary polycythaemia)

- A defect that arises in the stem cell and causes an over proliferation of red blood cells.
- Usually in the middle-aged and elderly.
- Often found by chance when an elevated Hb is recorded.
- There is an enlarged spleen and this may be the first finding.
- Sometimes it may only be diagnosed after an acute thrombotic event.
- Plethoric (ruddy) complexion.
- Diagnosis is confirmed by blood tests.
- About 60% of patients die from thrombotic events.
- Treatment is to lower the Hb often by repeated venesection (withdrawal of blood).
- Chemotherapy with hydroxyurea may help.
- Radioactive phosphorus is used in severe cases.
- Untreated cases − the mean survival is 2 years. May be increased to about 14 with treatment.

Myelofibrosis

Increased fibrous tissue is formed within the marrow cavity. This disturbs normal manufacture of red blood cells which now occurs in the spleen and liver. It may be a consequence of other myeloproliferative disorders such as polycythaemia and acute myeloid leukaemia.

Clinical features

- Weight loss − thin arms and legs with enlarged abdomen.
- Usually grossly enlarged spleen.
- Anaemia.
- There may be ascites.
- Purpura and bleeding may result from thrombocytopenia (low platelets).

Treatment

- Supportive and symptomatic.
- Blood transfusion may be necessary for severe anaemia.
- Death usually occurs from gradual marrow failure with bleeding and overwhelming infection.

The spleen

- Largest lymphoid organ in the body.
- Situated in the left hypochondrium.

- Main functions are destruction of old red cells and immunologic defence.
- Splenomegaly is enlargement of the spleen, and this can lead to hypersplenism — a decrease in the number of red cells due to pooling and destruction by the enlarged spleen.

Causes of splenomegaly

Haematologic

- Chronic myeloid leukaemia — may be massive and extend into right iliac fossa
- Other leukaemias
- Lymphomas
- Haemolytic anaemia
- Myelofibrosis

Infections

- Chronic malaria
- Schistosomiasis
- Septicaemia
- Glandular fever (infectious mononucleosis)
- Tuberculosis
- Brucellosis

Inflammation

- RA
- Sarcoidosis
- Systemic lupus erythematosus

Splenectomy

Removal of the spleen, performed mainly for:

- trauma,
- haemolytic anaemias,
- idiopathic thrombocytopenic purpura,
- hypersplenism.

The main short-term complication is thrombophilia, and the main long-term complication is overwhelming infection. The main infective organisms are *S. pneumoniae, H. influenzae*, and the meningococci. Vaccines against these bacteria must be given to all who undergo a splenectomy.

Prophylactic antibiotics need to be given for the first 2 years following the splenectomy. In children, antibiotics should be continued prophylactically until the age of 16 years. Some recommend lifetime antibiotics following splenectomy.

Platelets

Platelets are small disc-shaped structures, $1-2$ μm in diameter, present in the blood. Their functions are related to haemostasis (stopping bleeding).

Essential thrombocythaemia

- There is an overproduction of platelets, which may be functionally impaired. This is associated with other myeloproliferative disorders such as polycythaemia, chronic myeloid leukaemia and myelofibrosis.
- Normal platelet count is $250-400 \times 10^9$/L. Diagnosis is on a platelet count of $1000-2000 \times 10^9$/L.
- Thrombotic occlusion of arteries, leading to myocardial infarction, stroke or gangrene, is common.
- Treatment is aimed at reducing the platelet count by using cytotoxic drugs such as busulfan or cyclophosphamide or radioactive phosphorus.

Thrombocytopenia

This is a reduction in platelet count and is discussed under bleeding disorders.

Abnormal bleeding

Causes include the following:

- Inherited deficiencies of coagulation factors such as haemophilia.
- Acquired coagulation deficiencies that may occur in liver disease and when vitamin K absorption is reduced.
- Drugs such as anticoagulants, e.g., heparin and **warfarin.** Anticoagulant therapy needs continuous monitoring. Aspirin also increases bleeding time.
- Thrombocytopenia may cause bleeding, especially when the platelet count is below 40×10^9/L. Causes include blood disorders such as leukaemia (see p. 305).
- Abnormalities of the vessel wall such as vasculitis and scurvy.

Abnormal clotting

Causes of thrombosis fall into one of the following categories:

- Abnormalities in the vessel wall
- Alterations in the state of blood flow
- Alterations in the blood

Bleeding disorders

A bleeding disorder is suggested when the patient has unexplained (i.e., no history of trauma) bleeding or bruising or prolonged bleeding following injury, surgery or tooth extraction.

> **!** Haetasis is the process of stopping bleeding following damage to a blood vessel. It is a complex process that involves platelets, coagulation factors (increase blood clotting) and anticoagulation factors (decrease blood clotting).

Coagulation defects

- Inborn defects have been described in all coagulation factors but are mostly extremely rare.
- The two most common defects are haemophilia (factor VIII) and Christmas disease (factor IX). Both of these are transmitted as sex-linked recessive characteristics. This means that females carry the disease but only males actually have the full disease.
- They are both associated with an increased bleeding tendency.
- There is a wide range of severity.
- Bleeding may occur into any tissue of the body but the most common bleeding site is into the joints (*haemarthrosis*). The joints most frequently involved are knees, elbows, ankles, shoulders and hips.
- Haemarthrosis leads to the sudden onset of acute pain and swelling. Movement is restricted by the patient.
- Recurrent episodes lead to chronic degenerative joint disease with chronic pain, deformity and limitation of movement.
- The most common cause of death from bleeding is cerebral bleeding.
- Internal bleeding may also occur, leading to obstruction of the ureter and haematuria. Intestinal obstruction is one manifestation of bleeding into the bowel.

Investigations

- There is a prolonged APTT.
- The individual clotting factors then need to be measured.

Treatment

- Specialized units are best.
- The deficient clotting factor (found in plasma) is infused intravenously both as prophylaxis, before and after surgery, and to treat acute bleeding.
- Many patients have supplies of the missing factor at home and inject themselves at the first sign of bleeding.

- Tragically, many patients have been infected with HIV from contaminated plasma. Some clotting factors are now available synthetically (using recombinant DNA).

Von Willebrand's disease

- This is an inherited deficiency of von Willebrand's factor, which is essential for normal platelet adhesion in the damaged blood vessel lining. It also leads to low levels of factor VIII.
- It can occur in both men and women, and there is a broad range of severity from symptomless to severe.
- Presentation is usually with bleeding.
- Treatment is administration of vasopressin preparations and, if severe, the administration of cryoprecipitate or plasma.

Vitamin K deficiency

Vitamin K is needed for the synthesis of several clotting factors. A deficiency of this vitamin results in a bleeding tendency.

Causes

- Haemorrhagic disease of the newborn — synthesis is defective in premature infants. They are given the vitamin at birth to reduce the risk of cerebral bleeding.
- Intestinal malabsorption, e.g., Crohn's disease, coeliac disease.
- Hepatobiliary disease, e.g., liver failure, obstructive jaundice.
- Dietary deficiency.
- Oral anticoagulant use (warfarin inhibits the action of vitamin K).

Disseminated intravascular coagulation

This is not an illness on its own but is always secondary to an underlying disorder. It is an inappropriate activation of the coagulation pathways leading to the inappropriate deposition of fibrin—platelet thrombi in the arterial and venous tree. This leads to haemorrhage as clotting factors become exhausted. Both thrombin and plasmin are activated. This stimulates fibrinolysis (clot breakdown). This leads to:

- depletion of clotting factors,
- depletion of platelets leading to thrombocytopenia and increasing the bleeding tendency,
- loss of haemostasis,
- excessive bleeding.

A large number of conditions may lead to acute or chronic disseminated intravascular coagulation (DIC).

Risk factors for acute disseminated intravascular coagulation

- Infections/infectious diseases such as meningococcal septicaemia and malaria.
- Obstetric causes such as preeclampsia.
- Shock due to trauma, cardiac arrest, blood loss or extensive burns.
- Sixty per cent have septicaemia. This may be due to infections such as *Escherichia coli* 0157 or meningococcal septicaemia.

Acute DIC presents as a haemorrhagic illness:

- The patient is usually severely ill.
- Fever, acidosis and hypoxia and hypotension due to severe blood loss are present.
- Signs of adult respiratory distress syndrome.
- There may be extensive petechiae or bleeding into the skin. There may be skin necrosis of the lower limbs (purpura fulminans).
- There may also be bleeding into the eyes, alimentary, renal, respiratory or genital tracts.

Diagnosis

Made with the aid of laboratory testing:

- Platelet count is reduced.
- Prothrombin time is elevated.
- The activated partial thromboplastin time (aPPT) is prolonged.
- Presence of fibrin degradation products and a low fibrinogen level.

Treatment

- Treat the underlying condition.
- Restoration and maintenance of the peripheral circulation.
- Replacement therapy with plasma products and platelets.
- Use of heparin may control the thrombotic component but remains controversial.

Prognosis

The condition can be fatal. Infarction may destroy an organ and limb ischaemia may lead to loss of digits or worse. The underlying condition is important in determining the prognosis.

Chronic DIC reflects a compensated state and occurs most often in patients with malignant conditions or large aortic aneurysms.

Thrombosis

A thrombus is a solid mass formed in the circulation from the constituents of blood.

Arterial thrombosis

Usually, the result of atheroma, which tends to occur in areas of turbulent blood flow in the arteries, e.g., at the femoral bifurcation.

Venous thrombosis

- Unlike arterial thrombosis, this usually occurs in normal vessels (i.e., without atheroma deposition), often in the deep veins of the leg.
- It originates around the valves as red thrombi.
- There is a risk of propagation and embolization to the pulmonary vessels.
- The risk factors for venous thrombosis are shown in Box 5.2.

White blood cells

Leukaemias

These are neoplastic disorders of the blood-forming tissues. There is an un-regulated proliferation of white cells or accumulation of white cells in the bone marrow. These replace the normal cells:

- There may be proliferation at any stage of development from the stem cell.
- Normal cells are replaced by malignant cells, and this leads to a low white cell, haemoglobin and platelet count.

BOX 5.2 Risk factors for a deep vein thrombosis

Patient factors	Disease or procedure
Previous deep vein thrombosis	Surgery — especially pelvis or hip
Age	Trauma — especially pelvis or hip
Immobility	Malignancy
Obesity	Varicose veins
Pregnancy	Heart failure
High doses of oestrogens	Recent myocardial infarction
Thrombophilia	Infection
	Inflammatory bowel disease
	Polycythaemia
	Thrombocythaemia
	Nephrotic syndrome
	Systemic lupus erythematosus (SLE)

- There may also be damage to normal white cells so they cannot function properly. There is a fall in antibody production.
- There is infiltration of other tissues including the spleen, liver and central nervous system.
- Divided into acute and chronic forms.

Causal factors

- No evidence of inheritance pattern
- Some genetic disorders are associated with it, e.g., Down's syndrome
- Radiation
- Chemicals
- Therapeutic drugs — cytotoxics
- Viruses
- Philadelphia chromosome

Diagnosis

- Blood picture
- Bone marrow puncture

Classification

Acute leukaemias

- Uncontrolled clonal proliferation and accumulation of blast cells in the bone marrow and other body tissues.
- Clinical features are a result of anaemia, neutropenia and thrombocytopenia.

Acute lymphatic/lymphoblastic leukaemia

- Most common in childhood — peaks between 4 and 5 years
- More common in developed countries

Acute myelogenous leukaemia

- Common in middle to old age
- Males above 65 years with a minor peak under 5.
- Seven types, according to cell type predominating.

Chronic leukaemias

- Very few normal cells but the abnormal do differentiate to a degree and thus marrow failure is not a feature.
- Mass of cells produced give the clinical symptoms, e.g., splenomegaly, lymphadenopathy.

Differ from acute leukaemia in that:

- The time course is longer.
- The onset is more insidious.
- The cells are more mature.
- The treatments required are less intensive.

Chronic lymphatic leukaemia A disease of the middle-aged and the elderly. Onset is insidious with:

- lethargy,
- fever and sweating,
- loss of weight,
- infections,
- moderate enlargement of lymph nodes in neck, axilla and groin,
- splenic and hepatic enlargement.

It is often picked up at a routine blood count. Usually some anaemia, white cell count (WCC) $> 15 \times 10^9$/L, of which more than 40% are lymphocytes. Patients may not need any treatment in the early stages when asymptomatic.

Drugs used include ***fludarabine, cyclophosphamide, chlorambucil*** or ***bendamustine***. They may be given singly or a combination may be used. Growth factor injections may be given to increase the WCC.

Patients are very susceptible to infections which are often the cause of death.

Chronic myeloid leukaemia

- Deceptive to call it chronic.
- Usually associated with a chromosomal abnormality. The Philadelphia chromosome is present in 95% of patients.
- Treatment is by control of the proliferation by the use of busulfan or hydroxyurea.
- Median survival 35 months. Usually within 5 years of diagnosis there is a blast crisis and acute transformation occurs, i.e., to acute leukaemia.
- Allogenic bone marrow transplant is useful in the chronic phase in young patients who have a compatible donor. Should be done within the first year for the best chance.

Pathophysiology
Acute leukaemias

Cause morbidity and mortality through:

- deficiency in numbers of normal blood cells,
- invasion of vital organs with impairment of organ function,
- systemic disturbances shown by metabolic imbalances — hyponatraemia, hyperuricaemia — may be a symptom of the disease or its treatment,
- aetiology unknown, but may include viruses, chemicals and radiation.

Clinical features

- Result from bone marrow failure
- History usually short
- Symptoms of anaemia and malaise — pallor and tiredness
- Repeated acute infections — fever
- Bruising and bleeding
- Painful and enlarging lymphadenopathy
- Bone pain, especially in children
- Symptoms due to infiltration of tissues — splenomegaly, hepatomegaly.
- Headache, nausea, vomiting and blurred vision due to raised intracranial pressure (ICP) in patients with CNS involvement.

Treatment

- Induction of remission
- Consolidation
- Cranial prophylaxis
- Continuation/maintenance therapy

Relapse can occur in three sites — bone marrow, CNS, testicle.

Treatment should be carried out in specialist centres. Chemotherapy may include combinations of steroids, vincristine, asparaginase, methotrexate, daunorubicin and cytosine arabinoside.

Myelodysplastic syndromes

These disorders are characterized by the liability to develop acute myeloid leukaemia.

The lymphomas

Lymphomas are malignant tumours of the lymphoreticular system. They originate in one of the lymph nodes or other lymphatic tissues of the body. They are classified on histologic appearance (appearance of the cells under the microscope) into Hodgkin's disease and various subtypes of non-Hodgkin's lymphoma (NHL).

Hodgkin's disease

Hodgkin's disease is the most common of the lymphomas. It is potentially curable. Early peak incidence is in the early 20s and a later peak occurs in middle age after 45 years.

Clinical features

- Seventy per cent of cases arise as a painless enlargement of a lymph node in the neck, axilla or groin, and it spreads to adjacent groups of lymph nodes.
- Systemic features include fever, night sweats and weight loss.
- Other symptoms include pruritus, fatigue, anorexia and alcohol-induced pain at the site of the enlarged lymph nodes.
- On examination the affected nodes are usually painless and have a rubbery consistency.
- There may be enlargement of the liver and spleen (hepatosplenomegaly).
- Staging in Hodgkin's disease is shown in Box 5.3.

Investigations

- Blood count may show anaemia and a raised erythrocyte sedimentation rate (ESR).
- Liver biochemistry may be abnormal.
- Radiologic examination of the chest and CT scanning.

BOX 5.3 Staging in Hodgkin's disease and non-Hodgkin's lymphoma (Ann Arbor System)

Stage I	Involvement of one lymph node or extralymphatic organ
Stage II	Two or more lymph nodes involved on the same side of the diaphragm or with localized involvement of an extralymphatic organ on same side of diaphragm
Stage III	Nodal disease on both sides of the diaphragm or with extralymphatic site or spleen
Stage IV	Disseminated involvement of extranodal sites, e.g., bone marrow, liver and lungs

- Lymph node biopsy is needed to give a definite diagnosis.
- Bone marrow biopsy may show involvement in advanced disease.

Treatment

- Radiotherapy or a cyclical combination of cytotoxic drugs or a combination of both is used.
- The prognosis is related to the stage of the disease.
- In the early stages (I and II without beta symptoms), radiotherapy may produce a cure. There is a 25% relapse rate, and subsequent combination chemotherapy produces virtually 100% cure.
- In stages III and IV, with or without beta symptoms, 60% are disease-free at 5 years.
- Variations depend on the presence of adverse prognostic factors such as beta symptoms, age >40 years, bulk disease.
- Most relapses occur within 1–2 years of completion of combination therapy.

Non-Hodgkin's lymphoma

This is a group of disorders arising from many different cell types. There are several confusing classifications, but the simplest is high-grade or low-grade NHL.

Clinical features

- Rare before the age of 40 years and most common in the sixth decade.
- Presents in a variety of ways and almost any organ in the body can be involved.
- Peripheral lymph node enlargement is the most common presentation.
- Systemic symptoms as in Hodgkin's may occur.
- Bone marrow infiltration may occur and lead to anaemia, recurrent infections and bleeding.
- Investigations are similar to those for Hodgkin's.

Treatment

Low grade:

- Not usually curable unless early stage I.
- Staged as for Hodgkin's. With involvement of one gland, this may be excised and followed with radiotherapy. This is, however, very rare.
- Patients may survive for many years (mean 7–10 years) and experience remissions following radiotherapy or cytotoxic therapy.
- Interferon-alpha is also used in the management.

High grade:

- Rapid onset and 60%–70% of cases present in stage III or IV.
- Common in impaired immune surveillance such as following kidney or heart transplants and treatment for another malignancy or AIDS.
- Combination chemotherapy is used for all patients, irrespective of staging.
- Some radiotherapy may be used for localized glands.
- Seventy per cent in stages I and II are disease-free at 5 years.
- Forty per cent in stages III and IV are disease-free at 5 years.

Lymphadenopathy

This is enlargement of the lymph nodes and has many causes.

Local:

- Infection such as tonsillitis, tuberculosis
- Secondary carcinoma
- Lymphoma

Generalized:

- Infections:
  - Epstein–Barr virus (glandular fever)
  - Cytomegalovirus
  - Toxoplasmosis
  - Tuberculosis
  - HIV infection
- Lymphoma
- Leukaemia
- Drug reactions, e.g., phenytoin
- Systemic lupus erythematosus
- RA

Multiple myeloma

This is a cancer of the antibody-producing cells (plasma cells) in the bone marrow. Antibody may be present in the urine (Bence–Jones protein) and this is diagnostic of the disease.

It accounts for only 1% of all neoplasms and is more common in the elderly (mean age of presentation is 60–70 years) and rare in those <40 years old.

Myeloma is not a curable disease and the median survival from diagnosis is 2 years. Five-year survival is about 35%.

Clinical features

- Bone pain is the most common presenting feature.
- Anaemia, infections and bleeding occur as the bone marrow is infiltrated with the cancer cells and cannot produce sufficient blood cells.
- Renal failure may occur due to the deposition of antibody in the kidney tubules.
- Bone cells are involved and osteoporosis, hypercalcaemia and pathologic fractures may result.

Treatment

- **Bortezomib,** a proteasome inhibitor — may be used as monotherapy. It may also be given in combination with **melphelan** and **prednisolone.**
- Bone marrow transplantation.
- Localized bone pain may be helped by radiotherapy.
- **Interferon-alpha** is also used in the management.

5.4 THE GASTROINTESTINAL SYSTEM

The gastrointestinal system stretches from the mouth to the anus and is really a muscular tube that is adapted along its length to aid the digestion and absorption of nutrients.

Symptoms of gastrointestinal disease could include the following:

- *Dysphagia* — difficulty in swallowing.
- *Dyspepsia* — a term used to describe many different symptoms of indigestion such as heartburn, acidity and pain.
- *Heartburn* — a symptom of acid reflux. A retrosternal burning discomfort which sometimes is confused with coronary pain.
- *Flatulence* — excessive wind. This may present as belching, abdominal pain and the passage of flatus.
- *Vomiting* — associated with many gastrointestinal conditions, but also occurs in many other conditions. If it is without pain it is not usually GI in origin.
- *Haematemesis* — vomiting blood. May be bright red, contain dark clots or look like coffee grounds, showing that digestion in the stomach has commenced.
- *Constipation* — infrequent passage of stool or difficult passage of hard stool.
- *Diarrhoea* — the passage of increased amounts of loose stool, not small amounts of stool.
- *Melaena* — bleeding in the tract which leads to the passage of black, sticky and smelly stools composed of partially digested blood.

- *Steatorrhoea* — the passage of fatty stools, these are pale, bulky and usually float, making them difficult to flush away.

Vomiting

There are many causes of vomiting, and it is likely to accompany any severe illness:

- Gastrointestinal causes include appendicitis, gastric ulcer, hiatus hernia, oesophageal carcinoma, gastritis, food poisoning, excess alcohol, pyloric stenosis, intestinal obstruction, strangulated hernia and, rarely, severe constipation.
- Metabolic disturbances such as diabetic ketoacidosis, uraemia and hypercalcaemia.
- Drugs such as chemotherapeutic agents, antibiotics, digoxin and opiates.
- Alcohol.
- Cerebral causes, e.g., raised intracranial pressure, head injury, meningitis, migraine.
- Any severe infection.
- Myocardial infarction or other trauma to the body.
- Severe pain.

Management

- Ensure the patient has a vomit bowl and tissues at the bedside.
- Stay with the patient if he wishes this.
- Record the type of vomit and the amount.
- Observe for signs of dehydration.
- The doctor may take blood for electrolyte estimation.
- Further management will depend on the cause.
- An antiemetic may be administered. Examples are metoclopramide or ondansetron.
- If the vomiting is secondary to chemotherapy, ondansetron may be more effective.
- Fluid replacement intravenously may be needed if the patient cannot tolerate fluid orally.

Diarrhoea

This is the passage of loose, semi-solid or liquid stools which are passed at more frequent intervals than is normal for the patient. It may also be defined as the passage of >300 mL of liquid faeces in 24 h. It may be acute or chronic and is not always due to a problem in the GI tract.

Causes

- Food poisoning — *Staphylococcus aureus, Salmonella*, viruses, *Campylobacter, E. coli*, etc. — often accompanied by vomiting.
- Inflammatory bowel disease — ulcerative colitis, Crohn's disease.
- Broad-spectrum antibiotics leading to pseudomembranous colitis (see below).
- Other drugs such as laxatives, antacids or digoxin.
- Diverticular disease, malabsorption, thyrotoxicosis, faecal impaction with overflow, irritable bowel disease.
- If the patient has recently been abroad, tropical diseases may be responsible.

Management

- This depends very much on the cause.
- Barrier nursing may be needed if infective cause.
- Stool specimens may need to be collected.
- Careful recording of fluid intake and output, including diarrhoea.
- Observation for blood or mucus in the stools.
- Rehydration may be possible orally if vomiting is not present.
- Salts as well as water are needed, and preparatory brands of powder to be reconstituted are available such as **Dioralyte.**
- If vomiting is present, the patient may not be able to take oral fluids and an IV infusion may be in progress to prevent dehydration.
- Antidiarrhoeal drugs are not usually prescribed. They can actually prolong infection.
- Antibiotics are not usually needed but in persistent infective diarrhoea the microbiologist may be consulted.

Pseudomembranous colitis (*Clostridium difficile*-associated diarrhoea)

- This is sometimes known as antibiotic-associated colitis and is due to an infection of the large bowel with an overgrowth of *C. difficile* bacteria. These bacteria produce a toxin that causes the symptoms.
- Antibiotic exposure is the most common cause. Broad-spectrum antibiotics such as cephalosporins kill many of the normal flora in the bowel and allow *C. difficile* to take over.
- It is a problem mostly in hospital where risk factors include advanced age, antibiotic therapy, chemotherapy, medication that suppresses the immune system or HIV infection and recent surgery. It may also occur in the community.

- Symptoms usually develop 5–10 days after starting antibiotic treatment but occasionally can develop after only 1 day of antibiotic use or as long as 10 weeks after discontinuation of the antibiotic.
- It is recognized as a significant cause of morbidity and mortality, mostly in hospitalized patients.
- Severity of the disease is variable and ranges from mild self-limiting diarrhoea to severe colitis, toxic megacolon or colonic perforation.
- The patient may have abdominal cramps, pyrexia, watery diarrhoea and perhaps blood in the stools.
- Patients may be nonsymptomatic carriers of the bacteria in their bowel.
- Treatment depends on severity. The causal antibiotic or medication is discontinued, and the *C. difficile* infection is treated with **metronidazole** or **vancomycin.**
- Fluid and electrolyte losses are replaced as necessary.
- Steps should be taken to reduce the spread of *C. difficile* to other patients.
- Not all diarrhoea following the use of antibiotics is due to *C. difficile*. Most diarrhoea is due to alteration in bowel flora (the bacteria living in the colon) decreasing the absorption of carbohydrates.

Constipation

This is the infrequent passage of hard stools with straining and difficulty. It is often a problem in the immobile and the elderly where the faeces may accumulate in the rectum and overflow incontinence of loose faecal matter may occur.

Causes

- Simple constipation due to lack of dietary fibre or dehydration and lack of exercise.
- Secondary to disease of the colon, e.g., diverticular disease, cancer, Hirschsprung's disease, painful haemorrhoids and anal fissures.
- Drug-related − many analgesics, especially opioids, cause severe constipation. Antacids with an aluminium base and anticholinergic drugs slow down motility.
- Neurologic diseases affecting the bowel and bladder, e.g., multiple sclerosis.
- Metabolic diseases such as hypothyroidism.

Treatment

- Simple constipation usually responds well to an increased fluid intake and more fibre in the diet.

- Bulk-forming laxatives may be used. They relieve constipation by increasing the faecal mass and their full effects may not be felt for several days. Bran is an example as are *methylcellulose (Celevac)* and *ispaghula husk (Isogel, Regulan).*
- Stimulant laxatives increase intestinal motility and often cause abdominal cramps. They should never be used in intestinal obstruction. *Bisacodyl* and *senna* are examples.
- Glycerol suppositories act as a rectal stimulant.
- Osmotic laxatives such as *lactulose* act by retaining fluid in the bowel. Lactulose may take up to 48 h to act.
- Microenemas are often used and are made of sodium citrate.

The oesophagus

The oesophagus is a muscular tube, about 25 cm in length, that extends from the pharynx to the stomach, passing through the diaphragm. It is lined by a mucosa of stratified epithelial tissue and a submucosa containing glands. The muscle consists of both longitudinal and circular muscle layers that are responsible for peristalsis and the passage of food from the mouth to the stomach.

The most common congenital abnormality affecting the oesophagus is oesophageal atresia where the oesophagus ends in a blind pouch. It is often associated with a fistula between the oesophagus and the trachea (tracheo–oesophageal fistula), and in about 50% of cases, there are other congenital abnormalities present. The condition is usually diagnosed at birth and the treatment is surgical to restore continuity of the oesophagus and eliminate any fistula.

Dysphagia

This is the most common symptom of any disease of the oesophagus. It is difficulty in swallowing which depends on the action of many muscle groups, some voluntary and some involuntary. The passage of food from the mouth to the stomach is dependent on a wave of peristalsis which is also dependent on nervous control.

Causes

Neuromuscular disease:

- Motor neuron disease
- Myasthenia gravis
- Cerebrovascular accident that affects the 9th, 10th or 12th cranial nerves
- Achalasia
- Diabetic autonomic neuropathy

Obstruction:

- Foreign body
- Stricture due to acid regurgitation (reflux)
- Tumour
- Compression from outside by a mediastinal mass

Malignancy should always be ruled out in cases of dysphagia. A barium swallow or an endoscopy may be used for this purpose.

Achalasia

There is an absence of peristalsis and a failure of the lower oesophageal sphincter to relax. It is a disorder of neurotransmission but the cause is not known. Vitamin deficiency, viral infection and autoimmune disease have all been implicated.

Clinical features

- Develops slowly over a period of years.
- Food and liquid accumulate in the oesophagus, and dilatation occurs at the lower end.
- Dysphagia and regurgitation occur.
- Accumulation of food and fluids can lead to aspiration and chest infection.

Diagnosis

A barium swallow shows the dilated oesophagus. Endoscopy will also be done to exclude any type of tumour.

Treatment

Calcium channel blockers and nitrates may be used to aid sphincter relaxation. This is successful in about 10% of patients.

Balloon dilatation of the lower oesophageal sphincter is successful in the majority of cases.

If dilatation is unsuccessful, surgery may be possible.

Reflux oesophagitis (gastro-oesophageal reflux)

This is a very common condition caused usually by a failure of the lower oesophageal sphincter. If the sphincter is incompetent, this allows stomach contents to reflux into the oesophagus when the person is lying flat or when the stomach is full. The mucosa of the oesophagus is not as thick as the stomach mucosa and so the acid contents cause corrosion and burning, leading to inflammation. This can lead to bleeding and ulceration followed by stricture.

Sometimes, over a long period of time the mucosa may change and there may be an increased risk of malignancy.

Clinical features

- Heartburn, regurgitation and dysphagia.
- May be pain on swallowing hot or spicy food and drink.
- Posture is important and the symptoms worsen on bending or lying down and also following a large meal or the intake of large quantities of fluid.
- Ulcers may cause some bleeding.

Treatment

- Weight loss, if overweight.
- Help to stop smoking, if a smoker.
- Reduction in alcohol intake, if heavy.
- Small and regular meals. No meal just before bedtime.
- Sleep sitting up or raise the head of the bed.

Drug therapy

Antacids and alginates such as **Gaviscon** may be used to help protect the mucosa. Proton pump inhibitors, e.g., **omeprazole**, may be given to reduce the acid secretion in the stomach.

Gastric emptying can be helped with **metoclopramide**. **Mebeverine** may be given for muscle spasm.

If medical management fails, surgical procedures can be used.

Hiatus hernia

This is a herniation of part of the stomach through the diaphragm. It is relatively common and is one cause of reflux oesophagitis. Fig. 5.5 shows a hiatus hernia.

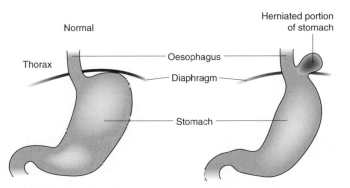

FIGURE 5.5 Hiatus hernia. *From Govan et al., 1993. Pathology Illustrated. Elsevier, reproduced with permission.*

In a *sliding hiatus hernia* the stomach herniates into the thorax when the patient is in the supine position. Standing causes the stomach to slide back into the abdominal cavity. The hernia is exacerbated by any factors that increase intra-abdominal pressure such as coughing, bending, straining and pregnancy.

In a *rolling or para-oesophageal hernia*, the fundus of the stomach herniates through the hiatus alongside the oesophagus. Reflux is less common but there is a danger of congestion, constriction and ulcer formation. The hernia may strangulate, which is a major complication.

Diagnosis is by barium studies and endoscopy.

The usual management of a sliding hernia (the most common type) is medical with weight reduction, antacids, proton pump inhibitors and sleeping in the sitting position all being important. Surgery is only contemplated when symptoms are severe. The hernia is reduced and the defect repaired. The operation is major as entry has to be made via the thorax.

Oesophageal tumours

These are usually malignant. Benign tumours of the oesophagus are rare. Ninety-five per cent are squamous cell carcinomas. This occurs worldwide and has a poor prognosis. It is the leading cause of cancer death in China but accounts for only 1%–2% of deaths in the West.

It has been linked to smoking, excess alcohol consumption, history of acid reflux and achalasia.

Clinical features

- Dysphagia, first with solids and eventually with liquids as well.
- Weight loss.

Investigations

- Endoscopy and biopsy.
- Barium swallow allows the length of the tumour to be assessed.
- CT scan to look for spread of the tumour into lymph nodes, mediastinum, lungs or liver.
- Endoscopic ultrasound.

Treatment

- May be curative or palliative depending on the age of the patient and the presence of metastatic disease. Some tumours are not resectable due to direct spread to the mediastinal structures, e.g., aorta, bronchus and diaphragm.
- Surgery is the best approach in the middle and lower oesophagus if the tumour is operable and the patient is well enough. Tumours in the upper

third of the oesophagus are extremely difficult to operate on due to the proximity of vital structures in the mediastinum.

- There is always the danger postoperatively of anastomotic leakage and stenosis. The leaks are difficult to manage and may be fatal.
- High-dose radiotherapy may sometimes produce long-term remission. It is used when surgery is not the best option, especially in the upper third of the oesophagus, or in those too unfit for major surgery.
- In inoperable cases the obstruction can be relieved by stenting when a wire mesh tube (stent) is inserted, via endoscopy, into the lumen of the oesophagus to hold it open.

Oesophageal bleeding

May be due to Mallory—Weiss tears. These are longitudinal tears in the lower end of the oesophagus due to prolonged or violent vomiting. Occasionally the bleeding can be very severe but is usually self-limiting. The tear may be repaired surgically if necessary.

Oesophageal varices

- These are enlarged, dilated and torturous veins that occur in portal hypertension, secondary to liver disease, often cirrhosis.
- They may lead to episodes of bleeding.
- Seventy per cent of patients with cirrhosis will develop varices, but only about one-third will bleed from them.
- Bleeding is likely from large varices and in severe liver disease.
- They are frequently the cause of life-threatening haematemesis when they rupture. This is usually painless but is extremely frightening for both the patient and the nurse.
- The mortality rate varies between 20% and 60% and has improved over the past 30 years. This is partly due to better high dependency care and partly due to the use of early warning scores.
- Patients with previous episodes of bleeding are at risk of subsequent episodes. Recurrent bleeding from varices has a worse prognosis.

Emergency treatment of bleeding varices

- The patient will need prompt correction of hypovolaemia with plasma expanders or a blood transfusion.
- Vasoconstrictor therapy may be used in an emergency to try to control bleeding. Vasopressin or glypressin may be used.
- Balloon tamponade may be needed to control bleeding. A Blakemore—Sengstaken tube is usually used. The inflated balloon presses on the bleeding veins.

- Endoscopic variceal band ligation or sclerotherapy with injection of a sclerosing agent may be used.
- Insertion of a wire mesh stent may be considered. The stent is expanded to the width of the oesophagus and presses on the veins to stop bleeding. It is removed within 2 weeks.

The stomach and duodenum

Peptic ulcers affect up to 10% of men and women in Britain within their lifetime and are the most common disorder of the stomach and duodenum.

Gastric ulcers occur in the stomach and duodenal ulcers (DUs) within the duodenum.

DUs are about four times common in men than women and are most common between 30 and 50 years of age.

The stomach has a thick protective mucosa but if this becomes thinner and less effective, the secretion of hydrochloric acid in gastric juice, with a pH of 1−2, and the enzyme pepsin will eat into the stomach lining and cause ulcers. The organism *Helicobacter pylori* is now known to be involved in gastritis and DU formation. More than 95% of those with DUs are infected.

Helicobacter pylori

- This organism is a Gram-negative spirochaete that produces urease.
- It is found in the gastric antrum and areas of the duodenum where it adheres to gastric epithelial cells under the mucous layers of the stomach.
- *H. pylori* is the most common cause of gastritis. It is thought to play a major part in the development of peptic ulceration and has also been associated with gastric cancer. The WHO has classified *H. pylori* as a definite carcinogen.
- *H. pylori* infection occurs throughout the world. The mode of transmission is still unclear but person to person is suspected. Fifty to sixty per cent of the adult population are infected.
- The natural reservoir of *H. pylori* is not known.
- Apart from human gastric mucosa, it is not known to thrive elsewhere.
- Ninety-five per cent of patients with DU are infected with *H. pylori*, and the bacterium is thought to be causal. If the infection is cured the DU disease does not recur.
- Only 15% of those with *H. pylori* develop DU disease − it is not known why.

Diagnosis

- Tests include C urea breath tests − very simple but not always accurate.
- Serological tests to detect antibodies to *H. pylori* are 90% sensitive, but antibody levels take up to a year to fall by 50% so this cannot be used to check if the infection has been eradicated.

- Stool tests can be done to diagnose and to monitor eradication.
- Although invasive, endoscopic mucosal biopsy and culture of the organism is the most certain diagnosis.

Treatment

- Acid inhibition combined with antibacterial treatment is highly effective.
- The organism is resistant to single antibiotic therapy.
- Triple regimens provide higher eradication rates (see Box 5.4). These consist of a proton pump inhibitor combined with two antibiotics for a 1-week regimen.
- Eradication of infection commonly results in long-term ulcer remission.

Gastritis

This is inflammation of the gastric mucosa. It can be acute or chronic. Acute gastritis is usually caused by drugs or chemicals causing injury to the protective lining of the stomach.

Alcohol, histamine, digitalis and certain metabolic disorders, e.g., uraemia, can all contribute to gastritis. Nonsteroidal antiinflammatory drugs such as aspirin also cause gastritis.

Clinical features

- Abdominal discomfort
- Epigastric tenderness
- Bleeding

Usually heals spontaneously over a period of days. Any causative drugs should be discontinued and antacids may be given to combat excess acidity.

Chronic gastritis is usually associated with *H. pylori* infection. It may be associated with atrophy of the gastric mucosa and tends to occur in the elderly. There may be autoimmune attack of the parietal cells in the stomach and an inability to secrete intrinsic factor that leads to pernicious anaemia.

BOX 5.4 An example of triple therapy: 1-week regimen

Clarithromycin 500 mg twice daily plus
Metronidazole 400 mg three times daily plus
Omeprazole 20 mg twice daily for 7 days

Peptic ulcers

The term *peptic* comes from the Greek 'to digest', and these ulcers occur as a result of the secretion of acid digestive juices.

They may occur at the following sites:

- Oesophagus — due to reflux
- Stomach — gastric ulcer
- Duodenum — DU

DU is much common (five times) than gastric ulcer, but the incidence has been decreasing since the 1950s. It is seen in all social groups, and 80% occur in men. It is now known that *H. pylori* is the most important factor in its aetiology.

Surgery for ulcers used to be extremely common but now most of them are treated medically with a regimen that includes eradication of *H. pylori*.

Most patients with a DU have excess acid secretion in the stomach. Those with a gastric ulcer have normal or low acid secretion usually.

The ulcers penetrate through the mucosa and into the muscle layer. DUs nearly always occur within 2—3 cm of the pylorus (where the chyme is most acidic).

Aetiology

- *H. pylori.*
- Smoking.
- Aspirin and nonsteroidal antiinflammatory drugs (NSAIDs).
- Alcohol.
- Stress — may lead to oversecretion of gastric acid due to stimulation of the vagus nerve. Ulcers tend to occur at times of high stress and anxiety.
- Zollinger—Ellison syndrome. This is a tumour of the pancreas that causes production of a gastrin-like hormone that stimulates the production of gastric juice, causing a hugely raised acidity in the stomach and the formation of multiple DUs.

Clinical features

- May be similar to other acute abdominal problems.
- The pain is in the epigastrium and may be intermittent. In DU eating relieves the pain and so there is no loss of appetite usually. In gastric ulcer eating usually exacerbates the pain and so the patient loses weight.
- Those with a DU tend to be overweight and male.
- Those with a gastric ulcer tend to be thin and even emaciated.

Investigations

- Fibreoptic endoscopy. This has superseded investigation with a barium meal. The ulcer can be seen, localized and biopsied.
- The mucosa can also be tested for the presence of *H. pylori*.

Treatment

Most (more than 80%) ulcers will heal with medical treatment. Treatment with either an H_2 antagonist, e.g., **ranitidine**, or a proton pump inhibitor, e.g., **omeprazole**, is used. If only this therapy is used the relapse rates are high but treating *H. pylori* infection as well has revolutionized the prognosis and reduced the relapse rate from 80% to 5%–10%. **Sucralfate** may be used to improve mucosal protection.

Occasionally surgery is still needed when:

- medical treatment fails to relieve symptoms (rare),
- there are complications such as uncontrolled haemorrhage or perforation,
- There is a possibility of malignancy – especially with a gastric ulcer that will not heal.

Surgery

1. Billroth I partial gastrectomy for a gastric ulcer – removes the area with the ulcer.
2. Highly selective vagotomy for DU – this operation reduces gastric acid secretion by dividing the part of the vagus nerve that controls acid secretion but retaining the part that controls motility of the stomach.
3. Gastrectomy – this is removal of the stomach and is only used in DUs due to Zollinger–Ellison syndrome or as an emergency in severe bleeding.

Side effects of partial gastrectomy

- Reduced gastric capacity – cannot eat normal-sized meals at first.
- Rapid emptying of stomach contents – dumping syndrome – causes transient hypovolaemia and faintness.
- Diarrhoea due to 'intestinal hurry'.
- Vitamin B_{12} deficiency due to lack of intrinsic factor.
- Recurrent ulceration of remnant (only 1%).
- Reduced iron absorption – may need supplements.

Complications of chronic peptic ulceration

- Perforation – causing peritonitis
- Bleeding – causing a haematemesis; the ulcer penetrates the gastroduodenal artery

- Pyloric stenosis due to scar tissue
- Malignancy (gastric ulcer)

Perforation

Usually a DU and so this is common in men. There is usually a history of indigestion but sometimes no history at all:

- Sudden and excruciating epigastric pain that rapidly spreads to the whole abdomen.
- Rigid 'board-like' abdomen that is due to generalized peritonitis.
- Shock — low blood pressure, rapid pulse, cold and clammy to the touch.
- Collapse.
- Patient lies very still as any movement causes pain.

Treatment

- Intravenous infusion to combat shock.
- Analgesia for the intense pain.
- Monitoring of vital signs.
- Antibiotics.
- Nil by mouth.
- Surgery — the perforation is oversewn.
- Medical treatment is commenced after the operation.
- If it is a gastric ulcer, there is a high risk that it may be malignant and some surgeons will do an immediate partial gastrectomy.

Haemorrhage

This may present as haematemesis or melaena and in some cases both may occur. There are many causes of bleeding from the upper gastrointestinal tract and these include:

- Peptic ulcer — 90%
- Oesophageal varices
- Drugs — aspirin, NSAIDs and steroids, causing acute erosive gastritis
- Tumours of the stomach
- Mallory—Weiss syndrome

Pyloric stenosis

This is a narrowing of the muscular outlet of the stomach, which causes delay in the passage of the stomach contents to the duodenum. This results in vomiting, which may be projectile and may include food eaten 24 h earlier.

The patient will lose weight and become dehydrated if the condition is not treated.

The patient does not usually give a history of ulcer pain, but just of episodic vomiting. An X-ray may show the hugely dilated stomach.

Causes

- Fibrosis and narrowing secondary to peptic ulceration
- Carcinoma of the antrum of the stomach
- Congenital pyloric stenosis in babies

Clinical features

- Vomiting — may be projectile, large amounts and containing undigested food.
- Rapid weight loss.
- Gastric peristalsis may be visible in some cases when the stomach is full.
- Mass may be felt in babies and in some cases of gastric carcinoma.
- Dehydration due to persistent vomiting.
- Electrolyte disturbance due to vomiting.
- Alkalosis.

Stomach cancer

Declining in incidence in the UK, it is associated more commonly with those of blood group A and occurs more frequently in men than women. There appears to be a connection with *H. pylori* infection and atrophic gastritis.

The decline is thought to be due to refrigeration, less use of preservatives and more fruit and vegetables in the diet.

Clinical features

- Often insidious in onset
- Increasing weakness and loss of energy
- Anaemia
- Loss of weight and anorexia
- Dyspepsia
- Pain
- Vomiting
- Perforation or haemorrhage may occur

There is a poor prognosis when diagnosed late, and it should be suspected in all cases of dyspepsia that start above the age of 40.

Endoscopy with biopsy is used for diagnosis.

Treatment

- Surgical when possible. A radical gastrectomy to include lymph nodes and the tail of the pancreas is more successful than less major surgery. This was pioneered in Japan.
- Often the surgery is palliative as when a laparotomy is attempted there may be secondary deposits in the liver. A partial gastrectomy may prevent obstruction occurring.
- Adjuvant chemotherapy or radiotherapy may be given. Immunotherapy is also being trialed.

The acute abdomen

This term relates to a patient whose symptoms are of acute onset and the patient will usually be admitted via A&E. Abdominal pain is often the most severe feature.

The patient may have a life-threatening condition that warrants emergency surgery or may have something simple such as severe constipation or even just gas in the bowel (wind).

Common causes of acute abdominal pain in adults

- Nonspecific pain that resolves without intervention
- Acute appendicitis
- Acute intestinal obstruction — strangulated hernia, adhesions, occlusion of the mesenteric artery
- Peptic ulcer — severe exacerbation of pain or perforation
- Gallstones — acute cholecystitis
- Acute pancreatitis
- Urinary tract infections (UTIs)
- Renal colic due to stones in the ureter
- Retention of urine
- Constipation
- Leaking or even ruptured abdominal aortic aneurysm
- Gynaecologic emergencies such as ectopic pregnancy

Peritonitis

This is inflammation of the peritoneal cavity, which includes the serosal covering of the bowel and mesentery, the omentum and the lining of the abdominal cavity. It is often localized at first as omentum is wrapped around inflammatory areas. However, this is often insufficient to prevent spread and generalized peritonitis results.

Sudden perforation of any abdominal organ leads to life-threatening peritonitis.

Common causes of peritonitis

Local

Localized peritonitis may occur in:

- appendicitis,
- Crohn's disease,
- diverticulitis,
- cholecystitis,
- salpingitis.

Appendicitis will be used as an example. Once the parietal peritoneum becomes involved, pain becomes localized to the affected area and is exacerbated by movement of the muscles in the abdomen.

The area will be tender when examined and the overlying muscles will contract – this sign is called *guarding*.

When the doctor removes his hand suddenly after applying pressure to the area, this sudden movement of the peritoneum causes intense pain which is known as rebound tenderness.

The doctor will also perform a rectal examination and anterior tenderness can be a sign of pelvic peritonitis.

There are usually signs of mild systemic toxicity that include low-grade fever, malaise, tachycardia and a slightly raised white cell count (*leucocytosis*).

Treatment This depends on the cause. If it is appendicitis, the appendix is removed but if it is salpingitis or diverticulitis, conservative treatment with antibiotics is usually used.

General

Generalized peritonitis may occur when:

- the peritoneum is irritated by noxious materials, e.g., bile, stomach acid, pancreatic enzymes or small bowel contents due to perforation;
- there is spreading intraperitoneal infection as in the rupture of an intra-abdominal abscess or faecal contamination in bowel perforation, trauma or an anastomotic leak.

The patient is seriously ill with generalized peritonitis. Inflammatory fluid moves into the peritoneal cavity and causes hypovolaemia. Alongside this toxaemia or septicaemia may be present.

The severity depends on the cause of the peritonitis and is most severe when contamination is by faeces, infected bile or pus. It is less severe if there is no infection, as in the early stages of a perforated DU.

The abdomen will be rigid and tender and because there is peristaltic paralysis, bowel sounds will be absent. A rectal examination by the doctor may reveal anterior tenderness and if so, pelvic peritonitis is indicated.

Treatment

- In generalized peritonitis, the patient is extremely ill and at risk of dying from toxaemia or sepsis. High doses of antibiotics are given intravenously.
- It is dangerous to operate in acute pancreatitis, but in the other causes, a laparotomy will probably be done urgently to clear the contaminating material and to find the cause, if not known.
- Intra-abdominal haemorrhage may occur in a ruptured ectopic pregnancy, leaking abdominal aneurysm or trauma to the liver or spleen. The blood causes peritoneal irritation that is similar to peritonitis, and diagnosis may be confirmed by peritoneal lavage. Saline is instilled via a peritoneal cannula and retrieval of bloodstained fluid provides the diagnosis.

Intestinal disorders

The small intestine extends from the duodenum to the ileum and most of the nutrients are absorbed here.

Small bowel obstruction

This may be complete or incomplete, simple or strangulated. A strangulated obstruction is a surgical emergency.

Small bowel obstruction (SBO) leads to dilatation of the intestine proximal to the obstruction as fluid from GI secretions and swallowed air build up. The dilatation stimulates secretions and even more fluid accumulates.

Causes

- Most common cause is adhesions or bands from previous surgery
- Strangulated hernia
- Volvulus
- Tumours
- Inflammatory strictures as in Crohn's disease
- Malignant tumours
- Intussusception (telescoping of the small bowel − common in children)

Management

- Nothing is given by mouth, and intravenous fluid replacement is used. The volume and type of fluid depend on the fluid and electrolyte balance. If there has been severe vomiting there may be serious fluid depletion.
- If the patient is vomiting, a nasogastric tube may be passed and the stomach contents aspirated. This will help to control the nausea and vomiting and will also remove swallowed air, reducing gaseous distension. It will also reduce the risk of inhalation of gastric contents, especially if anaesthesia is needed.
- Analgesia will be needed.
- If adhesions are the cause, the obstruction may relieve itself and no further treatment may be needed. If it does not, surgery will be required.
- Large bowel obstruction due to faecal impaction can be relieved by the use of enemas or the softening and manual evacuation of faeces.
- Operation may be necessary to relieve the obstruction. This will have to be immediate if strangulation is present and the blood supply to the bowel is threatened but may be delayed for a day or two if not, so that the patient can be stabilized and any necessary investigations can be done.

Strangulation of the bowel

This occurs when a segment of bowel becomes trapped, obstructing its lumen and disrupting its blood supply. If it is allowed to continue, there will be ischaemia of the bowel and infarction, perhaps leading to perforation.

Causes

- External hernia that may be inguinal, umbilical, femoral or incisional. The bowel becomes trapped outside the body and undergoes necrosis, often perforating within the hernial sac.
- A loop of bowel may become trapped within the abdominal cavity if there are fibrous bands or adhesions.
- A volvulus, where there is massive twisting of the bowel on its mesentery, may also be responsible.

Clinical features of bowel obstruction

- Vomiting — this may be large amounts and, depending on where the obstruction is, may be faecal in nature.
- Abdominal pain — usually colicky in nature and more severe in strangulation.
- Absolute constipation — no flatus is passed rectally. This happens in complete obstruction but not partial obstruction.
- Dehydration due to vomiting and a lack of intake.

- Abdominal distension due to gas. The lower the obstruction, the more the distension will be present.
- Abnormal bowel sounds — exaggerated, high-pitched and sometimes tinkling but completely absent in some cases.

Investigations and treatment

- Plain abdominal X-ray will show the gas-filled loop of bowel.
- CT scanning may help to distinguish the aetiology of the obstruction.
- Treatment is emergency surgery to relieve the obstruction. A resection of the bowel may be necessary.

Inflammatory disorders of the bowel

Inflammatory bowel disease is a term that incorporates both ulcerative colitis and Crohn's disease. These are both chronic and remittent bowel disorders that share some symptoms. Diarrhoea will be present in both, but recurrent bouts of abdominal pain are typical of Crohn's disease. There are periods of remission and relapse over many years.

Ulcerative colitis

First described in 1909, this is a chronic inflammatory disorder of the colonic and rectal mucosa and submucosa. It always involves the rectum and often extends proximally to involve varying amounts of colon. In about 20% of cases the distal end of the ileum may also be involved. Acute severe ulcerative colitis can be life-threatening and is a medical emergency that always requires hospital admission.

Clinical features

- There are recurrent acute exacerbations, and between these there may be remission or only low-grade activity.
- The acute exacerbations may last days to several months, and when they have subsided they may reappear in months or not for years.
- After many episodes of inflammation the epithelium may show abnormal cellular changes (*dysplasia*) and may even develop adenocarcinoma.
- There are both systemic and intestinal symptoms, depending on the severity of the attack.
- Diarrhoea, containing both mucus and blood, may be severe and the patient may have up to 20 loose motions a day.
- The diarrhoea may be preceded by abdominal cramps.
- Incontinence is a problem for many patients if there is any delay in getting to the toilet. This may interfere with the patient's social life and some fear leaving the house at all.

- Fulminant attacks may lead to dehydration, fluid and electrolyte imbalance and blood loss.
- High fever and tachycardia occur due to systemic illness.
- Anorexia, weight loss and lethargy.
- Chronic anaemia.
- Skin lesions — rare; erythema nodosum (tender red nodules on the shins).
- Arthropathy in about 20% of cases — a large joint problem similar to RA.
- Occasionally the inflammation may spread to the muscular bowel wall causing paralysis, dilatation and some necrosis. This is known as toxic megacolon and will lead to perforation unless an emergency colectomy is performed. There is sometimes a danger of perforation when toxic megacolon is not present.
- Some patients have inflammation that is confined to the rectum (*proctitis*).

Investigations

Typically a young adult (the most common presentation is between 15 and 25 years) with a history of several weeks of frequent loose stools. The attack may start as traveller's diarrhoea but does not settle.

Parasitic infections need to be excluded by the collection of stool specimens for microbiology.

Barium enema and endoscopy are used to assess the extent of the disease and to take biopsies.

Treatment

- A patient with a fulminant attack will be admitted to hospital and require intravenous fluid and electrolyte replacement. Some may need a blood transfusion.
- Radiographic exclusion of toxic megacolon (see below). This will show on a plain abdominal X-ray. Colonoscopy will not be done as there is a danger of perforation.
- Management varies not just between patients but also in the same patient for different episodes. Severity is classified as mild, moderate or severe. This is described in more detail in the NICE guidelines for ulcerative colitis. Oral and/or topical treatment with corticosteroids and aminosalicylates is used.
- Oral **mesalazine** with an enteric coating is used for long-term therapy and to try to prevent relapse. It is an aminosalicylate and appears to prevent the release of some of the inflammatory mediators and perhaps to neutralize some of the toxins present. Mesalazine may also be administered as a foam enema for local application.

- Local corticosteroid preparations in the form of suppositories, enemas or hydrocortisone foam may also be used but are less effective than amino-salicylates. Some patients may require both.
- If very acute, systemic steroids may be used as a short course and in severe cases may be given intravenously.
- Immunosuppressive drugs such as *azathioprine* are also used if there is little or no response to steroids. They may be used to allow a lower dose of steroid to be given. They do have adverse effects and skin rashes and nausea are common.
- *Infimixab* can be used for acute severe exacerbations where *ciclosporin* is contraindicated. Infimixab binds with TNF (tumour necrosis factor) which is an inflammatory mediator thought to be produced in ulcerative colitis and Crohn's disease. Within 2–6 weeks of the first infusion the patient should begin to feel better.
- Occasionally, antidiarrhoeal drugs such as *loperamide* may be given on the advice of a specialist but not in acute stage as they may increase the risk of toxic megacolon. A bulk-forming agent such as *methylcellulose* may also help to reduce the frequency of bowel motion.
- Surgical removal of the colon may have to be done as an emergency but may also be done when medical treatment fails or when there is a high risk of malignancy.

Crohn's disease

This was first described in 1932 by a doctor of the same name. The incidence has risen in the last 20 years in Britain, and the cause is not known.

It may affect any part of the gastrointestinal tract but usually the small bowel or the large bowel or both together are affected.

It differs from ulcerative colitis in that the inflammation involves the full thickness of the bowel wall. Chronic inflammation leads to oedema and the formation of ulcers and granulomas. Several different areas of the bowel may be affected, with bowel in between being normal (skip lesions).

The terminal ileum is the area most commonly affected so it used to be called terminal ileitis.

There are exacerbations and remissions, and different areas of the gastro-intestinal tract may be affected at each attack.

Clinical features

- Symptoms may be similar to ulcerative colitis, especially if the large bowel is involved, and vary according to the severity of the attack. Diarrhoea is usually less severe, containing blood less often. Abdominal pain, weight loss and lethargy are more typical, and there may be nausea and anorexia.

- There is often local tenderness if the terminal ileum is affected, but sometimes even with extensive disease the main feature is weight loss.
- Arthropathy can occur as in ulcerative colitis.

Complications

- Intestinal obstruction can occur due to a stricture and this may resolve spontaneously but may require surgery, especially if it is recurrent.
- The inflammation in Crohn's disease can spread to adjacent structures such as the peritoneum and peritonitis can occur. This may simulate acute appendicitis.
- There may be localized abscess formation following perforations, e.g., a pelvic abscess.
- Adhesions may follow from inflammatory spread.
- Fistulae may form between diseased bowel and other hollow parts:
  - Stomach — gastrocolic fistula: here the patient would have faecal vomiting
  - Urinary tract — leading to severe UTIs
  - Uterus or vagina — passage of faeces via the vagina.
- Perianal inflammation and sometimes recurrent perianal abscesses.

Investigations

Similar to ulcerative colitis for the large bowel but a barium follow-through will be done to investigate the small bowel or a 'small bowel enema' which is actually barium given via a nasogastric tube into the duodenum. Barium studies show typical narrowing of the bowel and ulceration.

Management

- Drug treatment is similar to ulcerative colitis and is usually effective in the acute stages, but there has not been success in maintenance drug therapy. Dietary therapy has given better results for long term.
- Topical steroid enemas and foams.
- High-dose oral steroids for the acute attacks. Less successful than in ulcerative colitis and of no use as maintenance.
- *Infimixab* is now recommended for severe Crohn's disease that has not responded to conventional treatment.
- Ustekinumab is also now available for patients with moderate to severe Crohn's disease. It has been previously used in the treatment of psoriasis and is a human monoclonal antibody treatment which stops cytokines (involved in the inflammatory response) being produced.
- Elemental diets that provide all nutrients in a simple molecular form to be absorbed in the proximal bowel have reasonable success but are expensive.

- There is evidence that food intolerance may play a part in acute exacerbations and so diet is important.
- Surgery may be needed especially when some of the complications above occur. This may be a resection of the small bowel or sometimes total colectomy if the large bowel is involved. This is because there may be several lesions (skip lesions) and recurrence is very likely. Some patients require surgery on more than one occasion for complications such as fistulae and abscesses.

Toxic colitis (toxic megacolon)

- This is an acute toxic colitis with dilatation of the colon. The dilatation may affect the whole of the colon or be segmental.
- It is a potentially lethal condition first observed as a complication of ulcerative colitis, but can complicate pseudomembranous colitis, radiation or other inflammatory conditions.
- Diarrhoea, abdominal pain, vomiting and fever may be present.
- Patients are usually very ill and may be dehydrated.

Stomas

Stoma comes from the Greek word for 'mouth' or 'opening'. It is the artificial opening of a tube (the colon or ileum) that has been brought to the surface of the abdomen as a colostomy or ileostomy to allow drainage of faeces or urine (urinary stoma).

It is usually performed when the bowel below the stoma is diseased and nonfunctioning. The faeces are collected in a removable plastic bag attached to the abdominal skin by adhesive.

A colostomy is fashioned to be flush with the skin, but an ileostomy has a 'spout' of bowel protruding for about 5 cm so that the irritant contents of the small bowel do not flow onto the skin. The enzymes present in the faecal content can cause destruction of the skin.

Stomas may be performed for:

- cancer of the colon – the most common reason for having a colostomy,
- diverticular disease,
- inflammatory bowel disease – ulcerative colitis or Crohn's disease,
- cancer of the bladder, trauma or intractable incontinence,

Types of stoma

Colostomy

Some colostomies are permanent and the stoma may be performed from any part of the large bowel, e.g., sigmoid (Fig. 5.6).

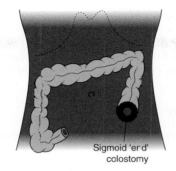

FIGURE 5.6   Sigmoid colostomy. *From Mallett, J., Bailey, C. Royal Marsden NHS Trust Manual of Clinical Nursing Procedures, fourth ed., reproduced with permission.*

Some stomas are temporary and divert the faecal output away from a more distal part of the bowel until it heals. When healing is complete, in weeks or even months, the colostomy is closed.

Temporary colostomies are most commonly formed from the transverse colon. A loop of bowel is pulled to the surface and held there with a glass or plastic rod, shown in Fig. 5.7. The distal loop of bowel has no functioning capacity and these stomas are sometimes called 'defunctioning' stomas.

Reasons for a temporary colostomy

- As an emergency measure in bowel obstruction.
- To allow a difficult anastomosis to heal.
- To allow a distal part of the colon to 'rest' in an inflammatory disease such as Crohn's disease or diverticulitis.

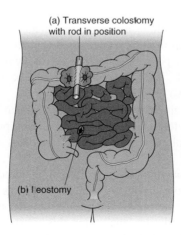

FIGURE 5.7   Transverse loop colostomy. *From Mallett, J., Bailey, C. Royal Marsden NHS Trust Manual of Clinical Nursing Procedures, fourth ed., reproduced with permission.*

Reasons for a permanent colostomy

- These are usually performed for cancer of the bowel.
- If there is no distal bowel remaining after a resection, as in an abdominoperineal resection of the rectum for a cancer of the lower rectum or anus.

Hartmann's procedure

- This is often performed for a cancer in the rectosigmoid region of the bowel.
- The cancer is resected but the colon is not joined to the remaining part of the rectum immediately as there is a high risk of infection and breakdown of the anastomosis.
- The proximal loop of bowel is made into a colostomy and the distal part is closed with staples or sutures.
- This means that the rectum is not functioning and although there will be no faeces passing through the anus, some mucus will still pass.
- When any inflammation has settled and healing has taken place, the bowel may be reconnected.
- Some patients are very elderly and find the colostomy functioning well. They may decide not to have another major operation and keep the colostomy instead.

Ileostomy

In this procedure the ileum is brought out onto the abdominal wall.

Reasons for an ileostomy

- Severe inflammatory disease of the large bowel as in ulcerative colitis.
- Familial polyposis coli — a rare disease that is genetically transmitted. Polyps first develop in adolescence and occur throughout the rectum and colon. Although the polyps are benign, invariably malignant changes occur in early adulthood. The whole colon should be removed and all close relatives should also be screened for the disease.
- An alternative to an ileostomy is a Park's pouch. A total colectomy is performed but the terminal ileum is made into a pouch and joined to the anus. The anal sphincter is preserved and thus continence is usually maintained.
- Psychological preparation of the patient is of utmost importance when a stoma is being considered and should begin as soon as possible. A specialized stoma care nurse will usually be responsible for this and will visit the patient to discuss the stoma, his lifestyle and coping with the stoma after the operation. The visits continue postoperatively and also when the patient is discharged. It is important to emphasize to the patient

that his lifestyle need not change just because he has a stoma. He may be horrified and extremely anxious at the thought, and it is important to involve his partner or close relatives in the discussions.

Early complications of stoma

- Sloughing or necrosis due to ischaemia (lack of oxygen due to poor blood supply) — this requires further surgery.
- Obstruction may occur due to faeces or oedema.
- Leakage onto the skin due to a badly fitting appliance may cause erosions. This may be due to poor siting of the stoma (e.g., over a crease in the skin) and if so may require further surgery to resite.
- Late complications include prolapse of the bowel, parastomal hernia and retraction of a 'spout' ileostomy. All these require further surgery.

Complications of large bowel surgery

Early complications include:

- Wound infections
- Pelvic or subphrenic abscess
- Leak or breakdown of the anastomosis
- Stoma problems, e.g., retraction

  Later possible complications include:

- Diarrhoea due to short bowel
- Impotence, if there has been damage to the pelvic parasympathetic nerves
- SBO due to adhesions

Colorectal polyps and carcinoma

Polyps

- Polyps are localized lesions protruding from the bowel wall. They are common in the colon and are actually benign neoplasms, but they have malignant potential.
- They should be treated as malignant until proven otherwise.
- The patient's first symptom is usually rectal bleeding or anaemia.
- Often there are no symptoms and the polyps are found in routine investigations.

Diagnosis and treatment

- Usually made by sigmoidoscopy. With a fibreoptic sigmoidoscope the colon can be examined up to the splenic flexure, which is the area of greatest occurrence.

- The polyps can be removed using diathermy and this may be done as an outpatient procedure. Histology will always be done.
- If the result shows malignancy and the polyp has been incompletely removed, then a resection will be needed.
- The patient will have to be followed up by endoscopy probably at 2-year intervals as there is a high risk of recurrence.

Colorectal cancer

There are about 42,000 new cases of colorectal cancer a year in the UK, and it is the second or third most common form of cancer in both sexes. It is slightly more common in males than females. Bowel cancer is most prevalent in the Western world and is rare in developing countries.

Colorectal cancer causes about 16,000 deaths every year in the UK with incidence increasing with age and more than 90% of deaths being in those above 55 years of age:

- The cancer is usually an adenocarcinoma that starts in the glandular mucosa.
- The cancer grows outwards at first but later may ulcerate and invade the bowel wall. Narrowing of the lumen of the bowel and intestinal obstruction may occur.
- The cancer spreads via the lymphatic system and also via the bloodstream.
- Lymphatic spread tends to occur first but sometimes there is spread via the bloodstream with no obvious lymphatic involvement.
- The spread via the blood is usually to the liver as the colon is drained by the hepatic portal vein.
- At the time of diagnosis, about 25% of patients already have widespread metastases.

Clinical features

- Symptomless anaemia
- Change in bowel habit
- Rectal blood loss
- Colicky pain
- Malaise, anorexia, weight loss
- Some patients may present with a bowel obstruction

Screening There is now an active screening programme in the UK for those without symptoms and aged between 60 and 74 years. Stool specimens are asked for and analysed for faecal occult blood every 2 years during this period. Those with positive tests are invited for colonoscopy. The accuracy of colonoscopy in the diagnosis of bowel cancer is greater than 90%.

About one-third of the cancers start in the rectum.

Diagnosis for those with symptoms

- Urgent colonoscopy
- Barium enema to show any polyps elsewhere in the colon
- CT scan or ultrasound of the liver to check for metastases

Cancer families Family history is the most common risk factor, after age, for cancer of the colon.

Some cancers are definitely familial and those with a family history may be screened by having regular colonoscopies.

Treatment

- Radical surgical resection. This may be an abdominoperineal resection of the rectum when the cancer is low in the rectum. The patient will have a permanent colostomy.
- A resection with an end-to-end anastomosis will be done for upper rectal or colon cancer.
- If the tumour is in the ascending colon, a right hemicolectomy may be performed and half the large bowel removed but no colostomy is needed.
- Pre- or postoperative chemotherapy or radiotherapy may be offered.
- Only about 1 in 10 patients with distant metastases at the time of operation survives 2 years.
- The metastases are usually in the liver and may be seen at operation or discovered after the operation if not found in the scan before surgery.

Appendicitis

The appendix is a short, thin, blind-ended tube, 7—10 cm long, situated in the right inguinal fossa and attached to the caecum (a pouch at the start of the large intestine). It has no known function in humans.

The most common abdominal emergency seen in A&E is acute appendicitis when the appendix becomes inflamed. This carries an overall mortality of about 1% and death is due to generalized peritonitis, being most common in the very young and the very old. The majority of patients do not fall in this category and are between 10 and 30 years of age.

The disease occurs only in the Western world and is probably linked to diet and lifestyle (low-fibre diets may be implicated here). Immigrants to this country become susceptible to the disease when they adopt our lifestyle.

Obstruction to the lumen of the appendix is the usual cause of appendicitis. This is commonly by faecaliths (small, hard masses of faeces). An appendix that is long, thin and retrocaecal is more prone to blockage than a short, straight appendix. Appendicitis may also be congestive, and there is no obvious obstruction but inflammation is present and may have been caused by ingested organisms.

Tumours of the appendix are extremely rare.

Disease process

- Resolution may occur and be complete but there is usually some scarring which makes the appendix more prone to future attacks of inflammation. This is recurrent appendicitis.
- The body may attempt to wall off the infection and an appendix abscess may result. This usually takes days to form.
- Gangrene and perforation may occur, especially in obstructive appendicitis.
- Perforation may lead to peritonitis (inflammation of the peritoneum) or local abscess formation, depending on the speed and efficiency of the body's defence mechanisms.
- Generalized peritonitis is more common in the very young and the very old where the body is less able to defend itself and the diagnosis is often delayed.

Clinical features

- Abdominal pain and tenderness in the central abdomen at first but then localizing in the lower right abdomen (right iliac fossa) over the appendix itself. The pain may be colicky at first but then becomes dull and constant.
- Unusual positions of the appendix may lead to pain in different sites, causing confusion in diagnosis.
- In congestive appendicitis development may be over a period of days and be preceded by a sore throat and flulike illness, especially in children.
- Obstructive appendicitis has an acute onset over less than 24 h usually.
- Anorexia, nausea and vomiting.
- Furred tongue.
- Slightly raised temperature usually.
- Diarrhoea or dysuria may sometimes occur due to irritation of the rectum or bladder.
- The white cell count is usually raised but may be normal, which can be misleading.
- The patient lies still because movement is painful.

Treatment

- Appendicectomy — removal of the appendix — is the treatment and should be carried out as soon as possible.

- If the patient is very ill with generalized peritonitis and dehydration, surgery may not be immediate and intravenous fluids and antibiotic administration take precedence.
- Wound infection is common and perioperative antibiotics are usually administered.

Complications

- The patient and relatives should be made aware of the possibility of complications before surgery as they may view this as a simple operation that is always straightforward.
- General complications of surgery include DVT, pulmonary embolus and pneumonia.
- Wound infection is very common.
- Pelvic abscess or other collection of pus intra-abdominally.
- Prolonged paralytic ileus may occur following removal of a very dirty appendix.
- Adhesive obstruction can develop months later and be the source of future problems.

The biliary tract

Gall stones

Gall stone disease is known as *cholelithiasis*. The gall bladder is a muscular sac that stores and concentrates bile, made in the liver. The bile is released when the gall bladder contracts on the arrival of a fatty meal in the duodenum. It emulsifies fats before their digestion by lipase enzymes. If bile does not arrive in the duodenum, fats are not digested or absorbed and loose, foul-smelling, fatty stools are passed (*steatorrhoea*). This leads to a lack of absorption of the fat-soluble vitamins (A, D, E and K). Lack of vitamin K leads to inadequate synthesis of prothrombin and problems with blood clotting. This is very important if surgery is necessary in these patients.

Bile leaves the liver via the common hepatic duct, which is joined by the cystic duct from the gall bladder to become the common bile duct. This joins the duodenum with the pancreatic duct at the ampulla of Vater, shown in Fig. 5.8.

Most gall stones in the Western world are predominantly cholesterol mixed with bile pigments and calcium salts (75%—90%). Some (up to 10%) are pure cholesterol. In Asia, however, gall stones are mostly bile pigment only. Radioisotope dating shows that the average gall stone is 11 years old when it is removed!

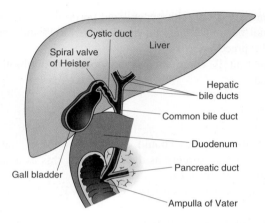

FIGURE 5.8 The biliary system. *From Govan et al., 1993. Pathology Illustrated. Elsevier, reproduced with permission.*

Gall stones develop insidiously, and in Britain at least 10% of the population probably have gall stones, but about 50% of those with gall stones remain symptom-free.

Gall stones are rare in childhood and increase in incidence with age. Women are affected four times as often as men, and it is said that the typical patient is fair, fat, fertile, female and forty! However, many do not fit this description.

The Western diet is believed to play a large part in the formation of gall stones because of its high-fat and poor-fibre content.

When a gallstone moves into the opening of the cystic duct it may block the outflow of bile. This results in pain when the gall bladder contracts and this is known as **biliary colic**. If the cystic duct remains inflamed it may cause acute inflammation of the gall bladder and this is **cholecystitis**.

Clinical features

- Most often the patient presents with pain in the epigastrium or the right hypochondrium. It is often not severe or well defined.
- May present with jaundice, if the gall stone passes into and blocks the common bile duct, thus obstructing the flow of bile into the duodenum. **Choledocholithiasis** is the presence of one or more gall stones in the common bile duct.
- Transient obstruction of the gall bladder by a stone may cause episodes of severe pain that are called **biliary colic.** These may be accompanied with nausea and vomiting.

- Biliary colic episodes (see below) are unpredictable and sporadic. The pain is localized in the epigastrium or right upper quadrant. It may be referred to the right scapular tip. It usually begins after a meal, especially a fatty one and is not relieved by vomiting, antacids, defaecation or changing position and may be accompanied by sweating, nausea and vomiting.
- If the infection persists, an abscess may develop and is called an **empyema** of the gall bladder.
- Obstruction of the pancreatic duct by a gall stone in the ampulla of Vater can trigger pancreatic enzymes and lead to **acute pancreatitis.**

Investigations

- Ultrasound will identify the presence of stones and the thickness of the gall bladder wall. It is not reliable in identifying stones in the duct, especially at the lower end.
- Gall bladder function can be demonstrated by an oral *cholecystogram*. A plain film is taken (control film) and may demonstrate the presence of stones, although only 10% of stones are radiopaque. Immediately after this a contrast medium is taken orally and is excreted by the liver, concentrating in the gall bladder. Twelve hours later, further films are taken. Filling defects can be identified that may be due to stones and the gall bladder may fail to opacify, which may mean a nonfunctioning gall bladder due to inflammatory damage.
- Endoscopic retrograde cholangiopancreatography (ERCP) involves the use of an endoscope to view the biliary duct system.
- Small gall stones can be removed by slitting the sphincter at the lower end and using a balloon catheter or Dormia basket to retrieve them. This may make a potentially dangerous operation unnecessary.
- Percutaneous cholangiography is used if ERCP is not available or is unsuccessful. A fine needle is inserted through the skin into an intrahepatic duct under X-ray control. Contrast medium is then injected and a stone may be identified as a filling defect.

Management

- *Cholecystectomy* (removal of the gall bladder) is the usual treatment for low-grade obstructive gall bladder disease.
- A low-fat diet is prescribed preoperatively and this may help to relieve symptoms, probably by not stimulating the gall bladder to contract as much. It may also lead to some weight loss and this is good in the overweight patient.

Biliary colic

This is caused by sudden and complete obstruction of the cystic duct by a stone. There is severe pain, rising to a crescendo in a few minutes and continuing relentlessly. The pain may last several hours and may end spontaneously or may be relieved by opiate analgesia.

- The patient may vomit.
- No fever is present.
- There is usually a history of similar attacks.

Management

- Patients may be managed at home with opioid analgesia.
- Ultrasound examination should be performed as soon as possible and a cholecystectomy will be done either as an emergency or booked electively.

Acute cholecystitis

This is acute inflammation of the gall bladder. The patient is unwell and often has a fever and is tachycardic. The right upper outer quadrant of the abdomen is tender.

The pain usually lasts for several days before subsiding.

Management

- Ultrasound may show stones and a thickened gall bladder wall.
- Analgesia in the form of *pethidine* or an alternative opioid is usually needed.
- Fluids should only be given orally.
- The patient may be nauseous and vomiting, and an intravenous infusion may be needed.
- An antiemetic may also be administered if needed.
- Antibiotics are usually administered and are given intravenously.
- Cholecystectomy will be needed and some surgeons keep the patient in hospital and perform the operation early. Others prefer to allow the acute episode to settle and bring the patient back for elective surgery in about 6 weeks.

Empyema of the gall bladder

This often presents with a swinging pyrexia, as do other abscesses. The gall bladder may become necrotic and perforate, leading to a subphrenic abscess or generalized peritonitis.

Immediate surgery is needed in empyema.

Bile duct stones

These originate in the gall bladder and pass down the cystic duct. Often they may be small enough to pass through the bile duct and into the duodenum.

They may produce some biliary colic and mild jaundice on their way. This means that recurrent gall bladder disease is common as there may be many stones in the gall bladder. The stone may become lodged in the narrowest part of the common bile duct, just before its entry into the duodenum. It may act as a sort of valve and lead to intermittent jaundice or may become lodged and lead to progressive jaundice. Some stones start off small and develop while actually in the bile duct system, becoming larger all the time.

Sometimes the stones in the bile ducts do not cause symptoms so the surgeon will investigate the bile ducts before surgery and will explore the common bile duct and remove any stones while removing the gall bladder. Following exploration of the bile duct, a latex T-tube drain will be inserted to allow drainage of bile and remain in situ for at least a week so that another cholangiogram can be done to ensure that all stones have been removed. If there are no stones in the common bile duct at operation, it will be closed without a T-tube drain.

Complications of biliary surgery

- Retained stone in the common bile duct.
- Biliary peritonitis caused by bile leaking into the peritoneal cavity.
- Bile duct damage.
- Haemorrhage.
- Ascending cholangitis. This is an infection ascending from the gall bladder and bile ducts upwards to involve the intrahepatic ducts. There will be swinging fever, intermittent pain and jaundice. Drainage is needed as an emergency.

Liver disease

This may be acute or chronic. There may be few signs of acute liver disease apart from jaundice and an enlarged liver. In chronic liver disease, there are many possible clinical features. These include the following:

- Spider naevi may be present on the chest and upper body. These are red spots with a spidery appearance that blanch on pressure.
- The hands may show palmar erythema.
- Asterixis may be present (a flapping movement of the hands).
- The liver may be enlarged at first but becomes small and hard later.
- Gynaecomastia (enlarged breasts) and testicular atrophy may occur in males.
- Clotting factor deficiencies lead to bruising and bleeding tendencies.
- The liver breaks down drugs so these will be metabolized more slowly.
- Jaundice.

- Ascites (fluid in the peritoneal cavity) — abdominal swelling may accumulate over many weeks or over a few days. If ascites is very severe, respiratory distress may occur.
- Mild abdominal discomfort may be present. There may be abdominal distension.
- Peripheral oedema sometimes.
- The patient will feel tired.
- Complications include portal hypertension and oesophageal varices (see p. 319). Seventy per cent of patients with cirrhosis will develop varices but only about one-third will bleed from them.
- Cerebral oedema with raised ICP may result in hypertension and bradycardia.
- Renal failure may occur as hepatic failure progresses.

Hepatic encephalopathy

This is a neuropsychiatric condition secondary to liver failure. It is not fully understood but is believed to be due to the liver failing to clear gut-derived toxins. These have an effect on the brain:

- It may occur in acute liver failure or in chronic liver disease.
- It is graded from Grade 0 (subclinical) to Grade 4 where the patient is in a coma:
  - Grade 0: there is normal mental status but small changes in memory, concentration and intellectual function.
  - Grade 1: there is mild confusion, irritability and disorders of sleep pattern.
  - Grade 2: there is drowsiness, personality changes and lethargy.
  - Grade 3: the patient is sleepy but rousable. Is unable to perform mental tasks and is disorientated.
  - Grade 4: there is coma but there may or may not be response to painful stimuli.
- Exact toxins still not known, but ammonia seems to play a major role and is produced by the breakdown of protein by intestinal bacteria.

Liver failure

The liver loses its ability to regenerate or repair. Presenting features include:

- Ascites
- Jaundice
- Encephalopathy
- Haemorrhagic diathesis

Fulminant hepatic failure

- Severe hepatic failure with encephalopathy that develops within 8 weeks of the onset of the underlying illness.
- It is rare but life-threatening and may complicate acute hepatitis due to any cause.
- There is massive necrosis of the liver tissue.

> ! Paracetamol overdose is the most common cause of fulminant hepatic failure in Britain.

- The patient is jaundiced.
- Mental state varies from slight drowsiness to total disorientation or unresponsive coma with convulsions.
- Signs of chronic liver failure such as ascites may be absent.
- Fever, vomiting, hypertension and hyperglycaemia occur.
- Complications include bacterial infections, gastrointestinal bleeding, respiratory arrest, renal failure and pancreatitis.

Subacute fulminant hepatitis

Development of hepatic failure is slower, over 8–26 weeks.

Chronic decompensated liver failure

The latent period is more than 6 months.

There are more than 600 liver transplants a year undertaken in the UK.

There are many causes of liver failure and some of these are described in the following sections.

The list below is not exhaustive.

- Toxins – alcohol, drug toxicity associated with a variety of drugs, e.g., co-amixiclav and statins, poisoning by mushrooms, herbal remedies, e.g., ginseng, illicit drugs, Reye's syndrome.
- Infections including viral hepatitis, cytomegalovirus and the Epstein–Barr virus.
- Cancer of the liver.

Cirrhosis of the liver

The liver structure becomes irreversibly destroyed by fibrosis. Normal tissue is replaced by scar tissue. Cirrhosis may be the final stage in many chronic liver diseases. It progresses slowly and does not cause symptoms in the early stages.

The liver gradually loses its ability to function normally, and some patients with hepatitis C (HCV) may have chronic hepatitis for 40 years before reaching this stage.

Causes

- Alcohol — the most common cause in the Western world.
- Posthepatitis — especially HCV in the Western world.
- Primary biliary cirrhosis — genetic autoimmune condition, 90% female.
- Nonalcoholic fatty liver disease. The risk factors for this are obesity, diabetes and hypertriglceridaemia.
- Haemochromatosis (increased iron absorption).
- Wilson's disease — inherited disorder of copper metabolism.

Treatment

Treatment is that for chronic liver disease, but the alcoholic must be advised to abstain from alcohol for life. If this is done, the 5-year survival is 90%.

Delirium tremens (withdrawal symptoms) may be treated with diazepam.

Follow-up shows that the majority of patients continue to abuse alcohol.

Neoplasms of the liver

Primary tumour (hepatocellular carcinoma)

- Most commonly occurs in patients who have had hepatitis B (HBV) or HCV and cirrhosis for many years.
- It is rare in the UK because of low rates of infection with HBV and C, but worldwide it is the fifth most common cancer in men and the eighth commonest in women.
- Vaccination for HBV and treatment for HCV should reduce these figures.
- Usually leads to death within 6—20 months. Surgical cure may be possible but in less than 5% of patients.
- Metastases may develop in the lung, brain or bone.

Secondary tumours in the liver

- These are metastases, most commonly from breast, colorectal, stomach, pancreas and lung.
- 30% to 70% of patients dying with cancer may have liver metastases on autopsy.
- The liver receives blood both from the systemic circulation and the portal circulation and so is extremely vulnerable. It is also the largest organ in the body.

- The patient will have lost weight, have pain over the liver and an enlarged liver (hepatomegaly). Ascites may be present.
- Jaundice occurs late, as the cancer blocks bile ducts, and is a very poor prognostic sign.
- Partial hepatectomy or laparoscopic liver resection may prolong survival if there is a single deposit.
- Chemotherapy may also be a treatment option but depends on the primary site.

Jaundice

This is a yellow coloration of the skin and the whites of the eyes. It indicates an excess of bilirubin in the blood:

- Obstructive jaundice occurs when the bile made in the liver does not reach the intestine due to an obstruction of the bile ducts which may be due to gall stones or cancer of the head of the pancreas.
- The urine is dark and the stools are pale.
- The patient may have pruritus (itching).

Conditions causing obstructive jaundice

- Stones in the common bile duct (see p. 341) — the patient will have pain and perhaps a history of gall stones. The jaundice may be progressive or fluctuating as the stone moves.
- Carcinoma of the head of the pancreas — the jaundice is progressive and painless.
- Other tumours such as metastases in the porta hepatis or carcinoma of the gall bladder (rare).
- Intrahepatic bile duct obstruction caused by liver secondaries or cirrhosis.
- As a reaction to certain drugs such as chlorpromazine.

! Biliary obstruction leads to poor fat absorption and so poor absorption of vitamin K (fat soluble). This vitamin is needed for the synthesis of prothrombin and the result is deficient blood clotting. Intramuscular vitamin K is given several days preoperatively, and this is usually sufficient to improve the prothrombin level.

Hepatocellular jaundice is due to liver disease such as hepatitis or cirrhosis, and the liver is unable to deal with all the bilirubin. In acute and chronic hepatitis the stools may be pale and the urine dark. *Haemolytic jaundice* is due to excessive production of bilirubin when there is excessive destruction of red blood cells. The urine and faeces have a normal colour.

> ! Patients with jaundice should always be assumed to represent a high risk for transmission of hepatitis.

Acute viral hepatitis

This may be due to several different viruses. The general features are similar but there is a difference in occurrence and prognosis between the various types.

Hepatitis A

- Transmitted by the faecal–oral route.
- Incubation is about 1 month and carriers have not been detected.
- It is usually a mild illness and flulike symptoms with myalgia (pain in the muscles) occur and tiredness. Mild jaundice occurs later.
- Progression to chronic liver disease does not occur.
- No specific treatment and admission to hospital is not usually necessary.
- Personal hygiene and hand washing are important in preventing spread.
- Immunization is recommended if travelling to certain countries.

Hepatitis B

- The virus is present worldwide with a low prevalence in the UK.
- Spread is by the bloodstream and sexually, e.g., transfusion of infected blood or blood products, contaminated needles with drug addicts, tattooists or acupuncturists, sexual intercourse particularly in male homosexuals. Transmission from mother to child during parturition can occur.
- Acute symptomatic disease or an asymptomatic disease may follow infection.
- Patients may become immune following the disease or they may become carriers.
- Symptoms similar to hepatitis A (HAV), but the illness may be more severe and there may be an immunologic syndrome with a rash and painful joints. Fever is unusual.
- The majority of patients make a full recovery but fulminant hepatitis occurs in 1%.
- Some go on to develop chronic hepatitis and cirrhosis or hepatocellular carcinoma.
- Some become asymptomatic carriers.
- Antiviral treatment may be effective in about one-third of patients. It is initiated by a specialist.
- Drugs include *interferon alpha (IFN-α), entecavir* and *tenofovir.* NICE has issued guidelines on treatment.

- Prevention is by avoiding risk factors and by vaccination.
- Vaccination is available for all healthcare personnel in the UK.

Hepatitis C

- Identified in 1988, HCV is bloodborne and was responsible for causing 70%−90% of posttransfusion hepatitis. From 1991 all donor blood has been screened for HCV, but a large percentage of those with haemophilia in the UK were infected.
- Transmitted intravenously, including by sexual intercourse.
- No vaccine is currently available for HCV.
- Incubation is usually between 6 and 9 weeks and the disease may be acute or chronic.
- Most acute infections are asymptomatic with only about 10% developing flulike symptoms with mild jaundice and a rise in serum aminotransferases.
- Some appear to clear the virus, but more than 75% of patients go on to develop chronic HCV infection.
- Most are not diagnosed until they present years later with abnormal liver enzymes or chronic liver disease.
- Cirrhosis develops in about 10%−20% after 20−30 years and some may develop liver cancer (see p. 348).
- Drug therapy depends on the genotype of the virus and is prescribed by specialists. *Peginterferon alfa* and *ribavirin* combined are used in those above 18 years of age. NICE has produced guidance.

Ascites

This is an excessive accumulation of fluid within the abdominal cavity and has many causes.

For clinical examination to detect ascites, there must be about 1500 mL of fluid present. Larger volumes will present as abdominal distension.

Ultrasound is used to detect small quantities and 500 mL can be detected.

Causes

- Cirrhosis of the liver is the most common cause of ascites. Cirrhosis leads to obstruction in venous drainage from the liver. It is seen in end-stage liver failure alongside peripheral oedema and sometimes pleural effusions due to hypoalbuminaemia.
- Malignancies of the GI tract − stomach, colon, pancreas and liver.
- Cancer of the ovary may lead to the peritoneum becoming 'seeded' with tumour deposits. The malignant cells produce a protein-rich fluid that contains malignant cells and may reach a volume of several litres.

- Severe congestive cardiac failure.
- Severe hypoalbuminuria.

Clinical features

- Abdominal distension
- Weight gain due to fluid retention
- Loss of appetite and nausea
- Discomfort
- Difficulty in breathing as expansion of the lungs becomes impaired

Management

- Treatment of the underlying cause.
- Restricted salt intake may be useful, but not if malignancy is the cause.
- Diuretics — **spironalactone** in cirrhosis as it increases sodium loss. May be combined with **furosemide.**
- Paracentesis may be needed. Fluid is removed from the peritoneal cavity using an aseptic technique. Removal of large volumes of fluid (<5 L) will be followed by administration of a plasma expander or human albumin solution.
- A transjugular intrahepatic portosystemic shunt (TIPS) can be used in patients who need regular paracentesis (more than three times a month).

The pancreas

The head of the pancreas is encircled by the duodenum and the tail lies in contact with the spleen. The pancreas is a fleshy gland with both endocrine and exocrine functions. The endocrine function is described on p. 414.

Pancreatitis

Inflammation of the pancreas.

Acute pancreatitis

- Acute inflammation of the pancreas associated with the release of enzymes that cause autodigestion.
- Associated with gall stone disease, excess alcohol consumption and some other rare causes, such as ischaemia and viruses, e.g., mumps and hepatitis. Associated with hyperlipidaemia.
- Full recovery of the gland usually.
- Mortality varies from 5% in mild cases to 30% in severe cases where there is necrosis and haemorrhage.

Clinical features

- Vary according to severity of the attack.
- Severe, sudden onset of upper abdominal pain that may radiate to the back.
- Pain usually decreases over 72 h.
- Nausea and vomiting usually accompany the pain.
- Diagnosis depends on the serum amylase. If this is raised more than four times the maximal normal value, acute pancreatitis is very likely. Amylase returns to normal in 3–5 days after the attack.

Management

- Nasogastric suction if severe vomiting.
- All feeding is stopped and in severe cases nothing at all is given by mouth.
- Analgesia with an opioid other than morphine. This is because morphine may have a spastic effect on the sphincter of Oddi. *Pethidine* may be used.
- Intravenous infusion to replace fluid and electrolytes.
- Severe cases will need treatment in ICU. Intravenous antibiotics will be given if necrosis is present.

Chronic pancreatitis

- Chronic inflammation that results in permanent damage.
- There may be endocrine or exocrine dysfunction.
- Still not clear whether acute and chronic pancreatitis are linked.
- Majority of cases are due to high alcohol consumption. The disease may arrest if the patient stops drinking.
- Patients who drink normal amounts of alcohol can also develop chronic pancreatitis. It may be excessive free radical formation that leads to the damage.
- Affects males more than females (4:1).
- Abdominal pain is the main symptom and may be almost as severe as acute pancreatitis.
- Some acute episodes appear to be precipitated by alcohol.
- Severe weight loss due to anorexia.
- Steatorrhoea (fatty stools) when lipase is reduced by 90%.
- Development of diabetes is common.

Management

- Stop drinking alcohol.
- Pain control, sometimes needing opioids, but simple analgesics, e.g., paracetamol, are also used.
- Surgery is occasionally used in specialized units for intractable pain.

Carcinoma of the pancreas

- Fourth most common cause of cancer death in the United States and UK, but only 10th most common site for new cancers.
- It is extremely difficult to diagnose in the early stages.
- Incidence increases with age and most are above 60 years old.
- Mostly adenocarcinomas from the ductal epithelium.
- Sixty per cent are in the head of the pancreas.
- Tumour spreads locally to involve the lymph nodes and the liver.

Clinical features

- Painless jaundice due to obstruction of the common bile duct.
- Most patients will have pain as the disease progresses.
- Weight loss.

Diagnosis

- Ultrasound is used.
- CT scan and fine needle biopsy may be done.
- If diagnosed early surgical removal may be possible. Often the tumour is discovered too late for resection to be done.

Management

- Five-year survival poor at about 5%. The median survival time is 4–6 months.
- Surgery is the only route for long-term survival.
- Twenty per cent of cases have a localized tumour, but resection with total pancreatectomy is not always possible due to the elderly age of the patients and comorbidities. After a successful resection, survival is still only 15%–20% at 5 years.
- Jaundice is usually relieved by a palliative bypass procedure, done endoscopically with the placement of a stent through the narrowest part of the common bile duct to allow drainage.
- Analgesia with long-acting morphine should be used.

Cystic fibrosis

- The most common cause of pancreatic disease in childhood.
- Inherited as an autosomal recessive condition. The most common inherited disease in white populations.
- A multiorgan disease with a basic defect in all exocrine glands and thick viscoid secretions.

- Diagnosis is by sweat testing. The sweat has a high sodium content.
- Pancreatic enzymes stagnate in the pancreatic ducts due to dehydration, and bile is concentrated to cause plugging.
- Pancreatic supplements are given and a low-fat diet.
- Reduced mucociliary clearance in the respiratory tract allows bacteria to colonize and results in lower respiratory tract infections with chronic production of sputum.
- May not present in the early years because can digest with only 5% of pancreatic function. Usually present with chest infections. Bronchiectesis may occur.

Management

- Respiratory disease is the main problem and physiotherapy may be needed twice a day.
- Antibiotics for exacerbations.
- Eventually respiratory failure may occur.
- Enteric-coated enzyme preparations are taken before meals.
- Liver disease is a complication in about 30% of cases in adulthood.
- Care is centralized at cystic fibrosis centres and this has resulted in an improvement in life expectancy from about 30 years in 1990 to an esti-mated survival of 40–50 years for a child born today.
- In future, it is hoped that there will be therapies to treat the basic defect. Gene therapy should be possible.

5.5 THE RENAL SYSTEM

The kidneys' main role is the elimination of waste material and the regulation of fluid and electrolyte balance by the formation of urine.

The functional unit of the kidney is the nephron, and there are approxi-mately one million nephrons in each kidney. Each nephron is able to produce urine.

Functions of the kidney

- *Excretory* – elimination of waste products and drugs
- *Regulatory* – control of body fluid volume and composition
- *Endocrine* – production of erythropoietin, renin and prostaglandins
- *Metabolic* – metabolism of vitamin D

Renal disease may be suspected from the following:

- Symptoms in the urinary tract.
- Hypertension.

- Elevated serum urea (from protein breakdown — usually excreted in the urine) or creatinine (from muscle breakdown and also excreted in the urine).
- Abnormalities in urinalysis.

Haematuria is blood in the urine. It may be caused by:

- infection of the urinary tract,
- stones (calculi),
- glomerulonephritis,
- neoplasms anywhere in the renal system,
- polycystic disease,
- trauma,
- warfarin excess.

If there is bleeding only at the end of micturition, this is more likely to have come from the prostate gland or base of the bladder.

Discoloured urine may be seen with:

- Porphyria (a disturbance in the metabolism of the breakdown products of haemoglobin, the porphyrins, which are excreted in the urine, discolouring it).
- Beetroot ingestion.
- Certain drugs (e.g., rifampicin).

Glycosuria is glucose in the urine. It may be caused by:

- diabetes mellitus,
- sepsis,
- renal tubular damage,
- corticosteroids.

Proteinuria is protein in the urine. It may be caused by:

- UTI,
- vaginal mucus contaminating the sample,
- diabetes with nephropathy,
- glomerulonephritis,
- nephrotic syndrome,
- CCF,
- hypertension,
- systemic lupus erythematosus (SLE) — a chronic inflammatory condition of connective tissue, affecting the skin and some internal organs,
- myeloma.

Urine output

In temperate climates the normal urine output is between 800 and 2550 mL in 24 h.

Anuria is failure of the kidneys to produce urine:

- The urine output is less than 50 mL in 24 h.
- Lack of production of urine has to be differentiated from an obstruction in the renal tract preventing the flow of urine.

- Can occur in a variety of conditions that result in a sustained drop in blood pressure.
- It is associated with increasing levels of urea in the blood.
- Haemodialysis may be required.

Oliguria is the production of an abnormally small volume of urine – less than 400 mL in 24 h. It may be due to:

- kidney disease – glomerulonephritis,
- dehydration – profuse sweating associated with physical activity and/or hot weather, diarrhoea,
- loss of blood or other body fluids,
- low cardiac output.

Uraemia is the presence of excessive amounts of urea in the blood. Accumulation of these waste products in renal failure results in:

- nausea,
- vomiting,
- headache,
- lethargy,
- hiccups,
- drowsiness,
- convulsions,
- coma and death if not treated.

The normal range for blood urea is 2.8–7.0 mmol/L.

Urinary tract infection

This is an infection of any part of the urinary tract as shown by the growth of microorganisms from a midstream specimen of urine (MSU).

A UTI is usually defined as the presence of >100,000 organisms per mL of urine and symptoms of genitourinary (GU) inflammation.

Pyelonephritis means the kidneys are involved. **Cystitis** means the bladder is involved. The principal danger is that a lower UTI can travel up towards the kidneys.

UTI is much common in women as their urethra is so much shorter and is nearer the anus.

Predisposing factors

- Urinary stasis which could be due to:
  - Obstruction to urine flow (enlarged prostate, renal calculi)

- • Poor fluid intake and/or excessive sweating
- • Infrequent voiding
- Trauma
- Instrumentation (catheterization, cystoscopy)
- Malformations of the urinary tract
- Diabetes mellitus
- Pregnancy

Causative organisms

The most common is *E. coli* which causes >70% of UTIs outside hospital but <41% in hospital. *Staphylococcus*, *Pseudomonas*, *Streptococcus faecalis* and *Proteus* are other examples.

Infections with less common organisms may occur in those who are immunocompromised, have underlying pathology or who are catheterized. These include *Klebsiella* and *Candida albicans*.

Clinical features of lower urinary tract infection

There are a range of symptoms and some may be asymptomatic:

- Frequency of micturition
- Pain on micturition — 'burning'
- Suprapubic pain
- Pyrexia
- Unpleasant smelling urine — *E. coli* infection smells of raw fish
- Frank haematuria (visible to the naked eye) sometimes

Clinical features of upper urinary tract infection and pyelonephritis

- Clinical features of lower UTI (sometimes)
- Loin pain and tenderness
- Headache, anorexia, malaise
- Pyrexia and rigors sometimes
- Raised pulse rate
- Nausea and vomiting
- Retention of urine sometimes

Management

- Urinalysis — contains blood and protein.
- Obtain MSU before commencement of antibiotics to identify the causative organisms.

- Commence antibiotic therapy — *trimethoprim* or *cephalexin* usually but may need to be changed if the microbiology report shows a lack of sensitivity to the antibiotic.
- Drink plenty — two cups an hour (>3 L daily). Cranberry juice may be useful in *E. coli* infections as it may prevent the bacteria being able to adhere to the bladder wall.
- Intravenous fluids may be needed if not able to tolerate oral fluids.
- Monitor urine output.
- Urinate frequently and not 'hold on' because of pain.
- Care of pyrexial patient.
- Analgesia if needed — pyelonephritis can be very painful.
- Repeated infections must be investigated to detect the cause.

Urethral syndrome or a bacterial cystitis

This occurs only in women and is the presence of urgency, frequency and dysuria (painful micturition) in the absence of readily identifiable bacteria in the urine.

It is induced by cold, stress, intercourse and nylon underwear.

The cause is unknown.

Chlamydia infection and tuberculosis must be excluded.

Renal stones and renal colic

Stones may be made of uric acid, cystine, xanthine, calcium oxalate or calcium phosphate and magnesium ammonium phosphate. The latter follows UTIs, especially those caused by *Proteus*. Passing low volumes of urine due to insufficient fluid intake encourages renal calculi.

Stones vary in size from small gravel-like stones to large staghorn calculi that fill the pelvis of the kidney.

Men are more commonly affected than women (3:1).

Clinical features

- Some large stones may be symptomless if in the kidney, whereas some very small stones can cause intense spasm and pain if in the ureter.
- Stones in the kidney cause loin pain.
- Stones in the ureter cause renal colic, which is a very severe pain that often radiates from the loin to the groin.
- Nausea and vomiting often occur with renal colic.
- The patient cannot lie still and tends to be writhing around in agony or walking about.
- There will be haematuria.

Management

- Pain is extremely severe and analgesia with opioids or a NSAID is immediately required.
- Antibiotics, if indicated. An antiemetic if need.
- *Tamulosin,* an alpha-blocker, may be useful to aid expulsion of the stone.
- Sieve all urine to 'catch' the stone.
- High fluid intake.
- Test urine for blood.
- Send an MSU for culture.
- Investigations − X-ray abdomen, ultrasound, IV urogram.

A small stone will pass spontaneously. A stone may take up to 3 weeks to pass. About one in five stones will not pass spontaneously.

Extracorporeal shock wave lithotripsy may be used. Shock waves are directed over the stone to break it up. The particles are then passed spontaneously.

Percutaneous nephrolithotomy is used for large stones including staghorn calculi.

Lasers may be used to break up the stone via ureteroscopy.

Open surgery is not usually needed, except where other measures fail or there are multiple stones.

Measures to prevent recurrence may need to be taken. These will depend partly on the type of stone, but the patient should be encouraged to raise his fluid intake, especially in summer.

Renal failure

This can present as either acute kidney injury (previously acute renal failure) or as chronic kidney disease (CKD). Those with chronic renal failure may have acute exacerbations where function deteriorates (acute on chronic renal failure).

Acute kidney injury (acute renal failure)

This is an acute failure of renal excretory function, occurring over hours or days, due to depression of the glomerular filtration rate. It may last for days or weeks and is accompanied by a rapidly rising serum urea, creatinine and potassium (K^+).

There is a fall of 25% or more in glomerular filtration rate (GFR).

! Acute kidney injury can cause sudden, life-threatening disturbances in the biochemistry of the blood and is a medical emergency.

Causes

Prerenal

This is a failure of blood supply to the kidneys. It occurs with hypovolaemia and hypotension:

- Haemorrhage
- Burns
- Diarrhoea
- Diuretics

Decreased cardiac output and hypotension is another cause:

- Myocardial infarction
- Massive pulmonary embolism
- Congestive cardiac failure

It also occurs with renal vasoconstriction:

- Sepsis
- Nonsteroidal antiinflammatory drugs

Systemic vasodilatation is also associated with:

- Liver disease
- Sepsis
- Drugs

The kidney is structurally normal but functionally compromised and functions normally rapidly if a good blood supply is restored. However, if severe or prolonged, these factors may lead to **acute tubular necrosis (ATN)**.

Renal

The cause may be renal when there are established structural abnormalities in the kidney:

- ATN, which is due to ischaemia of the medulla of the kidney and is secondary to poor renal circulation. It can be due to renal toxins including some drugs, e.g., aminoglycosides and lithium.
- All the prerenal causes mentioned above can lead to ATN.
- The outcome of the condition depends on the severity and duration of the ischaemia.
- Even relatively mild cases may last for up to 6 weeks.
- Glomerulonephritis.
- Drug-induced nephrotoxicity.
- Interstitial nephritis.
- Malignant hypertension.

- Blood transfusion.
- Preeclampsia and eclampsia.

Postrenal

This is more likely to lead to chronic renal failure:

- Bilateral ureteric obstruction.
- Bladder outflow obstruction, e.g., prostatic enlargement, stones, pelvic mass.

Presentation

- Oliguria (production of an abnormally small amount of urine: <400 mL in 24 h) may be present but not always.
- Early stages may be asymptomatic despite the accumulation of metabolites in the blood.

   There may be a rapid or slow rise in creatinine levels:

- Symptoms are commonly present when the blood urea rises above 40 mmol/L but may occur before this.
- Nausea and vomiting.
- Confusion.
- Loss of appetite.

   More than 90% with ATN show a full recovery of renal function but this is not the case for some other causes.

Management

Optimization of fluid balance

Both hypovolaemia and fluid overload must be avoided. Fluid intake has to be adjusted to ensure the following:

- In hypovolaemic patients, fluid replacement is essential.
- Urine output must be accurately measured hourly and the patient will be catheterized.
- Any other fluid losses such as diarrhoea, sweat and vomit must be charted.
- The patient may be weighed daily to monitor fluid balance.
- If the patient is overloaded, diuretics may be used and fluid intake should be limited.

   Specific measures depend on the causative condition.

Hyperkalaemia

Potassium levels rise in renal failure (hyperkalaemia), and patients will need to restrict their intake.

> ! Fruit and fruit juices are high in potassium.

Hyperkalaemia can lead to cardiac arrhythmias, and the patient will be attached to a cardiac monitor if the serum potassium rises.

Measures may need to be taken to reduce the serum potassium. Calcium resonium is an ion exchange resin that may be used either orally or rectally. In acute renal failure insulin and glucose bring down serum potassium levels faster and may be administered according to a standard regimen.

Acidosis

The pH of the blood is normally kept within the narrow range of 7.35–7.45. If there are excess hydrogen ions that are not being eliminated, the pH will fall and acidosis occurs. This happens in renal failure.

Dialysis

Ureic toxins can be removed by dialysis.

Indication for urgent dialysis

- Severe uraemia above 60 mmol/L.
- Severe acidosis pH < 7.1.
- Pulmonary oedema.
- Hyperkalaemia – K > 6.5 mmol/L (less if ECG changes are present).
- Uraemic pericarditis.

Chronic kidney disease (chronic renal failure)

This is a permanent, progressive reduction in GFR caused by loss of nephrons. It is progressive over a period of months to many years, depending on the underlying pathology.

CKD is common and underdiagnosed. Evidence shows that treatment may slow progression of CKD, but lack of symptoms in the early stages makes diagnosis difficult.

Strategies recommended by NICE (2) (2014) are aimed towards early identification and prevention of progression. Those with diabetes are especially targeted.

There are several recognized stages in CKD from 1 to 5. In Stage 1, there is loss of renal reserve. The GFR is >90 mL/min (normal is 120 mL/min). In Stage 5 the patient requires urgent renal transplantation and the GFR is <15 mL/min. Stage 3 has now been divided into 3A and 3B. The guidelines are available on the NICE website.

In the early stages the plasma urea and creatinine will not be raised, but there is impaired concentrating ability in the kidneys and this eventually leads to polyuria and thirst.

As the condition worsens there will be sodium and water retention. If end-stage renal failure (ESRF) or end-stage renal disease (ESRD) is reached, the patient requires renal replacement therapy in the form of dialysis or transplantation.

Some causes of CKD

- Diabetes mellitus
- Chronic pyelonephritis
- Glomerular nephritis
- Polycystic kidneys
- Hypertension
- Urinary tract obstruction as in prostatic disease
- Multisystem diseases that may involve the kidney, e.g., SLE and RA

Clinical features

The early stages may be asymptomatic. Most symptoms appear when the GFR is reduced to 10–15 mL/min.

Eventually the metabolism of the body becomes very disordered in chronic renal failure, uraemia results and most body systems are affected.

Gastrointestinal tract

- Anorexia
- Nausea
- Vomiting
- Hiccups

Skin

- Itching.
- Uraemic frost – if the urea is very high it may crystallize in the sweat: rare.

Blood

- Anaemia due to reduced erythropoietin and depression of the bone marrow by uraemic toxins.
- Tendency to bleed due to abnormal platelet function – mainly capillaries.

Cardiovascular system

- Hypertension, anaemia and fluid retention may lead to heart failure.
- Increased incidence of coronary artery disease due to abnormal fat metabolism.

Bones

Renal osteodystrophy is caused by:

- increased bone resorption and
- inadequate vitamin D production.

  And it may cause:

- bone pain and
- occasionally pathologic fractures.

Nervous system

- Accumulation of toxic metabolites leads eventually to uraemic neuropathy.
- Poor concentration, apathy, insomnia and irritation occur at first.
- Slurring of speech, tremors and seizures may occur eventually if untreated.
- Peripheral neuropathy may occur in the late stages of renal failure.
- In children, failure to grow is an important complication.

Management

The aim is to prevent any further decline in renal function:

- Treatment of underlying factors — hypertension, infection.
- Control of blood pressure with antihypertensive agents reduces the rate of progress of CRD.
- Removal of nephrotoxic drugs from medication.
- The client will be under the care of the dietician, and the risks and benefits of dietary protein restriction will be discussed.
- Patients may have a negative salt and water balance which needs correcting. High fluid intake allows excretion of metabolites despite inability to concentrate the urine. Until end stage is reached a normal fluid intake (1.5–2 L daily) is usually good. Dehydration should be avoided.
- Salt in the diet is kept to a minimum as it can cause increased blood pressure and fluid retention.
- Fluid restriction may be needed in patients with oedema.
- Potassium intake is restricted to reduce hyperkalaemia. Occasionally calcium resonium may be prescribed (see above).

- Anaemia can be treated with synthetic (recombinant) human erythropoietin.
- Patient education and involvement in care help to prepare for the future and the possibility of dialysis or transplantation.

End-stage renal failure

This is terminal renal failure and occurs when the kidney function is so poor that the patient requires dialysis or renal transplantation to survive.

Renal replacement therapy

The aim is to mimic the excretory functions of the normal kidney, including the excretion of nitrogenous waste such as urea and the maintenance of fluid and electrolyte balance.

Haemodialysis

The blood from the patient is pumped through a dialyser which is a collection of semipermeable membranes ('artificial kidney'). These bring the blood into close contact with the dialysing fluid and the biochemistry of the blood changes towards that of the dialysate due to diffusion of molecules down their concentration gradient. The concentration gradient is maintained by replacing used dialysis fluid with fresh solutions.

An adult of average size usually requires 4–5 h of haemodialysis three times a week, which may be performed in hospital or by home dialysis.

All patients are anticoagulated, usually with heparin, as contact with foreign surfaces activates clotting mechanisms.

Haemofiltration

This removes plasma water and its dissolved constituents such as K^+, Na^+, urea and phosphate by convective flow across a high-flux semipermeable membrane and replaces it with a solution of desired biochemical composition. It can be used for acute or chronic renal failure. High volumes need to be exchanged to achieve adequate removal, and in acute renal failure 1000 mL/h is exchanged. It is often performed on very sick patients in intensive care units.

Peritoneal dialysis

This is used for less severe renal failure. Continuous ambulatory peritoneal dialysis (CAPD) is being increasingly replaced by haemodialysis.

In peritoneal dialysis, the dialysate is fed into the peritoneal cavity via a flexible tube and the peritoneum itself acts as the semipermeable membrane. The catheter remains in place permanently.

In CAPD, 2-L exchanges are performed three or four times a day. This technique is easy to learn and in chronic renal failure the patient can use it at home.

Nightly intermittent peritoneal dialysis may be used to perform exchanges while the patient is asleep. Sometimes the dialysate is left in the peritoneal cavity during the day.

Bacterial peritonitis is the most common severe complication of peritoneal dialysis. Infection with *Staphylococcus epidermidis* is responsible for about 50% of cases. Treatment is with peritoneal antibiotics.

Back pain, malnutrition and constipation may also be problematic.

Transplantation

The only complete rehabilitation in ESRF is successful renal transplantation. Graft survival is 80% at 10 years in some units and may be up to 50% at 10–30 years. The replacement kidney can be obtained from cadavers or close relatives with ABO compatibility and close HLA matching.

Graft rejection is reduced by giving long-term immunosuppressive therapy with **corticosteroids, azathioprine, tacrolimus** and **ciclosporin**. These drugs must be taken for life and require careful monitoring.

Glomerulonephritis

This is an inflammatory response within the kidney due to the deposition of immune complexes in the glomerulus. The cause is often unknown but antigens derived from certain viruses or bacteria are sometimes involved.

Some causes of glomerulonephritis

- Beta-haemolytic streptococcus
- *Streptococcus viridans* (infective endocarditis)
- Mumps virus
- HBV virus
- Tropical infections, e.g., schistosomiasis
- SLE
- Malignant tumours
- Drugs, e.g., **penicillamine**

Clinical features

Glomerulonephritis presents in one of four ways:

- Asymptomatic proteinuria/haematuria
- Acute nephrotic syndrome (acute glomerular nephritis)
- Nephrotic syndrome
- Renal failure

Acute glomerular nephritis

This is often a poststreptococcal nephritis. It typically develops in a child, 1—3 weeks after a streptococcal sore throat. The antigens from the bacteria become trapped in the glomerulus, leading to acute glomerulonephritis.

There is an abrupt onset.

Clinical features

- Haematuria (macroscopic or microscopic)
- Proteinuria
- Hypertension
- Oedema — around eyes but may also in feet and ankles
- Oliguria
- Uraemia

Treatment

- Antibiotics to clear up any remaining infection.
- Good prognosis and spontaneous recovery usually takes place.
- Hypertension is treated with salt restriction, diuretics and vasodilators.
- Fluid balance is monitored by daily weighing and a fluid chart.
- Fluid restriction may be necessary if oliguria is present.
- In some cases due to SLE, steroids, e.g., prednisolone, may be given as immunosuppressants.

Nephrotic syndrome

This is not a disease but a triad of symptoms:

- Heavy proteinuria (>3.5 g/24 h)
- Hypoalbuminaemia
- Oedema — severe and affects the eyes, face, ankles and genitals

Blood lipids are usually raised.

All types of glomerulonephritis can cause the nephrotic syndrome. Other damage to the basement membrane in the glomerulus can also be responsible, e.g., advanced diabetic nephropathy.

When present as a secondary complication of renal disease, the prognosis is usually more severe.

Of those who have a remission, approximately 30% relapse within 3 years.

Treatment

- In children a renal biopsy may not be necessary as most cases are secondary to acute glomerulonephritis. In an adult, a renal biopsy is often undertaken to establish the cause.
- Oedema is treated with rest, salt restriction and diuretics.

- Diuresis must not be too vigorous or it may precipitate circulatory collapse.
- Steroids are usually given, especially in children.
- The diet is normal protein, low salt and low fat.
- Occasionally albumin replacement may be necessary.
- The underlying cause, if known, should be treated.

Urological tumours

Renal tumours in children

Wilms' tumour is thought to arise from embryonic renal tissue and accounts for more than 90% of tumours under the age of 20 years.

Renal cell carcinoma

This is the most common type of renal tumour in adults. Benign tumours are rare.

About 2% of all are malignant. Peak incidence is between 60 and 80 years. Males are affected more than females (2:1).

Clinical features

- Classic triad of features includes frank haematuria, loin pain and a loin mass. This is seen less now as ultrasound picks up the renal tumour when the patient is being investigated for nonspecific features such as weight loss, hypertension, anaemia, fatigue and peripheral oedema.
- Thirty per cent of patients have hypertension due to secretion of renin by the tumour.
- CT renal scanning is done with MRI or renal ultrasound if needed.
- Intravenous urogram (IVU) may be needed to show any obstruction to flow.
- Spread of the tumour is into adjacent structures such as the adrenal glands, liver, colon and spleen.
- The tumour may extend into the renal vein and from there to the vena cava.

Treatment

- Surgery — a radical nephrectomy for a unilateral tumour.
- Radiotherapy and/or chemotherapy may be used alongside surgery.
- Lung metastases are quite common. Sometimes a single tumour in the lung can be resected.

Transitional cell carcinoma of the renal pelvis and ureter

- Haematuria and renal colic are the presenting signs.
- Treatment is a nephroureterectomy.
- Postoperative radiotherapy may be given.
- Check cystoscopies as transitional cell carcinoma can recur around the ureteric orifice.

Carcinoma of the bladder

- Male:female ratio is 3:1. Median age is 68 years.
- 5000 deaths per year.

Noninvasive papillary tumour – bladder warts

- May be single or multiple.
- Haematuria is the first symptom is most cases.
- Five to ten per cent progress to become invasive.

Carcinoma in situ

- Confined to the epithelium.
- Thirty to fifty per cent progress to invasive. Most recurrences are in the first 2 years.
- Can be multifocal.

Invasive carcinoma

- Sixty per cent have no previous history of bladder tumours.
- Lymphatic involvement and spread via the lymphatics.

Risk factors

Associated with smoking and exposure to aniline dyes as well as urinary stasis.

Treatment

Cystoscopic resection and regular cystoscopic follow-up for superficial tumours.

For invasive tumours, options will depend on the tumour and include the following:

- Radiotherapy
- Cystoprostatectomy (removal of the bladder and prostate gland)
- Partial cystectomy

5.6 THE NERVOUS SYSTEM

The nervous system consists of:

- the central nervous system — the brain and spinal cord (Fig. 5.9) and
- the peripheral nervous system — somatic and autonomic nervous systems.

The brain

The brain is divided into the forebrain, midbrain and hindbrain. The forebrain is called the cerebrum and is the largest part. It receives and interprets sensory input and is responsible for motor output.

There are two cerebral hemispheres. A lesion of one hemisphere shows its effects on the opposite side of the body. The left is the dominant hemisphere in

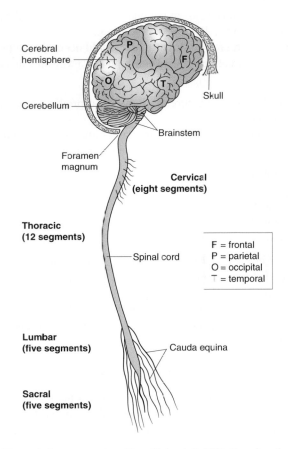

FIGURE 5.9   The central nervous system. *From Bickerstaff, 1978. Neurology for Nurses. Arnold, London. Reproduced by permission of Edward Arnold (Publishers) Ltd.*

all right-handed people and also in 70% of those apparently left-handed. The speech area is in the dominant hemisphere.

Clinical features of lesions of the cerebral hemispheres depend on the focus of a cerebral lesion. Abnormalities depend upon the following:

- The lobe affected by the lesion
- How large the lesion is
- How deeply it extends into the brain

Destruction of the motor area in the frontal lobe produces a *hemiplegia* — paralysis down one side of the body. A lesion in the occipital lobe will affect vision. A parietal lobe lesion will affect sensation on the opposite side of the body:

- *Aphasia* is loss of or defect in language and is caused by lesions that affect the speech area (usually the left frontoparietal region).
- *Dysphasia* is difficulty in speaking and is very common following a stroke if the damage is to the left side of the brain.
- *Dysarthria* is disordered articulation that could occur due to problems with facial muscles or weakness and is common in Parkinson's disease (PD), for instance.

An irritative lesion of the cerebral cortex can produce convulsions of the opposite side of the body.

The cerebellum is responsible for maintaining posture and balance. A lesion may produce the following on the same side of the body:

- Decreased muscle tone
- Reduced tendon reflexes
- Flexor plantar reflexes
- Intention tremor
- Marked ataxia

There are 12 cranial nerves that originate in the brain. Neurologic disease can affect any of these. The cranial nerves are detailed in Table 5.6.

Papilloedema is swelling of the optic disc seen through the ophthalmo-scope. It may be an early sign of a tumour in the brain but is also seen in oedema of the brain, accelerated hypertension, optic neuritis and subarachnoid haemorrhage (SAH).

Clinical signs of damage to nervous tissue

- Destruction leads to paralysis or loss of sensation.
- If there is damage to the motor system, weakness or wasting of the muscles will result. If damage is to the sensory system, tingling or pain may result.

TABLE 5.6 Cranial nerves – some lesions affecting their functions

Nerve number	Name	Controls	Lesion causes	Caused by
I	Olfactory	Smell	Loss of smell	Head injury Tumour of optic groove
II	Optic	Vision	Visual field defect or loss of sight	Compression in pituitary tumour or aneurysm Papilloedema Optic neuritis
III	Oculomotor	Eye movements	Unilateral complete ptosis, eye facing down and out, fixed and dilated pupil	Aneurysm, coning of the temporal lobe, tumour
IV	Trochlear	Eye movements	Diplopia	Isolated lesion rare
V	Trigeminal	Sensory for light and touch Motor for mastication	Sensory loss in face, reduced corneal reflex Pain in trigeminal neuralgia	MS, brainstem glioma and other tumours, aneurysm Trigeminal neuralgia – unknown cause
VI	Abducens	Eye movements	Convergent squint with diplopia	MS, compressed in raised ICP May be infiltrated by nasopharyngeal cancer
VII	Facial	Muscles of facial expression	Unilateral facial weakness	Bell's palsy, trauma, infection of middle ear, tumours, herpes zoster

Continued

TABLE 5.6 Cranial nerves – some lesions affecting their functions—cont'd

Nerve number	Name	Controls	Lesion causes	Caused by
VIII	Vestibulocochlear	Hearing, balance and posture	Deafness and tinnitus Vertigo Nystagmus	Ménière's disease Middle ear infection Noise Vestibular neuritis
IX	Glossopharyngeal	Sensation to throat and taste	Usually IX and X together	Glossopharyngeal neuritis – painful throat on swallowing – rare
X	Vagus phagus	Muscle of pharynx (gag), larynx and oesophagus Parasympathetic supply, swallowing, to heart and gut	Loss of gag reflex Depression of cough reflex Paralysis of vocal cords Difficulty in choking and hoarseness	Motor neuron disease Cancer of nasopharynx Polyneuropathy Brainstem infarct
XI	Accessory	Motor to trapezius and sternomastoid	Weakness of rotation of head and neck	Motor neuron disease Cancer of nasopharynx Polyneuropathy Brainstem infarct
XII	Hypoglossal	Motor to tongue	Unilateral weakness, wasting and fasciculation of the tongue	Motor neuron disease Cancer of nasopharynx Trauma to the neck

Motor neurons

Lesions may affect the upper motor neuron, between the brain and spinal cord, or the lower motor neuron, between the spinal cord and the muscle. Clinical features of upper and lower motor neuron disease are shown in Fig. 5.10 and Table 5.7.

Lesions of the peripheral nerves

These are mostly mixed nerves that carry both motor and sensory fibres. Each supplies a specific muscle group and has an area of skin from which sensation is carried. Damage to the nerve will lead to weakness in a group of muscles and a patch of analgesia and anaesthesia.

Sometimes many nerve endings may be diseased together and symptoms will be present in the periphery of all four limbs. This occurs in diabetic neuropathy, polyneuritis and other causes of peripheral neuropathy.

Lesions of the spinal cord

Complete destruction at any point causes paralysis and loss of sensation to all parts of the body supplied by nerves leaving or entering the cord below the level of the lesion. A lesion in the cervical spine will paralyse the arms, legs and the respiratory muscles if high enough.

If there is partial damage to the cord a variety of clinical features are present affecting both movement and sensation.

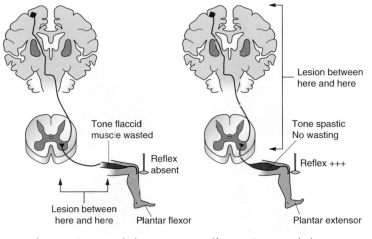

FIGURE 5.10 Clinical features of upper and lower motor neuron disease. *From Bickerstaff, 1978. Neurology for Nurses. Arnold, London. Reproduced by permission of Edward Arnold (Publishers) Ltd.*

TABLE 5.7 Some signs of upper and lower motor neuron disease

	Upper motor neuron	Lower motor neuron
Wasting	Slight	Very marked
Weakness	Could be any degree	Usually marked
Muscle tone	Increased (spastic)	Decreased (flaccid)
Tendon reflexes	Exaggerated	Absent
Plantar reflexes	Extensor	Flexor
Flexor spasms	Common	Do not occur
Fasciculation	Absent	Common if cells involved

Trauma

The skull provides very good protection but may be fractured by a severe blow. The fracture may be:

- simple,
- compound,
- comminuted,
- depressed (Fig. 5.11).

The type of fracture is of little consequence as it is the damage to the brain that is important.

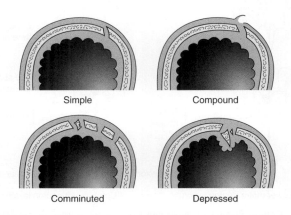

Simple   Compound

Comminuted   Depressed

FIGURE 5.11   Different types of skull fracture. *From Bickerstaff, 1978. Neurology for Nurses. Arnold, London. Reproduced by permission of Edward Arnold (Publishers) Ltd.*

Extradural haematoma

Follows trauma and is usually due to rupture of the middle meningeal artery following fracture of the temporal or parietal bone. There is a collection of blood in the potential space between the bone and the dura and it usually collects and enlarges fairly quickly (Fig. 5.12).

The patient may be knocked unconscious and classically recover full consciousness rapidly, but within a few hours start to deteriorate and:

- feel drowsy,
- develop paralysis down one side of the body,
- have one pupil dilated due to pressure of the expanding haematoma,
- require emergency surgery to remove the clot.

If left untreated, the patient may die. A large haematoma will require burr holes and evacuation. A small haematoma may be treated conservatively, and the patient is kept under close observation.

Mortality remains high if the patient is unconscious on admission.

The classical presentation above is not always present, and a haematoma in the skull may produce any of the following:

- Headache.
- Nausea or vomiting.
- Seizures.
- Raised ICP causing bradycardia and hypertension.
- CSF (cerebrospinal fluid) oozing from the nose (rhinorrhoea) or the ear (otorrhoea). This may follow a tear in the dura mater.
- Altered level of consciousness and a deteriorating Glasgow Coma Score.
- Weakness of the limbs.
- Unequal pupils.
- Focal neurologic deficits such as aphasia, ataxia or visual field deficits.

Subdural haematoma

A collection of clotting blood in the subdural space between the dura and the arachnoid mater. It may be acute and occur 3—7 days after the

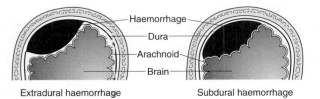

Extradural haemorrhage   Subdural haemorrhage

FIGURE 5.12 Extradural and subdural haematomas. *From Bickerstaff, 1978. Neurology for Nurses. Arnold, London. Reproduced by permission of Edward Arnold (Publishers) Ltd.*

initial injury, subacute (3–7 days after injury) or chronic (2–3 weeks after injury):

- Usually caused by a blunt head injury that may have been minor.
- Fine arteries between the arachnoid and the dura mater are damaged.
- May also be caused by tearing of the bridging veins in the subdural space. This occurs more commonly in infants and may be associated with non-accidental injury.
- Alcoholics are at risk because of low platelet counts and susceptibility to blunt head trauma.
- Anticoagulation therapy is also a risk factor.
- Tension on the bridging veins caused by cerebral atrophy puts the elderly more at risk.
- An acute SDH usually presents soon after a moderate to severe head injury.
- A chronic SDH may take 2–3 weeks to present. Blood collects slowly and symptoms tend to be gradually progressive.
- The patient may have forgotten the primary injury which may have been trivial (especially if taking anticoagulants).
- Increasing headache is usually present on presentation.
- There may be a history of anorexia, nausea and sometimes vomiting.
- An evolving focal neurologic deficit may be present, e.g., limb weakness.
- Personality changes and/or increasing drowsiness or confusion may occur.
- Treatment is by surgical evacuation of the clot.

Traumatic subarachnoid bleeding

- The vessels between the arachnoid and pia maters may be torn and bleeding into the subarachnoid space occurs.
- On recovering consciousness the patient will have severe headache and stiffness of the neck that gradually improve.

Subarachnoid haemorrhage

This is a spontaneous intracranial haemorrhage where the bleeding occurs into the subarachnoid space between the arachnoid and pia maters.

SAH only accounts for about 5% of all strokes but affects younger people and carries a 50% mortality.

The mean age is around 50 years and 10%–15% die before reaching hospital.

It is usually due to a weakness in the vessel wall. An aneurysm or bulge may be present in one of the cerebral arteries in the circle of Willis. It is called a *berry aneurysm* because of its shape and was thought to be congenital. It is now believed that hypertension and atherosclerosis may play a role in the occurrence of some berry aneurysms. SAH is due to berry aneurysms in 70% of cases, 10% are due to arteriovenous malformation and in 20% no lesion is found.

Risk factors include hypertension, smoking and excessive alcohol intake.

Clinical features

- The patient may be young and have a history of headaches or may rapidly develop a devastating occipital headache that spreads down the back of the neck. It may only last a few seconds or a fraction of a second and feels as though the person has been hit on the head. It is the severity of the headache that is typical.
- Vomiting occurs.
- *Photophobia* (dislike of the light) is present.
- Neck stiffness.
- Restlessness and irritability occur.
- Seizures may occur.
- There is often loss of consciousness.
- If small, the blood will be reabsorbed but if large, paralysis and death can follow.

Investigations

- CT scan.
- Cerebrospinal fluid (CSF) may be pink because of the blood it contains but lumbar puncture is only done if the CT scan is negative and no contraindications are found.
- Carotid and vertebral angiography to establish the site of bleeding before surgery.
- Needs to be differentiated from severe migraine and meningitis.

Management

- Immediate treatment is aimed at preventing further bleeding and reducing the risk of complications such as cerebral ischaemia.
- *Nimodipine* is commenced. This is a calcium channel blocker and is shown to reduce spasm of the cerebral blood vessels and thus ischaemia.
- Hypertension will be treated.
- Patients unconscious or with severe neurologic deficits have a poor prognosis.
- Neurosurgery may be performed to clip the neck of the aneurysm and prevent further bleeding. Insertion of an endovascular coil is replacing clipping in posterior circulation aneurysms as it is associated with a lower mortality.

Epilepsy

People who have epilepsy show a tendency to have recurrent seizures (also known as fits) with little or no provocation. Epilepsy is not a disease; it is a disorder or condition. A seizure is an altered chemical state of the brain leading to bursts of excessive electrical activity within it.

Some causes of epilepsy

- Head injury
- Brain infection, e.g., meningitis
- Stroke
- Brain damage — could be birth trauma or hypoxia
- Drugs and alcohol
- Biochemical imbalance
- Hormonal changes
- Cerebral palsy
- Brain tumour
- Fifty per cent have no known cause.

Causes of individual seizures

- Forgotten or incorrect medication.
- Lack of sleep
- Stress
- Excitement
- Boredom
- Alcohol
- Flashing lights (only 3%–5% of people with epilepsy are photosensitive)
- Drugs

Common types of seizure

Generalized

- Tonic-clonic — used to be known as grand mal.
- Absence — used to be known as petit mal.
- Tonic.
- Atonic.
- Myoclonic.

Partial (focal)

- Simple partial — no impairment of consciousness.
- Complex partial — with impairment of consciousness.
- Secondary generalized — starts as partial but evolves to tonic-clonic.

There are also *febrile convulsions* in children with a high temperature. *Pseudoseizures* are of behavioural or psychologic origin.

Management

Emergency treatment of a seizure is to ensure that the patient does himself no harm and that the airway is patent.

Anticonvulsant drugs are used for long-term treatment. Examples are **phenytoin, sodium valproate, lamotrigine** and **carbamazepine**. Ideally the epilepsy should be controlled with one drug.

Status epilepticus

This is when seizures follow each other for 30 min or longer without any recovery of consciousness or it may be a generalized convulsion lasting 30 min or more. It is a medical emergency and there is a risk of death from cardio-respiratory failure.

It is necessary to stop the fitting, and rectal **diazepam** or buccal **midazolam** may be used. The rectal route is easier when the patient is convulsing continuously. It may be extremely difficult to give a drug intravenously at this stage. If seizures continue, treatment includes intravenous **lorazepam** rather than diazepam, as it is shown to reduce the risk of status continuing.

In refractory status, patients may need to be anaesthetized and ventilated.

Parkinson's disease

This is the most common cause of progressive neurologic disorder in older patients. It is increasing in incidence alongside longevity. You will meet many patients with PD on care of the elderly wards.

It is a disorder of movement, and the main features are a tremor at rest and rigidity (Fig. 5.13).

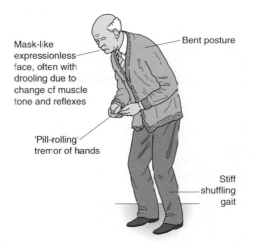

Mask-like expressionless face, often with drooling due to change of muscle tone and reflexes

Bent posture

'Pill-rolling' tremor of hands

Stiff shuffling gait

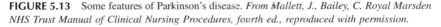

FIGURE 5.13 Some features of Parkinson's disease. *From Mallett, J., Bailey, C. Royal Marsden NHS Trust Manual of Clinical Nursing Procedures, fourth ed., reproduced with permission.*

It is due to a loss of nerves in an area of the brain called the substantia nigra. These cells are in the basal ganglia, an area of the brain that has a role in regulating motor function. The cells here use a neurotransmitter called *dopamine* and in PD there is a reduced ability of the cells in the substantia nigra to manufacture dopamine.

Dopamine is one of two transmitters produced and usually they are in balance. The other one is *acetylcholine* (ACh). When there is a reduction in dopamine, this means that the ACh has excessive action. The symptoms of PD are due to a decline in dopamine and a relative excess of ACh. PD is progressive but with the treatments now available, life expectancy is near normal.

The loss of cells from the substantia nigra and the progress of the disease occur at variable rates and to a variable extent. Some patients may become rapidly disabled in a few years and others may have a mild, slowly progressive disorder that does not need treatment for several years. The majority of cases fall in between these two extremes and the condition slowly becomes more incapacitating over a period of about 10 years.

Aetiology

PD is common worldwide but the aetiology is not completely understood. In Britain, it affects 1:1000 of the population and has a prevalence rate of about 1 in 200 above the age of 70. Males and females are equally affected. In two-thirds of cases the first symptoms occur between the ages of 50 and 60 years.

Most cases are idiopathic, i.e., the cause is not understood, but there are likely to be some environmental elements alongside a genetic risk of developing the disease.

Drug-induced Parkinsonism is caused by drugs that block the dopamine pathway or dopamine receptors. Such drugs are the antipsychotics such as **haloperidol** and some antiemetics such as **metoclopramide**.

Other causal factors include the following:

- Postinfective following encephalitis
- Intracranial tumours
- Ischaemia (lack of blood supply) in that part of the brain perhaps due to atherosclerosis
- Cerebral atrophy
- Trauma − often over a long period, e.g., boxing
- Toxic substances:
  - Copper: Wilson's disease
  - Manganese and mercury also when used in industrial processes
  - Carbon monoxide
  - MPTP: an impurity formed when opioids are manufactured illegally. In the 1970s, in California, there was an epidemic of young people with rapidly progressive PD following administration of illegal heroin.

Clinical features

It is believed that there is a long presymptomatic phase in PD and the dopamine produced by the brain is reduced by 70%–80% before any symptoms appear. The onset is thus insidious with a peak occurrence between the ages of 55–65 years.

Tremor

- Present at rest at first and reduced or eliminated by movement. It usually starts in one hand or arm and takes 2–3 years to spread to the other hand and arm.
- The tremor is rhythmic in nature and may be described as a 'pill-rolling movement'. It is less marked when the patient is involved in activity and is absent in sleep, but is increased by stress, fatigue and cold. It eventually spreads to include the lips, face, tongue and lower limbs.
- Although the tremor is rarely disabling it is very upsetting for the patient and a cause of embarrassment and anxiety. It may limit the amount of socializing the patient feels able to do and such activities as eating out may be curtailed.

Rigidity

- This may occur in virtually all skeletal muscle and throughout the full range of movement of the joints. Rigidity may be present in the limbs, trunk and neck.
- In the limbs it has a 'cogwheel' effect and also affects actions such as turning in bed. Satin-type sheets may help here.
- Fine movements such as fastening buttons become difficult.
- As the disease progresses there is a stooped posture, and the body and head are flexed forward. The acceleration present in the steps when walking may now lead to falls.

Bradykinesia (slowness or poverty of movement) and akinesia (lack of spontaneous movement)

These are present as a slowness of voluntary movement and reduced automatic movements:

- At first this leads to a difficulty with fine movements such as fastening buttons.
- The hands no longer swing on walking or hand swinging is reduced.
- The writing becomes smaller.
- When the legs are affected this leads to a 'shuffling gait'. The patient starts walking slowly but then speed builds up — *festinating gait.*

- Hesitation at doorways and difficulty in entering.
- Need to make a deliberate effort to initiate all movement.
- As spontaneous movement declines there is a mask-like expression.
- The eyes do not blink and there is a staring expression.
- The speech becomes a monotone and dysarthria occurs. Speech is weak and slurred.
- There is difficulty in eating and increased salivation. This is embarrassing and tends to lead to a desire to eat alone.
- There are slow reaction times.
- Later the cough reflex may be lost and chest infections occur.
- Fatigability of repeated movements.
- Difficulty in performing two movements at once, e.g., rising from a chair and shaking hands.

Postural instability

This makes turning difficult and there is poor balance on standing and moving. This may result in frequent falls.

Parkinson's disease dementia

This is dementia occurring more than 1 year after the diagnosis of PD. It is similar to Alzheimer's disease but is also associated with frequent visual hallucinations and fluctuations in lucidity. It is difficult to treat as some of the drugs used in PD are dopamine agonists and may worsen the problem.

Common problems

- Constipation due to lack of exercise and problems with chewing and swallowing as well as actual problems in defecation, sometimes due to spasm of the sphincter.
- It becomes difficult to cut up food, and eating a meal takes a long time.
- As there is loss of control of hand movement, it may be difficult to prevent spillage.
- Excessive salivation adds to the embarrassment of the patient.
- Due to muscular rigidity and paucity of movement, there are problems with chewing and swallowing, so the patient needs encouragement to eat and a diet that can be easily managed.

Communication

- The same person is still there inside a body that feels as though it will no longer do what is asked of it.
- This means there is still a strong desire to communicate and show facial expressions such as smiling.

- The presence of a mask-like expression and the inability to respond rapidly to conversation, together with a monotonous slow voice, mean that the patient may become introverted and avoid company.
- Education of those around the client will enable them to understand the condition and so promote better communication.

Depression

This may accompany the disease and may be partly due to the chronic nature of the illness and its effect on social activity. Doctors may treat this with antidepressant drugs with reasonable success in some patients.

> ! Always remember that the client with PD usually has an active mind locked inside a body that will not allow communications such as facial expression and talking clearly.

Drug treatment of Parkinson's disease

> ! No drugs alter the course of the disease but symptoms do improve dramatically initially.

The aim is to increase the amount of available dopamine in the brain.

The drugs are not used until necessary to avoid unnecessary side effects of the medication. There is also a problem that some medication is very effective for a period of time but then effectiveness decreases.

Selegiline prevents the breakdown of dopamine in the brain and is often used as the first-line treatment. It may delay the need for levodopa for several months.

The introduction of *levodopa* in the 1960s revolutionized the treatment of PD. Although it is dopamine that the brain is lacking, it cannot be given as treatment as it does not pass the blood—brain barrier and remains in the peripheral circulation. Levodopa is the precursor of dopamine, and it does get into the brain. It is converted into dopamine by an enzyme in the brain tissue. It is given with an agent to prevent its conversion to dopamine in the peripheries. This reduces the side effects of the drug. *Madopar* or *Sinemet* are the usual tablets.

Multiple sclerosis

Multiple sclerosis (MS) is a chronic inflammatory disease of the central nervous system with unknown cause. Areas of discrete demyelination develop at many sites in the brain and the spinal cord. It is one of the most common causes of neurologic disability amongst people under the age of 50. The disease usually presents between 20 and 40 years of age. It affects 1 in 2000 of the population in this country but less than 1 in 100,000 in equatorial regions. The highest incidence in the world is in Orkney and Shetland.

Lesions develop at different sites at different times, usually with some capacity for regeneration and restoration of function. Remyelination is never complete and the new myelin is thinner than the old.

The sizes of the plaques vary and ongoing disability is variable. Nerve conduction in the affected axon is slow and inefficient.

The disease usually takes the form of relapses and remissions but in some cases a slowly progressive deficit occurs.

Aetiology

- Cause is not known.
- Believed to be an autoimmune disorder.
- Common in females than males − ratio 1.5:1.
- Increased incidence in close relatives − about 10-fold.
- More common in temperate than equatorial regions. Those who move to a low-risk area before puberty acquire low risk. If they move after puberty, they do not.
- Higher consumption of animal fat in high-risk areas.
- Some antibodies, e.g., to the measles virus, are higher in those with MS. *Chlamydia* has been questioned as a possible cause.

Clinical features

- The onset may be acute or insidious and because of the highly variable distribution of the plaques, signs and symptoms are varied.
- A common first symptom is blurring of vision due to a lesion affecting the optic nerve. Colour vision may be affected. Recovery usually occurs in 4−8 weeks and 5 years later, the patient often has difficulty remembering which eye was affected.
- Twenty-five per cent of patients present with visual symptoms.
- Thirty per cent of those with optic neuritis have no other evidence of MS and do not go on to develop the disease.
- Brainstem demyelination may cause diplopia, vertigo, facial numbness and dysphagia.

If a lesion affects the spinal cord it most often interferes with the legs and may cause:

- Heaviness, dragging or weakness of arms or legs.
- Loss of pain and temperature sensation.

- Tingling, numbness, sense of coldness, sense of skin wetness in arms or legs.
- Bladder or bowel dysfunction:
  - Spastic bladder: frequency, urgency, precipitance of micturition, ultimately incontinence.
  - Spastic bowel: constipation.
- Remissions may last for many years and their length is unpredictable.
- Fatigue and depression both may be problems as the disease progresses. Intellectual function is usually preserved.
- Features are often worse in hot weather, after a hot bath, during fever and after exertion.

Prognosis

- Seventy-five per cent relapse and remit.
- Twenty per cent have no significant disability after 5 years.
- Average life expectancy is 20—30 years.
- Five per cent of cases are rapidly progressive and fatal within 5 years.
- Poor prognostic factors are late age of onset, development of dementia and early ataxia.
- There is relative protection from the disease in pregnancy but an increase in the proportion of attacks in the postnatal period.

Investigations

- MRI identifies the plaques readily but may still not be conclusive in the early stages of the disease.
- CSF examination is not usually needed but cells and protein are often raised.

Treatment

- A potentially disabling disease with no curative treatment. Wide variations in severity and course of the disease. Research is building momentum; however, and there are new disease-modifying therapies beginning to become available. Some, e.g., laquinimod, are in their final stages of testing and may hold new hope for MS sufferers.
- Treatments include drugs that aim to modify the disease process, steroids to prevent relapse, drugs to ease symptoms and therapies to minimize disability.
- NICE have produced guidelines for the treatment of multiple sclerosis in the community. These are available at their website (www.nice.org.uk). They advise that linoleic acid 17—23 g/day may reduce the progression of disability. Linoleic acid is found in sunflower, corn and soya.

- Corticosteroids in an acute episode may promote remissions and probably relieve oedema and inflammation in the plaques. They have no effect on the long-term outcome of the disease and do not protect against a further relapse.
- Drugs to modify the disease process are immunomodulatory agents. They include interferon beta-1a, interferon beta-1b, **glatiramer** and **natalizumab.**
- Interferon is a naturally occurring protein in the body which protects us against viruses and has been manufactured in several forms using genetic engineering. It has been shown to reduce disability progression and exacerbations in some patients. Side effects include flulike symptoms and the injection should be given at bedtime. Beta-interferon by injection has been used in relapsing and remitting disease, defined as at least two attacks of neurologic dysfunction over the previous 2 or 3 years followed by a reasonable recovery and who are able to walk unaided.
- Glatiramer acetate is an immunomodulating drug licensed for reducing the frequency of relapses in ambulatory patients with MS who have had at least two clinical relapses in the past 2 years.
- Natalizumab is a more recent treatment and is reserved for patients with more advanced and very active MS. It is a monoclonal antibody that inhibits the migration of white cells into the CNS.
- None of these drugs cure MS. They may slow progression slightly and reduce relapses.
- Treatment is always by a specialist according to guidelines from the Association of British Neurologists.
- There is a website for patients (www.msdecisions.org.uk) to help patients decide what the best therapy is for them.
- There is debate as to the effectiveness of cannabis in MS.
- Other treatment is symptomatic and supportive.
- Muscle relaxants, e.g., **baclofen**, benzodiazepines and **dantrolene** reduce the pain and discomfort of spasticity.
- Infection may be associated with worsening disability, and immunization against influenza should be offered.

Motor neuron disease

This is a progressive degenerative disease of unknown cause which affects the upper and lower motor neurons in the brain and spinal cord. It leads to progressive paralysis and eventual death:

- The cause is unknown and it affects 6 in 100,000 of the British population. Links to an abnormality of mitochondrial function have been made and there is one rare familial form of the disease.
- Pathology is not inflammatory and there is no evidence to indicate an immune mechanism.

- Searches for toxic factors have been fruitless.
- Onset is uncommon before the age of 40 years, and men are affected about twice as frequently as women.
- The mean survival is 3 years; 20% may live 5 years or more, but it is doubtful if this is the same disease.
- The sensory system is not involved.
- There is degeneration of the anterior horn cells of the spinal cord and the lower motor neurons in the cranial nerves.
- Upper cranial nerves controlling eye movements and motor nerves to the bladder and bowel sphincters are spared.
- The disease has a focal onset but becomes more generalized with time.

There are three main patterns of presentation.

Amyotrophic lateral sclerosis

- This is the classical form of the disease. It is usually focal with one group of muscles affected first. The onset is in the limbs usually.
- It is a disease of the lateral corticospinal tracts and produces a spastic paralysis.
- There is a mixture of upper and lower motor neurone features.
- Amyotrophy means atrophy of muscle which would be unusual in other forms of spastic paralysis.

Progressive muscular atrophy

- This is rarer and gives lower motor neuron symptoms.
- Wasting may begin in the small muscles of one hand and then spread through the arm. May begin unilaterally but soon spreads to both sides.
- Fasciculation is common and fibrillary twitching occurs.
- Cramps may occur.

Motor neurone disease with bulbar onset (progressive bulbar palsy)

- Bulbar − relating to the medulla oblongata. Palsy − paralysis.
- Lower motor neuron degeneration only may occur here. More usually both upper and lower motor neuron degeneration occurs.
- Results in dysarthria, dysphagia, choking and regurgitation of fluids as common symptoms.
- This form is common in women than men for an unknown reason.

Prognosis

- Remission is unknown.
- The disease progresses, spreading gradually and causing death.

- Survival for more than 3 years is most unusual.
- Awareness is preserved and dementia is unusual.
- Sphincter disturbances do not usually occur. If they do, it is very late in the disease.
- There is progressive respiratory paralysis and, together with aspiration pneumonia, this is the usual cause of death.

Treatment

- The only drug to help is *riluzole*, and this may prolong life by 2–4 months. NICE has issued guidance on its use.
- Patients remain alert, and drug treatment to alleviate distress is indicated.
- Antispasmodics may help with the pain due to spasticity.
- Antidepressants may help with associated depression.
- Noninvasive ventilation may be used overnight in sleep and has proved extremely helpful.
- Most patients die in their sleep as a result of increasing hypercapnia.

Delirium (acute confusional state)

This is a clinical syndrome where impaired consciousness is associated with abnormalities of perception or mood. It involves abnormalities of thought and perception as well as levels of awareness. Impairment of consciousness is variable and often fluctuates. It is usually acute in onset and intermittent.

It can be avoided in many cases, and lack of awareness leads to missed diagnosis and a poor outcome.

Confusion is often worse at night and there may also be hallucinations and delusions. Restlessness and aggression may be present.

It can present in hypoactive or hyperactive forms. The hypoactive form may be difficult to recognize and may be confused with apathy and depression. The patient becomes withdrawn, quiet and sleepy.

Delirium is a common complication of hospitalization in the elderly and also has a higher prevalence in those with a malignancy or HIV. Hip fracture and operative procedures following this may lead to delirium as may ICU admission.

Treatment with certain drugs may be linked to delirium. These include anticonvulsants, opioids, anxiolytics, hypnotics, steroids, anti-Parkinsonism medications and anticholinergics.

Management

Clear communication and involvement of family and carers will help.

The environment should be kept stable including light and temperature.

Drugs used to treat delirium may lead to worsening of the delirium but the use of antipsychotics such as *haloperidol* or *olanzapine*, short term (usually 1 week or less) can help in selected patients.

NICE have produced clinical guidance on the treatment of delirium. This is available on their web site at www.nice.org.uk.

Dementia

This is a chronic or persistent disorder of mental processes and is due to organic brain disease. It is marked by memory loss and disorders, personality changes, impaired ability to reason and disorientation. Consciousness is not affected but social functioning is impaired.

It affects up to 10% of those aged 65 years or above and 20% of those above 80 years of age. It is very low below the age of 55 years.

There are many causes but the most common is Alzheimer's disease, accounting for nearly 70% of cases. Other causes include vascular dementia, alcoholism, hypothyroidism and PD.

Alzheimer's disease

This is a degenerative condition of the brain, the cause of which is still not clear. There is a gradual reduction in neurons in parts of the brain and the deposition of amyloid plaques.

Clinical features

- Insidious onset (slow) that progresses over several years.
- Memory loss is usually the first sign.
- Slow disintegration of personality and intellect occurs.
- Difficulty with performing familiar tasks such as preparing a meal.
- Problems with language and word use.
- Disorientation to time and place.
- Poor and decreased judgement, e.g., may wear lots of jumpers on a hot day.
- Problems with abstract thinking.
- Misplacing things — putting things in unusual places.
- Changes in mood and behaviour — can show rapid mood swings.
- Changes in personality — may become very dependent on one person.
- Loss of initiative and desire to do things — may sit for hours in front of the television.
- All aspects of cortical function are eventually affected.

Investigations

- CT scanning will demonstrate cerebral atrophy and will exclude some other possible causes that could be curable, e.g., depression, adverse drug reactions and metabolic changes or nutritional deficiencies.

- There is no single diagnostic test. The patient needs a comprehensive assessment.
- Examination of the brain at autopsy will confirm.

Care and management

- It is important to always respect individuality. NICE have produced guidance for the care of those with dementia (www.nice.org.uk).
- The promotion of independence is vital and both patients and carers will need support appropriate to their needs.
- Although there is no cure for the disease, medical and social management can help all concerned.
- For those close to the patient it is hard to see their relative changing into perhaps an unrecognizable person with a different personality and weak intellectual ability.
- Management should be in the community if at all possible and support should be given to carers.

Medication in Alzheimer's disease

Anticholinesterase (AChE) inhibitors are drugs that prevent the breakdown of acetylcholine in the brain and may slow down the decline in some patients and improve memory.

Drugs include *donepezil* (Aricept), *rivastigmine* (Exelon) and *galantamine* (Reminyl). NICE has produced guidance on the use of these drugs in Alzheimer's disease. They are prescribed in mild to moderate Alzheimer's disease. Treatment should be initiated by a specialist. Benefit should be assessed by cognitive assessment after 3 months. The drug should be discontinued if the patient is not responding.

Memantine is an NMDA antagonist and is an alternative where AChE inhibitors are not tolerated.

Infective and inflammatory disease

Meningitis

This is inflammation of the meninges and underlying subarachnoid CSF. It may be caused by bacteria, viruses, fungi, drugs and contrast media or blood (following SAH). Usually refers to infection by microorganisms, which reach the meninges by direct spread from the ears or nasopharynx, via a cranial injury or by spread in the bloodstream.

Bacteria causing meningitis include:

- Group B streptococci
- *Neisseria meningitidis* (meningococcus)

- *Haemophilus influenzae*
- *Streptococcus pneumoniae*
- *Myobacterium tuberculosis*

Viral meningitis is more common and usually less serious than bacterial.

It occurs in all age groups but more commonly in infants, young children and the elderly.

There is no licensed vaccine against serogroup B meningococcus which is now the most common cause of bacterial meningitis (and septicaemia) in the UK.

Clinical features

Headache, neck stiffness and fever constitute the meningitic syndrome:

- Acute bacterial meningitis has a sudden onset with rigors and a high fever.
- Severe headache, photophobia and vomiting are often present.
- Should be considered for all patients who have a headache and fever.
- Consciousness is not usually impaired, although the patient may be delirious.
- A petechial rash is evidence of meningococcal meningitis and septicaemia.
- Drowsiness and loss of consciousness signal complications such as venous sinus thrombosis, severe cerebral oedema or cerebral abscess.
- Mortality is about 15% even with treatment. The earlier the antibiotics started, the better the prognosis.
- In fulminant meningococcal septicaemia there are often large ecchymoses (bruises) and gangrenous skin lesions may occur.

Invasive meningococcal disease

May present with meningitis, septicaemia or both.

Generalized nonblanching, petechial rash in an ill child is suggestive of meningococcal septicaemia. If this is present without meningitis, there will be no stiff neck, back rigidity, bulging fontanelle, photophobia or seizures.

There may be cold hands and feet, fever, altered consciousness and skin mottling.

Urgent intravenous antibiotics are needed. Benzylpenicillin is the drug of choice, unless the patient is allergic to this. Antibiotic treatment is now started by paramedics, such is the urgency.

Diagnosis

- Confirmed by lumbar puncture unless there are signs of raised intracranial pressure.
- The CSF is cloudy due to the presence of pus. It is also sent for protein and glucose level tests as well as microscopy. White cells in the CSF will be

raised, protein will be raised and glucose may be low in the presence of bacteria.
- Blood cultures before antibiotic therapy.

Management

- If the diagnosis is suspected, intravenous antibiotics must be started immediately.
- Treatment is started with *cefotaxime* or *benzylpenicillin.* Those allergic to penicillin are given *chloramphenicol.*
- Subsequent antibiotic treatment depends on the CSF microscopy which tells us what the bacteria are sensitive to.
- In bacterial meningitis dexamethasone (a steroid) is given with, or soon after, the first dose of antibiotic. Steroids have been shown to reduce some of the complications of meningitis including deafness. There is no evidence that they reduce mortality.
- All cases of meningitis must be notified to the local public health authority.

Meningococcal prophylaxis

Oral *rifampicin* is given to very close contacts to eradicate nasopharyngeal carriage of the meningococcus.

Viral meningitis

Usually a benign and self-limiting disease that lasts 4—10 days. Headache may continue for several weeks, but there is no long-term damage.

Encephalitis

This is inflammation of the brain parenchyma (functioning part of the brain) which may be caused by a virus or bacteria. In HIV infection, opportunistic organisms (e.g., *Toxoplasma gondii*) are important. It may occasionally be due to other conditions such as toxins and autoimmune disorders.

Acute viral encephalitis

Most viral infections in childhood are able to cause encephalitis. Herpes simplex is the most common causal virus in the UK. Others include herpes zoster (chickenpox), mumps, measles and the Epstein—Barr virus (glandular fever).

Clinical features

- Headaches and drowsiness
- Flulike illness

- Similar symptoms to meningitis — neck stiffness, fever, headache, vomiting
- Sometimes severe with hemiparesis and dysphasia, seizures and coma
- Prognosis is poor if the patient is in a coma
- Herpes simplex when severe has the worst prognosis

Investigations

- Viral serology.
- CT scan — shows oedema.
- EEG may show slow wave activity.

Treatment

Herpes simplex, if suspected, is immediately treated with intravenous *aciclovir*.

Anticonvulsants and sedatives may be needed in some cases.

Cerebral abscess

The causes are shown in Box 5.5, but often no direct cause is found.

Intracranial abscesses are uncommon, but are life-threatening.

Causative bacteria may be *streptococci, staphylococci* and *enterobacter.* Sometimes a chronic abscess may be due to tuberculosis.

Clinical features

- Fever
- Seizures
- Focal neurologic signs
- Raised intracranial pressure

BOX 5.5 Causes of a cerebral abscess

Direct spread of microorganisms	Spread in bloodstream
Skull fracture	Lung in bronchiectasis
Focus of infection in paranasal sinuses	Heart in endocarditis
Focus in middle ear	Bone in osteomyelitis

Care and management

- Intravenous antibiotics
- Surgical drainage

Intracranial tumours

These make up 10% of all tumours and 20% of childhood cancers. Primary brain tumours do not usually metastasize outside the brain but spread by local infiltration and may seed into the subarachnoid space or ventricles. They carry significant mortality and have the effects of any space-occupying lesion (SOL). Neurones cannot replicate and so primary brain tumours affect the connective tissue in the brain. Many brain tumours are metastases from primary tumours elsewhere in the body, e.g., breast, lung.

Primary tumours

High grade

- Gliomas:
  - Astrocytoma — the most common
  - Oligodendroglioma
  - Glioblastoma multiforme (GBM)

Low grade

- Meningioma — the most common
- Neurofibroma
- Pituitary tumours
- Acoustic neuroma

Secondary tumours

From:

- Lung
- Breast
- Prostate
- Thyroid
- Colon

Clinical features

- Headache
- Altered mental function
- Convulsions

- Focal neurologic deficit
- Raised ICP may produce:
  - Early morning headache
  - Vomiting
  - Papilloedema
  - Hypertension
  - Bradycardia
  - Decreased conscious level

Investigations

- CT or MRI scanning.
- Biopsy or CSF examination for histology.
- If cerebral metastases are suspected then investigate for the primary tumour, e.g., chest X-ray.

Management

This will depend on the tumour and the prognosis. Dexamethasone is a steroid that reduces cerebral oedema and is given to all patients with raised ICP or focal signs. It can produce outstanding improvements, with the unconscious patient often recovering consciousness.

Surgery is the best treatment where possible.

If surgery is not possible, radiotherapy should be considered — it may be curative for some tumours and prolongs survival in others.

Chemotherapy gives relief in some tumours and is important alongside radiotherapy in palliative care.

Astrocytoma

- Differ in histologic grade — a low-grade tumour has a 5-year survival of about 50%, high grade has 5%.
- Surgery — may be repeated in low-grade tumours.
- Radiotherapy mostly in unresectable low-grade tumours.
- Chemotherapy — CCNU, a fat-soluble drug that crosses the blood–brain barrier, is the basis of treatment.

Glioblastoma multiforme

This is the most common brain tumour in adults and carries a very poor prognosis.

The mean age of occurrence is 55 years.

Surgery is used but the tumour is usually infiltrative, and so complete removal is not possible.

Radiotherapy improves survival.

Temozolomide is an antineoplastic drug used in the treatment of newly diagnosed GBM in adults.

Analgesia, anticonvulsants, anticoagulants and corticosteroids are also used.

Survival at 1 year is about 30% in a high-grade tumour.

Meningioma

- Tumour of the meninges of the brain.
- Very slow growing and usually benign.
- Interval to recurrence following surgical excision is about 4 years.
- Surgery is usually the mainstay of treatment, and radiotherapy is limited to those patients in whom surgical excision was incomplete or recurrence occurs.
- Prognosis is usually very good.

Hydrocephalus

This is an excessive amount of CSF occupying the ventricles in the cranium. It may occur when there is obstruction to the flow of CSF and is very rarely due to an increased production of CSF. In children, it is due to a congenital malformation of the brain, meningitis or haemorrhage. In adults it may be due to:

- late presentation of a congenital defect,
- cerebral tumour,
- SAH,
- meningitis,
- head injury.

Clinical features

- Headache
- Vomiting
- Papilloedema
- All caused by raised ICP
- May also be nystagmus

Treatment is usually surgical with the insertion of a shunt to drain the CSF.

Diseases of voluntary muscle

These are the myopathies. Weakness is the dominant feature. Some may be congenital, e.g., muscular dystrophy, some are inflammatory and some may be associated with drugs, toxins and endocrine weakness.

Muscular dystrophy

This is the most common myopathy.

Duchenne muscular dystrophy is the most common form of the disease with an onset in childhood.

Weakness occurs in myopathy with reduced muscle strength.

Acquired myopathies

These are secondary to other diseases especially metabolic or endocrine disease.

Thyroid disease, parathyroid disease, corticosteroids and biochemical causes such as potassium deficiency (hypokalaemia) may cause a generalized flaccid weakness if severe.

Drug-induced myopathy

This may occur when the patient is taking statins to reduce their plasma cholesterol.

Myasthenia gravis

This is an acquired autoimmune disease, where antibodies attack and destroy the nicotinic acetylcholine receptors at the neuromuscular junction. This leads to skeletal muscle weakness and fatigue that improves with rest. The thymus gland is enlarged in about 70% of those under 40 years and a thymic tumour is found in about 10%.

Clinical features

- Fatigability.
- Proximal limb muscles, eye muscles and muscles of mastication and facial expression are those most commonly involved.
- In 65% of cases the eye muscles are the first to be involved.

Care and management

- The anticholinesterase drug ***pyridostigmine*** is used in the early stages.
- The dose is determined by the patient's response.
- In those under 45 years with severe disease, thymectomy may be performed.
- Immunomodulating drugs such as azathioprine and corticosteroids do lead to improvement in some cases.

5.7 THE ENDOCRINE SYSTEM

The endocrine system, alongside the nervous system, is responsible for control and communication within the body. The glands are ductless and release their secretions directly into the bloodstream to act upon a target organ that may be far away from the gland itself.

The pituitary gland

Although it is normally only the size of a pea, the pituitary gland secretes many vital hormones, the majority of which are important in the control of other endocrine glands. It is often known as 'the leader of the orchestra' or the master endocrine gland and is attached beneath the hypothalamus in a bony cavity (sella turcica) at the base of the skull. Pituitary hormones are shown in Table 5.8.

TABLE 5.8 Pituitary hormones

Hormone	Function
Anterior pituitary	
Growth hormone (GH or somatotropin)	Stimulates the growth of long bones Increases protein synthesis
Adrenocorticotrophic hormone (ACTH)	Controls secretion of corticosteroid hormones from the adrenal cortex
Melanocyte-stimulating hormone (MSH)	Stimulates the production of melanin
Thyroid-stimulating hormone (TSH)	Stimulates the production of thyroid hormones by the thyroid gland
Gonadotrophins 1. Luteinizing hormone (LH) 2. Follicle-stimulating hormone (FSH)	Stimulates ovulation, corpus luteum formation and the production of progesterone Stimulates androgen synthesis in the testes Stimulates the ripening of follicles in the ovary Stimulates the formation of sperm in the testes
Prolactin	Stimulates milk production after childbirth
Posterior pituitary	Hormones are synthesized in the hypothalamus but stored and released from the pituitary
Vasopressin (antidiuretic hormone − ADH)	Increases the reabsorption of water by the kidneys and so prevents excessive water loss from the body Also constricts the blood vessels
Oxytocin	Causes contraction of the uterus in labour Stimulates the flow of milk from the breast

Diseases of the posterior pituitary gland

These are rare and are usually related to antidiuretic hormone (ADH) secretion.

Diabetes insipidus

- This is due to insufficient ADH.
- Leads to polyuria and polydipsia.
- It is most often due to a lesion in the hypothalamus or posterior pituitary gland. This would include tumours, aneurysms, thrombosis and infections.
- The person has either partial or total inability to concentrate the urine.
- Total urine output varies between 4 L and 12 L per day.
- Usually there is an acute onset and dehydration may develop rapidly if fluids are not replaced.

   Clinical presentation:

- Polyuria
- Nocturia
- Thirst — especially a desire for cold drinks
- Low urine osmolality
- High plasma osmolality

   Treatment:

- Replacement therapy with a synthetic vasopressin analogue — desmopressin (DDAVP) — may be needed.
- Oral hydration is often sufficient.

Pituitary tumours

These are usually benign, slow-growing adenomas. Symptoms may arise due to:

- over- or under secretion of the hormones secreted by the pituitary gland,
- pressure on the surrounding tissues,
- infiltration of the tumour.

Overproduction

The tumour secretes the hormone of the cell type from which it arose. This is no longer beneficial to the body and is not under control of normal feedback mechanisms:

- Growth hormone excess results in acromegaly or gigantism.
- Prolactin excess.
- Cushing's disease from excess adrenocorticotrophic hormone (ACTH).

Underproduction

- This is due to pressure on the cells by the growing tumour.
- Leads to hypopituitarism.
- Progressive loss of hormones.
- Luteinizing hormone and follicle-stimulating hormone are usually affected first, resulting in menstrual irregularity and amenorrhoea.
- Growth hormone (GH) loss may be silent except in children.
- Thyroid-stimulating hormone (TSH) and ACTH are usually last affected, resulting in hypothyroidism and Addison's disease.
- ADH secretion is affected if the tumour extends to the hypothalamus.

Local effects

- Headaches.
- Visual loss with field defects. This is caused by pressure on the optic chiasma (where the optic nerves from the eye cross over in the brain). It can lead to blindness.
- Obesity and altered appetite and thirst due to involvement of the hypothalamus.
- Seizures.
- Early puberty may occur in children due to hypothalamic involvement.
- Hydrocephalus may result from an interruption in the flow of CSF.

Diagnosis

- Radiographic examination of the skull and CT scan in conjunction with contrast material.
- Laboratory evaluations.

Treatment

Surgery and radiation therapy are used.

Hypersecretion of growth hormone

- In a child, this leads to gigantism. In an adult, this leads to acromegaly.
- Relatively rare disorder.
- Fifteen per cent of pituitary tumours do secrete growth hormone, and the most common cause of acromegaly is a pituitary adenoma.
- Occurs more frequently in women than men.
- Slow progressive disease which, if untreated, results in a decreased life expectancy.
- There is an increased risk of hypertension, LVF and diabetes mellitus.
- Headache and other symptoms of an SOL may be present.

Diagnosis
Measurement of serum GH.

Treatment
Removal of the tumour or treatment with radiation therapy.

Thyroid gland
The activity of the thyroid gland affects the whole body. It is involved in the control of body metabolism and its hormones govern cellular oxygen consumption and thus all heat and energy production. It produces the hormones thyroxine (T_4) and tri-iodothyronine (T_3). Thyroxine is the hormone produced in the greatest quantity and its release is stimulated by TSH from the pituitary gland.

Goitre
A goitre is an enlargement of the thyroid gland and may be due to either increased or decreased activity of the thyroid or a lack of iodine needed to synthesize thyroid hormones. It is common in women than men.

The thyroid may enlarge at puberty and in pregnancy, but this is often associated with normal activity (*euthyroidism*) and does not warrant treatment.

It is often first noticed as a cosmetic defect and is usually painless. Large goitres can cause dysphagia (difficulty in swallowing) and difficulty in breathing when they compress the oesophagus or trachea.

Endemic goitre was common in areas where iodine content in the soil was low. It was so common in Derbyshire that it became known as 'Derbyshire neck'. Iodine is now added to foods, e.g., table salt, and endemic goitre is virtually unknown.

Hyperthyroidism (thyrotoxicosis)
This is due to increased activity of thyroid hormones, whatever the cause. It leads to:

- an increased metabolic rate,
- heat intolerance,
- increased tissue sensitivity to stimulation by the sympathetic nervous system.

Causes

- Excess thyroid hormones are produced by the thyroid gland:
  - Graves' disease — autoimmune and familial
  - Toxic nodular goitre

- Thyroid cancer
- Increased TSH secretion
- Drugs — amiodarone
- Acute thyroiditis
- Ectopic thyroid tissue (outside the thyroid gland)
- Ingestion of excessive thyroid hormone

Clinical features

All forms of thyrotoxicosis share some common characteristics. These are shown in Fig. 5.14.

Endocrine

- Enlarged thyroid gland (97%—99% of cases).
- Increased breakdown of cortisol.
- Hypercalcaemia (see p. 209) and decreased parathyroid hormone levels.
- Decreased sensitivity to insulin due to increased degradation of insulin.

Gastrointestinal

- Weight loss despite increased appetite.
- More frequent passage of less-formed stools due to increased peristalsis.
- Decreased blood lipid levels due to malabsorption of fat.

Skin — due to the hyperdynamic circulation

- Excessive flushing and warm skin
- Heat intolerance
- Sweating
- Fine, soft hair and sometimes temporary hair loss

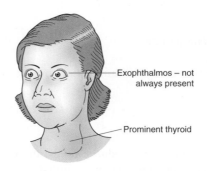

FIGURE 5.14   Some features of thyrotoxicosis. *From Govan et al., 1993. Pathology Illustrated. Elsevier, reproduced with permission.*

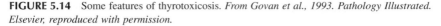

Cardiovascular

- Tachycardia at rest (raised sleeping pulse rate)
- Increased cardiac output
- Palpitations and AF, especially in the elderly

Respiratory

- Breathlessness

Nervous system

- Hyperactivity and restlessness
- Insomnia
- Short attention span
- Tiredness
- Fine tremor

Eyes

- In Graves' disease there is exophthalmos — protrusion of the eye balls.
- Elevated upper eyelid — leads to lack of blinking and staring expression.
- Oedema of the conjunctiva.
- Retro-orbital inflammation and oedema, probably caused by antibodies, lead to protrusion of the eyes.

Graves' disease

This is the most common form of hyperthyroidism and is an autoimmune disorder where antibodies bind to the TSH receptor and stimulate the production of thyroxine. It is associated with other autoimmune disorders such as myasthenia gravis and pernicious anaemia. It affects more women than men, mostly between the age of 20 and 40 years.

The thyroid is enlarged (goitre) and there is exophthalmos. The condition may relapse and remit.

Diagnosis of hyperthyroidism

Clinically, a mild case may be difficult to differentiate from an anxiety state. Diagnosis may be obvious but treatment will never be started without biochemical tests, some of which are shown in Table 5.9. TSH is suppressed, T_3 and T_4 are raised.

TABLE 5.9 Thyroid function tests	
Test	Results
Total thyroxine (T$_4$)	Low in hypothyroidism Raised in thyrotoxicosis
Total T$_3$	Raised in thyrotoxicosis
TSH (thyroid-stimulating hormone) (immunoradiometric assay)	Suppressed in thyrotoxicosis Hypothyroidism Hypothalamic-pituitary disease

Ultrasound may be used to determine the size and shape of the gland and whether there is any tracheal compression present.

Treatment of hyperthyroidism

Three possible treatments are available:

- Antithyroid drugs — most cases initially
- Radioactive iodine
- Surgery

Beta-blockers can be given for rapid symptom control as many of the symptoms are mediated via the sympathetic nervous system. Propranolol 40–80 mg every 6–8 h may be used but should be avoided in asthma. The beta-blockers are stopped when a euthyroid state is obtained. If patients cannot tolerate beta-blockers, calcium channel blockers may be used.

Antithyroid drugs

Carbimazole 10–20 mg every 8 h inhibits the formation of thyroid hormones. It is also an immunosuppressive agent. Improvement may not be seen for 10–20 days, although synthesis is reduced rapidly, thyroxine has a long half-life of 7 days (this means it is only eliminated slowly from the body).

Beta-blockers are used for more immediate symptomatic control.

The production of thyroxine may be blocked totally by carbimazole and a replacement regimen of thyroxine tablets, 0.1 mg daily, given. This is continued for 18 months and then reviewed.

The major side effect of carbimazole is a potentially fatal, but reversible, agranulocytosis (1 in 1000 patients within 3 months of commencement of treatment). Regular white cell counts (every 3 months) must be done during drug therapy. Patients must come for a FBC if they develop a sore throat.

As an alternative, the dose of carbimazole may be reduced after 4–6 weeks, according to the levels of thyroid hormones. Review in 2–3 months and reduce again. Gradually over 12−18 months the dose is reduced to 5 mg daily and then when the patient is euthyroid on this, it is discontinued.

About 50% of patients will relapse and a repeat course of carbimazole or other forms of treatment, including surgery, will be considered.

Radioactive iodine therapy

- Administered orally in doses 100 times higher than those used for scanning.
- Can be used in patients of any age.
- The radioactive iodine is rapidly taken up by the gland, and emission of radiation then destroys it.
- Very simple but results are slow to take effect and unpredictable.
- Late underactivity of the gland may occur, requiring thyroxine.
- Small theoretical risk of inducing malignancy.
- Absolutely contraindicated in pregnancy due to damage to the fetus.

Surgery

Subtotal thyroidectomy

Indications for surgery:

- When quick and effective cure is required, especially in the young with Graves' disease.
- When antithyroid drugs have been unsatisfactory due to persistent side effects or noncompliance.
- More effective in some types of nodules and goitres.

Preoperative care:

- Vocal cord function is assessed by indirect laryngoscopy. This looks at the function of the recurrent laryngeal nerve, which can occasionally be damaged in the operation.
- There may be a change in voice quality after any thyroidectomy, and the patient should be warned of this.
- Whenever possible, patients should be rendered euthyroid before surgery.
- If they are thyrotoxic, there are anaesthetic risks such as cardiac arrhythmias.
- Also, when the gland is manipulated in the operation, there can be a massive release of thyroid hormone into the bloodstream. This precipitates a thyroid crisis, which may be lethal.
- Thyroid activity is reduced by antithyroid drugs such as carbimazole in the weeks before surgery. Beta-blockers may also be used if control is difficult.
- Antithyroid drugs increase the blood flow to the thyroid and so are stopped 10−14 days before surgery. Potassium iodide (Lugol's iodine), 60 mg three times daily, is given by some surgeons to reduce the vascularity of the gland, although its efficacy is unproven.

Partial thyroidectomy The aim is to remove enough of the gland to render the patient euthyroid while leaving enough of the gland to prevent hypothyroidism.

Complications of thyroid surgery

- In theatre, uncontrolled haemorrhage is possible, but rare.
- Unilateral or bilateral damage to the recurrent laryngeal nerve in the operation presents as a laryngeal obstruction after tracheal extubation. It necessitates the performance of an immediate tracheostomy.

Immediate postoperative complications:

- Major haemorrhage may cause severe blood loss and tracheal compression. This presents as a rapid swelling of the neck and a large volume of blood loss via the wound drain.
- To avoid suffocation from bleeding, a clip or suture-removing pack must always be at the patient's bedside for emergency reopening of the wound.
- Emergency surgical exploration is essential to find the bleeding point.
- Laryngeal oedema – presents as stridor and may necessitate intubation.
- Thyrotoxic crisis – abrupt onset of extreme agitation and confusion, hyperpyrexia, profuse sweating and rapid tachycardia or arrhythmia. It requires emergency treatment with beta-blockers, intravenous hydrocortisone and potassium iodide.
- The mortality is 10% from coma, pulmonary oedema or circulatory collapse.

Late postoperative complications:

- Hypoparathyroidism due to erroneous removal of the parathyroids, normally embedded in the four poles of the thyroid. This presents with muscle cramps, paraesthesia and tetany within 36 h of operation.
- Unilateral recurrent laryngeal nerve damage – presents as hoarseness and defective cough.
- Superior laryngeal nerve damage leads to a change in quality of the voice.

Long-term complications:

- Hypothyroidism.
- This may be overlooked, as it develops slowly and insidiously. Loss of energy, weight gain, depression and an intolerance of cold weather are symptoms. Treatment is with thyroxine for life.

Thyroid cancer

This is relatively uncommon (1% of all malignancies) and is responsible for about 400 deaths each year in the UK. The incidence rate has increased by

about four-fifths in the last 10 years but almost 9 in 10 people diagnosed
survive 10 years or more (Cancer Research UK, 2018). Types of thyroid cancer
are shown in Table 5.10.

- Thyroidectomy is usually the treatment and this may be followed by
  radioactive iodine, which will be taken up by any remaining cancer cells
  and metastases.
- Replacement thyroxine will be needed.

Hypothyroidism

This is a reduced level of thyroid hormone and is sometimes called myx-
oedema because of swelling under the skin. It is the most common disorder of
the thyroid gland.

Aetiology

- Autoimmune thyroiditis. Antithyroid antibodies are produced and result in
  defective secretion of thyroid hormones. This leads to an increased production of TSH and, often, a goitre. It is then called Hashimoto's disease.
  Sometimes the gland atrophies without producing a goitre. There may be a
  history of autoimmune disorders, and 10% of patients also have pernicious
  anaemia.
- Loss of tissue following partial thyroidectomy.

TABLE 5.10 Types of thyroid cancer

Cell type	Frequency	Characteristics	Spread	Prognosis
Papillary	70%	Young people Slow growing	Local Sometimes lung and bone metastases (secondaries)	Good, especially in young
Follicular	20%	Common in females	Metastases to lung and bone	Good if resected
Anaplastic	≤5%	Aggressive	Locally invasive	Very poor
Lymphoma	≤2%	Variable		Sometimes responds to radiotherapy
Medullary cell	5%	Often familial	Local and metastases	Poor

- Disorders of the pituitary gland may cause a lack of TSH and so low secretion of thyroid hormones.
- Peripheral resistance to thyroid hormone may be the cause.

Clinical features

- Onset is insidious and the disease may be advanced before it is recognized. It may be confused with depression.
- Diminished energy and also physical tiredness.
- Intolerance to the cold; cold skin.
- Diminished sweating.
- Increase in weight with decrease in appetite.
- Constipation.
- Hoarseness of the voice.
- Dry and rough skin; dry, brittle hair. Reduced nail growth.
- Slow thought processes and confusion; memory loss.
- Slow pulse rate.
- Slow respirations may lead to hypoventilation and carbon dioxide retention.

Investigations

- All suspected cases should be investigated.
- Thyroid hormone levels. There is a low level of thyroxine, which stimulates pituitary secretion of TSH.
- Anaemia may be present.
- ECG shows a slow rate and flattened or inverted T waves.
- Rise in titre of thyroid antibodies.

Treatment

Thyroxine is given in doses of 25–50 µg a day, starting with a low dose and raising it every 14 days until normal levels of TSH are achieved. The average daily maintenance dose is 250 µg. The patient should be warned that treatment is for life.

Parathyroid glands

Parathormone (PTH) from the parathyroid glands controls the concentration of calcium and inorganic phosphorus in the blood. It raises the plasma calcium by removal of calcium from bone, by increasing intestinal absorption of calcium and reducing renal excretion. It increases the synthesis of vitamin D and lowers serum phosphate by enhancing its excretion.

In health, parathormone levels rise as plasma calcium levels fall.

Hyperparathyroidism

Causes

- Parathyroid adenoma.
- Conditions causing hypocalcaemia, e.g., chronic renal failure.

Clinical features

- If mild, may be asymptomatic.
- Symptoms are related to hypercalcaemia. They include malaise, anorexia, nausea and vomiting. Drowsiness or confusion may occur.
- Peptic ulceration and acute pancreatitis.
- Kidney involvement may present with renal colic from stones, haematuria or polyuria from tubular damage.
- Bone pain suggests involvement of the bones and backache is common.

Investigations

- Plasma calcium is high and plasma phosphate is low.
- Alkaline phosphatase is raised, reflecting increased osteoblastic activity.
- Radiologic changes may include demineralization.

Treatment

Surgical removal of the tumour.

Hypoparathyroidism

- This is a failure of secretion and is rare.
- Major causes are postnatal and postsurgical following thyroidectomy.
- Idiopathic hypoparathyroidism may be associated with autoimmune disorders such as Addison's disease.
- Clinical features are caused by hypocalcaemia.
- Tetany occurs, which is characterized by carpopedal spasm. This is Trousseau's sign and may be provoked by inflating a sphygmomanometer cuff to just above systolic pressure for at least 2 min.
- Treatment of tetany is with intravenous calcium and long-term oral calcium, and an active metabolite of vitamin D are needed.

Adrenal glands

The adrenal glands are small, triangular in shape and situated on the superior poles of each kidney. They have an outer cortex and an inner medulla.

The adrenal medulla secretes adrenaline (epinephrine) and noradrenaline (norepinephrine).

The cortex secretes steroid hormones — glucocorticoids (cortisol), mineralocorticoids (aldosterone) and some sex hormones (mostly androgens).

The secretion of aldosterone is under the control of the renin–angiotensin system. The secretion of glucocorticoids is controlled by ACTH from the anterior pituitary gland, controlled in turn by cortisol release factor (CRF) from the hypothalamus. Cortisol is secreted in response to circadian rhythm, stress and other factors.

Glucocorticoid hormones

Cortisol is the main hormone:

- Essential to life, although it is not known why.
- Secreted more in stress.
- Influences metabolism of most body cells.
- Concerned with the metabolism of carbohydrates, fats and proteins.
- Glucocorticoids have an antiinflammatory and immunosuppressive action, and it is for these actions that they are used therapeutically. All their other actions then become unwanted side effects.
- There are a number of synthetic compounds with similar action, e.g., prednisolone.

Addison's disease — adrenal insufficiency

An uncommon condition in which there is destruction of the adrenal cortex resulting in a deficiency of corticosteroid production.

Aetiology

- Eighty per cent result from antibodies being produced against adrenal cortex antigens.
- Associated with other autoimmune conditions such as Hashimoto's thyroiditis, Graves' disease and Type 2 diabetes mellitus.
- Rarer causes include tuberculosis, surgical removal, haemorrhage (in meningococcal septicaemia) and malignant infiltration.

Clinical features

- Insidious onset with lethargy, depression, anorexia, muscular weakness and weight loss.
- May also present as an emergency with vomiting, abdominal pain and hypovolaemic shock.
- Important signs are hypotension caused by salt and water loss and hyperpigmentation caused by increased secretion of ACTH, stimulating

melanocytes to produce melanin, which is responsible for skin pigmentation.
- There may be hypoglycaemia.

Investigations

- Serum urea and electrolytes.
- Adrenal antibodies are detected in most cases of autoimmune adrenalitis.
- Chest radiography will show TB.
- Diagnosis may be made by using the tetracosatrin (synthetic ACTH) test.
- Treatment should not wait for any results if it is an emergency. Hydrocortisone 100 mg should be given immediately after taking a sample of blood for measurement of plasma cortisol (will be low) and ACTH (will be high due to loss of negative feedback).

Treatment

- Lifelong replacement with steroid tablets.
- In normal individuals, steroids are released in stress of any type, e.g., infection, trauma and surgical operations. In Addison's disease, the dose of steroid must be increased in any of these situations.
- The patient must carry a steroid card and wear a MedicAlert bracelet in case of accidents.

Cushing's syndrome

Caused by persistently and inappropriately raised levels of glucocorticoids.

Aetiology

- Most cases result from the administration of steroids for the treatment of medical conditions, e.g., asthma.
- Spontaneous Cushing's syndrome is rare but may result from a pituitary adenoma, ectopic ACTH-producing tumours (e.g., small-cell lung cancer), adrenal adenoma and very rarely adrenal hyperplasia.

Clinical features

- Obese with central fat distribution affecting the trunk, abdomen and neck (buffalo hump).
- Moon face and plethoric complexion.
- Protein catabolism causes the skin to be thin and to bruise easily.
- Purple striae on the abdomen, breasts and thighs.

Investigations

- Raised plasma cortisol level is confirmed by the low-dose dexamethasone suppression test. Dexamethasone, a potent synthetic glucocorticoid, is given in a low dose, 0.5 g every 6 h, orally for 48 h. This will suppress the serum cortisol in normal individuals by 48 h.
- Raised 24-h urine level of free cortisol.

Treatment

- Surgical removal of any tumours, if possible.
- *Metyrapone* is an inhibitor of cortisol synthesis and may be useful if removal is not possible.
- Reduction of steroid dose in iatrogenic cases.

Phaeochromocytoma

A rare, benign (usually) tumour of the adrenal medulla in which one or both of the catecholamines are secreted in excess.

Hypertension (may be paroxysmal) is the most common sign, along with headache, pallor, sweating, palpitations and apprehension.

The treatment is surgery where possible, under alpha and beta blockade using phenoxybenzamine and propranolol, started before the operation. These drugs can be used in long-term treatment where surgery is not possible.

Diabetes mellitus and the pancreas

This is a syndrome characterized by a persistently raised blood glucose level associated with a deficiency of or resistance to insulin. In health the normal range for fasting blood glucose is 4.0–5.4 mmol/L. This rises up to 7.8 mmol/L after eating.

More than 3.5 million people in the UK have been diagnosed with diabetes but the figure is more likely to be 4 million when undiagnosed cases are included. More than 420 million people worldwide have diabetes (WHO, 2017).

Less than 15% of those with diabetes in the UK have Type 1 diabetes. The remaining 85% have Type 2 diabetes.

Box 5.6 shows the classification of diabetes by the WHO.

Action of insulin

- Insulin is a hormone secreted by the beta cells of the islets of Langerhans in the pancreas.
- Its secretion is dependent upon the level of glucose in the blood.
- After a meal when glucose levels rise, insulin is secreted.

BOX 5.6 Classification of diabetes mellitus (WHO)

Type 1 diabetes — beta cell destruction and eventually insulin dependent

Type 2 diabetes — usually non-insulin-dependent; may be predominantly insulin resistant or predominantly secretory deficit.

Other specific types of diabetes:

- Secondary to pancreatic disease, e.g., chronic pancreatitis, pancreatectomy
- Secondary to endocrine disease, e.g., Cushing's syndrome, acromegaly
- Drug induced, e.g., steroids, thiazide diuretics
- Associated with genetic syndromes
- Gestational diabetes
- Impaired fasting glycaemia and impaired glucose tolerance

- Insulin is necessary to allow glucose to enter the body cells and be used for energy. If there is excess glucose, insulin encourages its storage as glycogen in the liver and muscles and triglycerides in the adipose tissue.
- If there is insufficient insulin, the body cannot use its glucose which will then accumulate in the blood and spill over into the urine.

Diagnosis

- Random blood glucose measurement above 11.1 mmol/L.
- Fasting blood glucose level above 7.0 mmol/L.
- HbA1c measurement. Normal level is below 6.0% (42 mmol/L). Prediabetes is between 6.0% and 6.4% (42–47 mmol/L). Diabetes is above 6.5% (48 mmol/L).
- Oral glucose tolerance test (GTT) if borderline.

If the person has symptoms of diabetes, only one laboratory measurement is needed for diagnosis. If there are no symptoms then two measurements are needed.

Oral glucose tolerance test

- Normal blood glucose ranges from under 6 mmol/L when fasting to 7.8 mmol/L after food. The subject should have fasted for at least 10 h, but no longer than 16 h. Blood glucose is measured before and 2 h after the ingestion of 75 g glucose dissolved in water (may be given as Lucozade).
- A normal fasting blood glucose measurement would be <6.0 mmol/L.
- A fasting blood glucose level above 7.0 mmol/L is diagnostic of diabetes.
- Another blood sample is taken 2 h after the ingestion of glucose.
- A normal blood glucose at this point would be <7.8 mmol/L.
- If the measurement rises above 11.0 mmol/L, this is diagnostic of diabetes mellitus.

Type 1 diabetes mellitus

Used to be called insulin-dependent diabetes mellitus (IDDM):

- The pancreas ceases to produce insulin. The person is dependent on insulin by injection and without this, they would eventually die.
- Autoimmune disorder, the causes of which are not entirely understood. The insulin-producing cells in the pancreas are attacked by beta cell antibodies and eventually are totally destroyed.
- Certain individuals have a genetic predisposition towards the disease but an environmental trigger factor is needed. This is likely to be a virus.
- The onset of the disease has its highest incidence around 11−12 years of age. It can occur at any age but is uncommon above the age of about 40 years.

Clinical features

- Polyuria (passing lots of urine)
- Thirst
- Polydipsia (drinking lots)
- Weight loss
- Lack of energy

Without treatment the body has to use fat for energy and as it cannot use any glucose without insulin, the fat breakdown forms ketones. Ketones are acidic and accumulate in the blood. They will also be present in the urine.

On diagnosis the patient will require treatment with insulin, which will be lifelong. Ideally the patient will not need admission to hospital.

Insulin therapy

The normal production of insulin by the pancreas has to be mimicked as closely as possible by the administration of insulin by injection.

Insulin cannot be given orally as it is inactivated by gastrointestinal enzymes. It is usually given by subcutaneous injection and the injection site is rotated on a systematic basis, using the thighs and the abdominal wall. Some patients also use the upper arms or buttocks.

The patient may have to inject himself up to four times daily and for some, this is the worst aspect of their illness. New, very fine insulin needles have now made the process practically painless.

Types of insulin

- Insulin used to be extracted mainly from the pancreas of pigs (porcine) and also from cows (bovine), but human insulin is now the norm and is made using genetic engineering.

- Insulin syringes now come disguised in various forms, such as pens, that children can take to school. For information on the devices available, contact the diabetes specialist nurse linked to your hospital.
- Soluble (fast-acting) insulin is the type that would be used in an emergency and at the time of surgical operations on those with diabetes. This is a clear fluid. It may also be given intravenously in an emergency.
- There are also modified insulins available that are longer acting and so need to be administered less frequently. These are used for injecting twice daily (isophane insulin).
- Newer fast-acting insulin analogues such as insulin aspart (NovoRapid) are faster acting than soluble insulin and may be injected at the start of a meal.
- Long-acting insulin analogues such as insulin glargine (Lantus) give a flat basal insulin level over 24 h.
- Biphasic insulins are a mixture of soluble and isophane insulins in various quantities. Mixtard 30/70 is 30% soluble and 70% isophane, suitable for twice-daily injecting.

Types of insulin are shown in Table 5.11.

Fingerprick glucose monitoring

- Those with Type 1 diabetes will be used to monitoring their own blood glucose using test strips and a blood glucose meter. This simple machine measures the level of glucose in a spot of blood. They may have been taught to adjust their insulin according to their results.
- It is essential that those involved in this procedure have been trained.
- Great care has to be taken when obtaining blood from the finger of a diabetic person. The side of the finger should be used rather than the fleshy area of the finger tip. It will be easier to obtain blood from a warm finger.

Type 2 diabetes mellitus

Used to be called noninsulin-dependent diabetes mellitus (NIDDM):

- This is usually an inability of the body to use the insulin adequately (insulin resistance) but sometimes may be due to insufficient production of insulin.
- These patients are not dependent on insulin for their survival. May be receiving some insulin to help control their diabetes, but can live without it.
- The symptoms of Type 2 diabetes develop insidiously, and patients may be diagnosed on having a routine blood or urine test. They may have had the disorder for years and not known about it.
- Early diagnosis and treatment is vitally important to prevent long-term complications. These are exactly the same in Type 1 and Type 2 diabetes (see below).

TABLE 5.11 Types of insulin

| Types of insulin | Brand names | Following subcutaneous administration | | | Description |
		Onset	Peak	Duration	
Quick-acting insulin					
Recombinant human insulin analogues	Insulin lispro (*Humalog*) Insulin aspart (*NovoRapid*) Insulin glulisine (*Apidra*)	5–20 min	30 –60 min	2–5 h	Amino acid structure slightly altered to make action faster and of shorter duration
Soluble insulin (insulin injection; neutral insulin)	Human sequence insulins: *Actrapid, Humulin S, Velosulin, Insuman Rapid* Highly purified animal insulins: *Hypurin Bovine Neutral Hypurin Porcine Neutral Pork Actrapid*	30–60 min	2–4 h	4–8 h	Structure as in the human body

Intermediate-acting					
Isophane insulin (Isophane protamine, Isophane NPH)	Insulatard, Humulin I, Insuman Basal Pork and Bovine Isophane, Pork Insulatard	1–2 h	5–8 h	12–18 h	Soluble insulin and the protein protamine in equal amounts
Long-acting					
Insulin zinc suspension	Hypurin Bovine Lente	1–2 h	6–20 h	Up to 36 h	Combined with zinc for longer action
Basal insulin analogue	Glargine (Lantus) Detemir (Levemir)	90 min	Flat profile	24 h	Amino acid structure changed – long action for basal level
Biphasic insulins					
Biphasic isophane	Human Mixtard 10, 20, 30, 40, 50 Pork Mixtard 30 Hypurin Pork 30/70 Humulin M3, Insulin Comb 15, 25, 50	Mixture of fast-acting soluble and intermediate-acting isophane. Mixtard 10 is 10% soluble, 90% isophane. Reduces the number of injections. Often twice daily			
Biphasic insulin lispro	Humalog Mix 25	25% insulin analogue and 75% insulin lispro protamine			
Biphasic aspart	Humalog Mix 50 NovoMix 30	50% of each 30% analogue and 70% aspart protamine			

- Incidence increases with age and as people are living longer, so the disease is getting more common.
- Type 2 runs in families.
- The disorder is closely linked to obesity. A healthy diet and body weight together with exercise will reduce the incidence of Type 2 diabetes.
- Type 2 diabetes may be controlled by diet alone. If this is not possible, oral hypoglycaemic agents are prescribed to bring down the blood glucose.
- The condition is progressive and the patient may eventually require insulin for good blood glucose control.

The aims for Type 1 and Type 2 diabetes are similar:

- To maintain a blood glucose that is within the normal range if possible and thus prevent or reduce the complications of diabetes.
- Thorough communication and education to encourage patients to have control of their own disorder.
- To help the person lead a normal and active life.
- Two landmark trials — The Diabetes Control and Complications Trial (DCCT) in Type 1 diabetes and the United Kingdom Prospective Diabetes Survey (UKPDS) for Type 2 diabetes — showed that there is a close link between poor blood glucose control and the development of complications in diabetes. Also highlighted in this research was the importance of blood pressure control in the prevention and control of complications.

Medication in Type 2 diabetes

> ! Although diet alone may be sufficient in some patients, oral hypoglycaemic agents are usually needed. There are several types of drug available and these are shown in Table 5.12.

Metformin is the first-line drug for Type 2 diabetes. It does not stimulate insulin secretion and does not lead to weight gain. It has also been shown to reduce the incidence of cardiovascular events in Type 2 diabetes.

Drugs that stimulate insulin secretion include sulphonylureas such as gliclazide. These drugs can cause hypoglycaemia and do result in some weight gain.

> ! There are also newer drugs available.
> - Glitazones reduce insulin resistance.
> - Incretin mimetics help the body to produce more insulin.
> - Gliptins block the action of DPP-4. This is an enzyme that destroys the hormone incretin. SGLT2 inhibitors reduce the amount of glucose absorbed by the kidneys and bloodstream.

TABLE 5.12 Some oral hypoglycaemic agents and their actions

Type of drug	Name	Mode of action	Special features	Side effects
Sulphonylureas	Gliclazide (*Diamicron*) Glibenclamide (*Daonil*) Tolbutamide Glimepiride (*Amaryl*) Glipizide	Augment insulin secretion Need residual pancreatic activity	May rarely cause hypoglycaemia – especially in elderly – may last many hours – treat in hospital Can encourage weight gain	Usually mild and infrequent Gastrointestinal, e.g., nausea, diarrhoea, constipation
Biguanides	Metformin	Decreases gluconeogenesis Increases peripheral use of glucose	Drug of choice in obese Very little danger of hypo	Anorexia, nausea, diarrhoea, metallic taste, lactic acidosis
Glitazones	Pioglitazone (*Actos*) Rosiglitazone (*Avandia*)	Reduce peripheral insulin resistance	Used with other oral hypoglycaemics Not with insulin	Check liver function tests Higher incidence of fractures in females
Meglitinides	Repaglinide (*Prandin*) Nateglinide (*Starlix*) Senaglinide	Stimulate insulin release	Rapid onset, short duration of action	Hypoglycaemia Rashes
	Acarbose (*Glucobay*)	Enzyme inhibitor – delays digestion of starch and sucrose	May be used in combination with oral drugs or insulin	Flatulence, soft stools, diarrhoea

Often patients need a combination of tablets to control their diabetes.

The diet in diabetes

On diagnosis, the client will see a dietitian.

Contrary to popular thinking, the diet in diabetes is one that can be eaten by the whole family. It is a 'healthy eating' diet. The diet should:

- meet the patient's overall daily energy requirements; these depend partly on age, sex and level of activity,
- be low in fat, especially saturated or animal fat,
- give about 50% of calories in the form of carbohydrate, aiming to increase the complex carbohydrate in the diet (this is found in foods such as pasta, potatoes and bread) and reduce the fast sugars such as sucrose. Foods with a low glycaemic index (GI) should be eaten,
- contain at least five portions of fruit and vegetables daily.

If you wish to know more about the diet in diabetes you should contact your hospital dietitian or diabetes specialist nurse. The Diabetes UK website is excellent (www.diabetes.org.uk).

Hypoglycaemic medication in Type 2 diabetes

> **!** There are several different types of medication that help to lower blood glucose. These are shown in Table 5.12.

Diabetic emergencies

Hypoglycaemia

This occurs when the blood glucose falls below 3.0–3.5 mmol/L. It does not occur in the patient with diabetes who is diet controlled, but may occur if someone with Type 2 diabetes is on certain oral hypoglycaemic agents, such as tolbutamide or gliclazide. It is most common in those receiving insulin.

Causes

- Too much insulin (either accidental or deliberate).
- Missing or delaying a meal or snack.
- Excessive exercise with no reduction in insulin.
- Alcohol.

Clinical features Some symptoms are due to the release of adrenaline (in an attempt to raise blood glucose) and others are due to the lack of glucose reaching the brain:

- Pallor
- Trembling
- Sweating
- Feeling 'lightheaded'
- Blurred vision
- Tachycardia
- Increasing confusion − sometimes aggression
- Incoherent speech

An attack of hypoglycaemia may occur very rapidly, and if the nurse notices a change in behaviour of a patient with diabetes and he becomes irritable or lethargic, he should seek help immediately. Prompt action may mean that oral instead of intravenous glucose may be given.

Treatment

- Glucose may be given orally if the client is awake and fully conscious.
- If he is unconscious intravenous dextrose will be administered.
- Glucagon 1 mg may be given intramuscularly if intravenous dextrose is not available. This is a hormone produced by the pancreas that causes the release of glucose from stores in the body.

Diabetic ketoacidosis

- DKA occurs following a raised blood glucose and insufficient insulin in Type 1 diabetes but may rarely occur in ketone-prone Type 2 diabetes.
- It is a biochemical triad of ketosis, hyperglycaemia and acidaemia.
- Most cells cannot use glucose in the absence of insulin. Fat stores have to be used for energy with the production of ketones.
- Compared to hypoglycaemia, deterioration is slow.
- Hyperglycaemia is present and ketones are heavily present both in the urine and on the breath.
- Polyuria is present and at first polydipsia but as the acidosis increases, nausea and vomiting may occur, making drinking impossible.
- Dehydration will now increase, leading to a lowering of blood pressure and a rapid, thready pulse.
- The respirations become deep (Kussmaul's breathing) and the ketones can be smelt on the breath (they smell of acetone, which is nail varnish remover, or pear drops).
- Without treatment, drowsiness and coma will follow.

- Diabetic ketoacidosis is a medical emergency and urgent intervention is needed.

Diagnosis

- Ketonaemia of 3.0 mmol/L or more or significant ketonuria.
- Blood glucose above 11 mmol/L or known diabetes mellitus.
- Bicarbonate less than 15.0 mmol/L and/or venous pH less than 7.3.

Causes

- Untreated diabetes, i.e., undiagnosed patient.
- Illness, e.g., UTI or throat infection. Infection increases the body's insulin requirement, but the patient may actually omit his insulin as he has no appetite for food.
- Omission of insulin in illness, for example when vomiting. It is of vital importance that insulin is never totally stopped when the patient is ill.

Treatment

- Assessment of the patient's conscious level half hourly.
- Half-hourly monitoring of vital signs — blood pressure, pulse and respirations.
- An intravenous infusion of normal (0.9%) saline helps to combat the dehydration.
- Bloods will be taken for blood glucose measurement and urea and electrolytes. An arterial sample will be taken for blood gases to assess the level of acidosis.
- Portable ketone meters allow bedside monitoring of blood ketones. It is essential that ketones are reduced.
- Insulin therapy will be commenced with a short-acting insulin such as Actrapid or Humulin S.
- Insulin will be given according to the blood glucose measurements which may be taken hourly at first.
- A dextrose infusion may also be given alongside the normal saline, to prevent hypoglycaemia, as the patient responds to the insulin.

Hyperosmolar nonketotic state

Severe hyperglycaemia (usually above 40 mmol/L) without ketosis but no precise definition is appropriate. It is the metabolic emergency associated with Type 2 diabetes:

- Patient may present with undiagnosed diabetes and may be severely dehydrated and comatose.

- Often precipitated by consumption of glucose-rich drinks such as Lucozade or lemonade.
- Certain medications such as thiazide diuretics or corticosteroids could precipitate the coma.
- Usually elderly patients.
- Treatment includes fluid replacement and insulin.

Long-term complications of diabetes

These may be divided into small-vessel and large-vessel diseases.

Small-vessel disease (microvascular)

This type of disorder only happens in diabetes. It is much more common when there is poor control of blood glucose levels. The incidence of complications also rises with the length of time the patient has had diabetes.

Retinopathy. The small vessels at the back of the eye are affected and if untreated, eventually this can lead to blindness. All diabetics need an annual eye check. Treatment with photocoagulation can prevent blindness.

Nephropathy. This is damage to the kidney. There will be albumin in the urine and usually a raised blood pressure. If the damage continues chronic renal failure can follow. Renal failure is the cause of death in 10% of patients with diabetes.

Neuropathy. This is damage to the peripheral nerves, which may lead to sensory loss and is one of the reasons why extreme caution is needed when dealing with the feet of those with diabetes. The chiropodist should be consulted on a regular basis and the nurse should never attempt to cut the toe nails of the client with diabetes.

Damage to the skin of the feet in the presence of both neuropathy and poor circulation is one of the reasons why amputations are so common in patients with diabetes.

Large-vessel disease (macrovascular)

CVD is the cause of death in approximately 70% of patients with diabetes:

- CVD — may lead to angina and heart attacks.
- Cerebrovascular disease — may lead to stroke.
- PVD — may lead to severe pain on walking and contribute to poor healing of any injuries to the foot.

All of these occur in the nondiabetic population but are much more common in those with diabetes due to a more rapid development of atherosclerosis. In patients with diabetes, stroke is twice as common and myocardial infarction is 3–5 times more likely.

In those with diabetes all CVD risk factors should be aggressively tackled. This includes hypertension, smoking, lipid abnormalities and stress. Aspirin is used as an antiplatelet drug and ACE inhibitors are prescribed.

Surgery in diabetes

- Long-acting or intermediate-acting insulin should be stopped the day before surgery, and soluble insulin is substituted.
- During surgery an infusion of insulin and glucose is given. The infusion is maintained until the patient can eat.
- Glucose levels are checked and potassium levels are monitored.
- Oral hypoglycaemic agents should be discontinued 2 days before surgery and soluble insulin is substituted if necessary.

5.8 DISEASES OF THE BONES AND JOINTS

Bone is a collagen-based matrix with mineral laid upon it. Its strength depends upon both these components. The minerals are calcium, phosphorus and magnesium. Vitamin D, parathormone and calcitonin (produced by the thyroid gland) are important in bone mineralization. The new bone is deposited by the osteoblast cells and old bone is resorbed by the osteoclast cells. Bone is not static and is constantly remodelling throughout life.

Osteoporosis

This is the most common metabolic bone disease in which there is a loss of bone mass per unit volume. Bone composition remains normal. This leads to reduced strength and the weakened bone fractures easily. Damage is particularly likely to occur to the femoral neck, the dorsal vertebrae and the distal radius. The trauma precipitating this damage may be very minor.

Women lose bone mass more rapidly than men, and in the UK more than two million women are thought to have osteoporosis.

Aetiology

Most examples are the result of progressive decrease in bone mass with age:

- Bone formation and resorption are balanced in adulthood. With ageing, the balance swings towards bone resorption and whether this reaches a critical point or not depends largely on the bone mass achieved as an adult. The bone mass is greater in men than women and also greater in blacks than in whites.
- Changes in body oestrogen levels also cause more bone resorption in women after the menopause as oestrogen prevents bone resorption. As

women also live longer, on average, than men they have more problems with osteoporosis.

- Exercise throughout life helps to maintain bone mass, and immobility for any reason may precipitate premature osteoporosis.
- Occasionally direct causes can be found, such as Cushing's syndrome, diabetes, thyrotoxicosis, chronic renal failure and use of drugs such as glucocorticoids and long-term heparin.
- Other risk factors include low body weight, cigarette smoking, excess alcohol intake and family history.
- Elderly patients, especially if they are housebound or live in care homes are especially at risk.

Clinical features

- Asymptomatic osteoporosis is common.
- Backache is common.
- The vertebrae may collapse due to typical crush fractures and there may be an exaggeration of the curvature of the thoracic spine.
- Collapse of vertebrae may lead to loss of height.
- Fragility fracture − a bone fracture that occurs after a minor fall (equivalent to a fall from the height of an ordinary chair or less). Hip fracture is common.

Investigations

- Conventional X-rays are not very sensitive for detecting decreased bone density.
- Dual-energy X-ray absorptiometry (DEXA) is used to measure bone density, usually of the lumbar spine and proximal femur.
- DXR is a simpler and newer technique but appears to be less sensitive.
- Ultrasonic measurement of bone can be used to assess fracture risk but tends to underdiagnose osteoporosis.
- Blood levels of calcium, phosphate and alkaline phosphatase are normal.

Prevention of osteoporosis and fractures

- Adequate intake of calcium and vitamin D is needed. Dietary supplements should be used where necessary.
- Prophylaxis is preferred and a good diet, with plenty of calcium and low alcohol intake, will help.
- Smoking should be discouraged as it is associated with lower bone density.
- Moderate alcohol intake only.

- Regular exercise against gravity is recommended (30 min of weight-bearing exercise three times weekly).
- Home risk assessment and falls prevention in the elderly by the use of hip protectors.

Drug treatment

- Bisphosphonates are drugs that reduce bone turnover but are not suitable for everyone. Examples are **alendronate** and **risedronate**.
- **Teriparatide** is a fragment of parathyroid hormone and stimulates bone formation. Treatment should be instigated by a specialist.
- **Strontium ranelate** inhibits bone resorption and stimulates new bone formation.
- **Raloxifene** is a selective oestrogen receptor modulator (SERM) and reduces postmenopausal bone loss. There is a slightly increased risk of VTE and a slightly decreased risk of breast cancer when taking this drug.
- Early oestrogen replacement during the menopause (HRT) is used where other therapies are contraindicated. It should not be used for long periods (5 years maximum) and is most beneficial early in the menopause. When HRT is discontinued bone loss resumes and may even be accelerated.

Vitamin D deficiency

- Results in rickets in children and osteomalacia in adults. It is uncommon in the UK but may occur in Asian women and the elderly as a result of dietary lack and failure to be exposed to sunlight.
- May also occur in malabsorption from any cause including previous gastric surgery and coeliac disease.
- Rare causes include long-term use of anticonvulsants, liver and renal failure.
- The main function of vitamin D is to ensure an adequate concentration of calcium for bone formation. Deficiency leads to a failure of calcification. Soft bones lacking in tensile strength result but there is no interference with bone bulk.

Childhood rickets

The bones become distorted and there may be pain and weakness. It leads to the stunting of growth and bowing of the lower limbs. There may be a pigeon deformity of the chest and delay in closure of the anterior fontanelle.

Distortion of the pelvis in females may lead to difficulties with childbirth.

Osteomalacia in adults

May produce pain and tenderness as well as spontaneous fractures. Muscle weakness is also present. Plasma calcium may be low and tetany may ensue.

Treatment

- Prevention is better than cure!
- Education and living standards are important and susceptible populations should be targeted.
- A good diet with vitamin D and calcium supplements should be given.
- Exposure to sunlight is also important.
- Patients on long-term anticonvulsants should receive supplements.

Paget's disease of the bone

- This is known as osteitis deformans and is common in the elderly (up to 10%).
- There is a familial tendency to develop the disease although its aetiology is not known.
- British cases are clustered in the northern part of the country.
- There is an increased turnover of bone in some areas of the skeleton. This results in abnormal architecture of the bones, with the legs and axial skeleton (including the skull) most commonly affected.
- Often the patient is asymptomatic but constant localized bone pain may occur and this is unrelieved by rest.
- The features may be distorted, and the affected areas may feel warm.
- Complications are due to compression by the bony overgrowths and include blindness and deafness.
- Simple analgesics and physiotherapy are used.
- Bisphosphonates are used for treatment and may be given intravenously or orally.

Osteomyelitis

This is infection in the bone. It may be bloodborne or occur from direct spread of microorganisms. Predisposing conditions are shown in Box 5.7. It is difficult to treat and may result in extensive physical disability.

Acute osteomyelitis is usually caused by *Staphylococcus aureus* but other organisms include *Pseudomonas aeruginosa*, *Salmonella*, streptococci, *Candida* and mixed aerobic and anaerobic organisms.

There is fever, pain and tenderness over the affected bone. Blood culture or needle biopsy is done for diagnosis but treatment may be possible from the clinical picture alone.

BOX 5.7 Acute osteomyelitis — predisposing conditions

Direct spread	Bloodborne
Open fractures	Skin sepsis and ulcers
Penetrating trauma, e.g., animal bite	Intravenous drug abuse
Replacement joints	Chronic urinary tract infection
Penetrating ulcer, e.g., in diabetic neuropathy	Sickle cell disease
	Chronic diverticulitis

Chronic osteomyelitis usually results from untreated or undertreated acute osteomyelitis. There is bone erosion and areas of cystic degeneration. Necrosis of bone follows and there may be intermittent flare-up of the disease over a period of years with fever, local pain and sinus formation.

Treatment

- Antibiotics and drainage of inflammatory exudates.
- Evaluation is by bone scanning and MRI.
- Chronic osteomyelitis may require a combination of surgery and antibiotic therapy.
- Hyperbaric oxygen is sometimes used.

Bone tumours

Many different types of tumours involve the skeleton, but primary bone tumours are rare and occur mainly in the young. Benign lesions may cause pain with expansion and predispose to pathologic fractures.

Secondary metastases in bone are common, especially from malignancies of the breast, bronchi, prostate, thyroid and kidney.

The rate is low below 15 years (3% of all malignancies), adolescents have the highest rate and the lowest rate of all is between 30 and 35 years. Above 35 years, the incidence slowly rises due to metastases in bone.

Osteosarcomas

These malignant bone-forming tumours account for about 38% of bone tumours. Occurrence is 3:2 times more common in males. Sixty per cent occur under 20 years and a secondary peak occurs in the 50—60 age range, mostly in those with Paget's disease.

Ninety per cent of these tumours are located in the metaphyses of long bones, especially the femur. Fifty per cent occur around the knee joint.

Clinical features

- Pain and swelling.
- Pain slight and intermittent at first but becomes more intense and of longer duration. It is often severe at night and analgesia becomes necessary.
- Usually there is a coincidental history of trauma.
- Sometimes may present with a fracture.

Diagnosis

Early recognition is essential for a reasonable prognosis. Many could be diagnosed early but often the individual does not seek medical attention. There may be vague symptoms that could be related to minor trauma or inflammatory conditions.

Radiologic studies including plain X-ray, CT scan and an MRI enable diagnosis and often staging to be done. MRI may also be used to follow the progress of the tumour with treatment.

Treatment

Surgery is the treatment of choice. Amputation used to be the rule but now chemotherapy may be given first and limb salvage made possible by removal of the tumour while preserving the limb.

Chemotherapy is usually given both pre- and postoperatively using combinations of drugs.

Ewing's sarcoma

- Originates from cells within the bone marrow space.
- Mean age of diagnosis is 15 years of age. Rare after 30 years of age. The incidence has not changed above 30 years.
- Most common in the mid-shaft of long bones or in flat bones.
- Most common complaint is pain and swelling, but fever may be present with malaise and anorexia.
- The tumour breaks through the bone and may form a soft tissue mass. It is most common in the femur and pelvis but can occur in any bone.
- It metastasizes early to nearly every part of the body. Metastases are present in about 25% of cases at diagnosis. Common sites are the lungs and other bones.
- Bone scan, chest X-ray and chest CT are used to detect metastases.
- Biopsy is used to establish the diagnosis.

- Chemotherapy is usually the first line of treatment. Preoperative chemotherapy is used before surgery or radiotherapy or a combination of both. Chemotherapy is then continued for 12−18 months afterwards.

Inflammatory joint disease

Commonly termed arthritis, this is characterized by inflammatory damage and destruction of the synovial membrane or articular cartilage in the joints. There are also systemic signs of inflammation including fever, malaise, anorexia and a raised white cell count.

Rheumatoid arthritis

This is a classic autoimmune disorder with self-perpetuating inflammation occurring in the joints and resulting from immune reactions. It can be described as a nonsuppurative, noninfectious, proliferative synovitis. There are a wide variety of extra-articular features of the disease as well.

The first tissue to be affected in the joint is the synovial membrane that lines the joint cavity. Eventually it may lead to the progressive destruction of articular cartilage. The result is a progressively disabling arthritis with pain, joint deformity and loss of movement.

More than 70% of patients present with a bilateral and symmetrical polyarthritis, usually of insidious onset. All synovial joints may be affected but some are more commonly affected than others (Fig. 5.15). There may be extra-articular involvement of other tissues and in this way the disorder resembles systemic lupus erythematosus and other multiorgan autoimmune disorders. These patients tend to have a poorer prognosis.

The trigger factor is unknown and various agents have been suggested including some of the enteric bacteria and the Epstein−Barr virus. The precise triggering may vary from person to person.

Incidence

- Predominantly female − 3:1.
- Occurs in 2% of the population worldwide.
- Just as common in tropical countries as in cold, damp Britain.
- Does not appear to have occurred in ancient times.
- May commence at any age from 10 to 70 years. Highest incidence is in the 70s.
- Two to four times higher incidence in women than men.
- Genetic factors seem to be vitally important in determining a predisposition.
- Early diagnosis and treatment with disease-modifying antirheumatic drugs (DMARDs) should reduce joint destruction and disability.

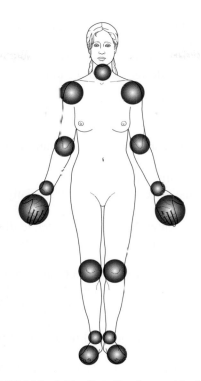

FIGURE 5.15 Joints affected by rheumatoid arthritis.

Aetiology

> ! The joint damage of RA is autoimmune in nature. appearing in genetically predisposed individuals, after exposure to an unknown trigger.

Normally the immune system does not attack 'self'; any part of self is tolerated. In autoimmune disorders something has gone wrong with this mechanism and the body starts to make antibodies to certain body proteins. In diabetes, it is to the islets of Langerhans and so this is organ-specific. In RA there is a more generalized reaction, which may cause systemic problems as well as those in the joints. Quiescent episodes may cause a reduction in the inflammation and pain but there will always be some lymphocytes in the synovium (i.e., some inflammation).

Those with rheumatoid factor present are seropositive. In 20% of cases the client may be seronegative and not have the rheumatoid factor. The rheumatoid factor does not always mean RA. It is present in some other diseases, e.g.,

SLE, TB and in some elderly clients whose relatives have RA but who have no evidence of the disease.

There are changes in the synovial fluid. An increase in volume occurs, the turbidity increases, mucin decreases and the numbers of white cells in it are increased.

Clinical features

- Polyarthritis with pain and swelling in symmetrical small joints (e.g., fingers and toes).
- Morning stiffness in affected joints.
- May have additional general symptoms, especially tiredness, irritability and depression.
- Usually of insidious onset, but RA is a systemic disease, and in the minority of patients it may begin with acute fever, weight loss and excessive fatigue.
- Gradually the disease spreads: fingers to hands and wrists, toes to feet and ankles, elbows, shoulders and knees can be affected.
- The joints take on a characteristic deformed appearance. There is difficulty holding cutlery and problems with walking and even dressing.
- There are periods of exacerbation and remission throughout the course of the disease.
- Because RA is a systemic disorder there may be other changes throughout the body.

Subcutaneous nodules in 25% of cases. Usually in those positive for rheumatoid factor. Most common in the elbows adjacent to the olecranon process, but also at the back of the skull and the Achilles tendon. May occur at any subcutaneous site that is exposed to contact or pressure. Nodules are rounded, firm masses in the subcutaneous tissue varying in diameter from less than 0.5 cm to several centimetres. There is an outer layer of granulation tissue containing lymphocytes and an inner zone of fibrinoid necrosis.

Vasculitis. This occurs at many sites and can involve any major organ. Usually in patients with high titres of rheumatoid factor. Small-vessel vasculitis involves arterioles, venules and capillaries and leads to localized purpura and petechiae. Severe digital vasculitis is rare. Presents with pallor, cyanosis and coldness of the distal digits. Pain and ischaemic ulcerations with necrosis of the finger ends occur. Dry gangrene will result unless treated. Amputation may be indicated.

Fibrinous pleurisy and fibrosis of the lungs. At autopsy 50% of all RA patients have had pleural involvement. Less than 20% will actually experience symptoms and less than 5% will have pleural effusions. Chronic bronchitis may be secondary to RA but this is controversial. Those with RA who smoke appear two to three times more likely to develop chronic bronchitis.

Cardiac involvement. Pericarditis is the most frequent manifestation. At autopsy about 40% show some evidence of previous pericardial involvement. Very few experience any symptoms. If they do, it is likely to be chest pain.

Neuropathy. Usually relatively mild distal sensory neuropathy showing as paraesthesia. Decreased touch sensation in the feet.

Carpal tunnel syndrome. This may occur due to compression of the median nerve by proliferative tenosynovitis of the wrist. The symptoms may precede the onset of RA by years in some cases.

Eye changes. Keratoconjunctivitis (dry eyes) and scleritis commonly. Those with scleritis will get severe pain, photophobia and impairment of vision. Ten per cent will develop keratoconjunctivitis from decreased tear secretion.

Splenomegaly. This is often associated with leucopenia and known as Felty's syndrome. There are often high titres of rheumatoid factor. Skin ulceration and recurrent infections are likely to occur.

Anaemia. Mild normocytic hypochromic anaemia due to poor erythropoiesis and the type that commonly occurs in chronic illness. May be aggravated by blood loss from NSAIDs.

Fatigue, malaise and depression. Fatigue is a common symptom and can precede the onset of joint synovitis by many months.

Investigations

- Immunologic investigations show a positive rheumatoid factor in about 80% of patients.
- Anaemia may be present (see above).
- Platelet and white cell count may be raised.
- The ESR may be raised.
- Radiologic changes — may not be present very early in the disease.

Management

- NICE has published guidelines on the standards of care for people with RA. These can be found on their website.
- Main objective is to reduce the occurrence of joint destruction and pain as well as to enable the patient to lead as normal a life as possible.
- An increasing range of DMARDs are now available and need to be given as early as possible in the disease. This means referral to a rheumatologist as soon as possible so that treatment will be initiated in the first few months of the disease process.
- Patients with RA need an MDT involved in their care.
- Physiotherapy forms an important part of the care, with exercises to try to maintain joint movement and strengthen weak muscles.

- Occupational therapists are involved and provide splints for joint protection as well as aids and appliances to increase independence.
- Pain specialists may be able to advise suitable form of analgesia and nondrug management, e.g., trans-electrical nerve stimulation (TENS).

Drug therapy

There is no curative treatment.

Several classes of drug are used, including DMARDs, analgesics to control the pain, NSAIDs, corticosteroids and cytokine modulators.

DMARDs include *azathioprine* and *ciclosporin* (immune modulating drugs that help to suppress the immune response), *methotrexate* and *sulfasalazine.*

NSAIDs such as *ibuprofen* or *naproxen* are the mainstay of treatment. They improve the symptoms and signs of RA, decreasing pain and also inflammation but do have gastrointestinal side effects and so are prescribed with a proton pump inhibitor (PPI) such as *lansoprazole* to decrease acid secretion. They have little or no effect on the underlying disease process and do not prevent joint destruction. Paracetamol or codeine phosphate can also be used.

Osteoarthritis

This is a common degenerative disease affecting the whole joint. It affects more than 10% of all adults, both men and women. The prevalence increases with age. By the age of 75 years, 85% of people have some osteoarthritis (OA) of at least one joint.

OA occurs worldwide in all climates.

Any joint can be affected but it most commonly affects the weight-bearing joints, especially the knees, and interphalangeal joints of the hands. It is also common in the hip joint.

It may be:

- Primary — a degenerative disease and the result of wear and tear on the joint.
- Secondary — attributable to other causes, e.g., joint injury in athletics or trauma.

Excessive joint loading may be a contributing factor:

- Obesity
- Postural defect
- Malformed joint
- Long-term occupational or athletic stress on a joint

Clinical features

Not everyone with structural changes in their joints has any symptoms:

- Joint aches and stiffness arising gradually in middle age.
- Increase with activity and decrease with rest.
- No systemic signs or symptoms.
- As the degeneration increases, the pain becomes more persistent and stiffness increases.
- Rest and night pain occur with advanced disease.
- Limitation of movement in the affected joint.
- Most serious loss of mobility is from hip and knee involvement.
- No systemic features such as a temperature or a rash.
- Advanced disease can be seen on a plain X-ray.

Management

No arrest of the process:

- Analgesia is helpful, paracetamol is first used with topical NSAIDs. If paracetamol is insufficient the NSAIDs may be prescribed with a PPI such as *omeprazole.*
- Physiotherapy and the use of activities that reduce strain can help.
- Intra-articular corticosteroid injections may be considered.
- Joint replacement often becomes necessary.

Fractures

A fracture may be a complete break in the continuity of a bone or it may be an incomplete break or crack.

Clinical features

The clinical manifestations vary according to the type of fracture and the site:

- When a fracture occurs there will be soft tissue injury as well and blood vessels and nerves may be damaged. Neurovascular assessment is needed. There may be impaired sensation and numbness.
- Typically fractures are painful and there is loss of function. The pain is due to muscle spasm and is worse on movement.
- Deformity (unnatural alignment) occurs at the fracture site.
- Swelling is caused by the fracture haematoma and soft tissue oedema.
- Tenderness, muscle spasm and pain are usually present.
- There may be angulation at the fracture site with shortening of the limb and rotational deformities.

- Crepitus may occur. This is abnormal movement at the fracture site. The broken bone ends grind against each other.
- Shortening may occur due to overlapping of fragments and muscle spasm.
- Sometimes reasonable function may be retained as in a stress fracture or an impacted fracture. This may lead to the doctor missing the fracture.

It may be the case that the fractures sustained by a patient are only a small part of the damage, and in cases of multiple injuries other trauma is more important. Maintaining the airway is always the first priority. There may be spinal injuries or head injuries also.

Diagnosis

X-ray of the whole length of the bone, including the adjacent joints, should be done.

Causes

Trauma

Sudden injury is the cause of the majority of fractures. They occur in previously healthy bone:

- May be direct trauma, e.g., hitting the ulna with a stick. The fracture occurs at the site of the injury.
- May be indirect trauma, e.g., a fall on the hand may fracture the clavicle. Force was applied at a site remote from the injury.

Stress

The bone is fatigued by repeated stress, e.g., a fractured tibia in an athlete, ballet dancer or military recruit. This type of fracture is often due to new strenuous and repetitive activity when gains in muscle strength occur more rapidly than gains in bone strength.

Pathologic

This occurs when a bone is already weakened by disease. The trauma needed may be quite trivial or the fracture may occur spontaneously. Examples of diseases are osteoporosis, cancer metastases in bone, bone cysts and Paget's disease.

Classification of fractures (Fig. 5.16)

Closed or simple fractures

There is no communication between the site of the fracture and the exterior of the body.

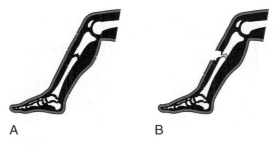

A   B

FIGURE 5.16 Open and closed fractures. (A) Closed or simple fracture. There is no communication between the fractured bone and the body surface. (B) Open or compound fracture. There
is a wound leading down to the site of fracture. Organisms may gain access through the wound
infect the bone. *From Adams, Hamblen, 1999. Outline of Fractures, reproduced with permission.*

Open or compound fractures

The overlying skin is broken and the wound leads down to the site of the
fracture. This means infection may enter the bone. The skin break may be a
small puncture or the bone may protrude right through the skin. Infection in
the bone is called *osteomyelitis* (see p. 402) and may be difficult to eliminate.

> ! All fractures are either open or closed.

A fracture is comminuted when there are more than two fragments to the
bone. This type of fracture may be difficult to align.

Patterns of fracture

Complete fracture

The bone is completely divided into two separate fragments. Different fractures are shown in Fig. 5.17.

The fracture is often described in terms of the pattern seen on the X-ray as:

- Transverse — occurs straight across the bone and is usually caused by an
  angulation, not twisting, force. Unlikely to become displaced after
  reduction.
- Oblique — occurs at a 45 degrees angle to the shaft of the bone and is more
  difficult to stabilize at reduction.
- Spiral — encircles the bone and is usually caused by a twisting force and
  prone to redisplacement following reduction.

Incomplete fracture

Occurs more frequently in the more flexible, growing bones of children. The
bone is not completely broken into two parts.

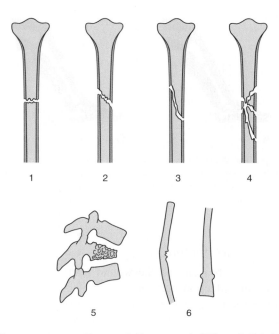

FIGURE 5.17   Common patterns of fracture. 1, Transverse; 2, Oblique; 3, Spiral; 4, Comminuted; 5, Compression; 6, Greenstick. *From Adams, Hamblen, 1999. Outline of Fractures, reproduced with permission.*

A *greenstick* fracture occurs in children, especially under the age of 10. Their bones have elasticity and buckle. If the force applied is strong enough, a complete fracture will occur in a child.

A *hairline* fracture occurs when little force has been applied.

An *impacted* fracture may occur in adults. The bone fragments are jammed into each other. This is common in a fractured neck of femur.

A *crush* or *compression* fracture may occur in cancellous bone when it has been compressed beyond the limits of tolerance, e.g., heels (calcaneum), as a result of falling from a height, or vertebrae.

Complicated fracture

There is accompanying damage to neighbouring structures such as nerves, blood vessels or tendons, e.g., a fractured humerus may damage the brachial artery.

Depressed fracture

A segment of bone is depressed below the level of the bone. This is usually due to a sharply localized blow and is common in skull fractures.

Displacement

This is present if the bone ends have moved from each other. Reduction of a fracture is realignment of the bone ends. It is only necessary if there is some displacement.

Dislocation

A dislocation is loss of congruity between the articular surfaces of a joint. Sometimes a fracture dislocation occurs when the joint is dislocated and at least one of the bones involved is fractured.

A Pott's fracture is dislocation of the ankle joint with fracture of the tibia or fibula.

Treatment

This depends very much on the type and site of the fracture.

First aid

Immobilization by the use of a sling, a splint or traction will lessen the pain. Great care must be taken with spinal injuries.

Uncomplicated fractures

There are three fundamentals of treatment for fractures:

- Reduction
- Immobilization
- Preservation of function

Reduction. This is realignment of the bone fragments. It is not always necessary either because there is no displacement or because the displacement is immaterial to the final result. Reduction may be carried out in three ways.

Manipulative reduction. Closed manipulative reduction is usually done under general anaesthesia but local or regional anaesthesia may sometimes be used. Most fractures can be realigned by this method. The skin is not opened and the bones are moved back into place.

Mechanical traction. This is necessary when there are strong muscles exerting a displacement force, as in a fractured femur. It aims to draw the bone fragments back to their normal length. It may be done rapidly under general anaesthesia or more slowly by prolonged traction without anaesthesia.

Operative reduction. Reduction takes place with direct vision of the bones at an open operation. This is done when an acceptable reduction cannot be maintained by closed methods and is common when there is nerve or articular surface involvement. The fragments will be fixed internally to ensure maintenance of their position.

Immobilization. Some fractures require rigid splinting to maintain their position until union of the bone can occur but others do not and immobilization can do more harm than good in some cases.

Immobilization is done to:

● prevent displacement of the bone fragments,
● prevent movement that may interfere with union,
● relieve pain.

A fracture that has required reduction will always require immobilization to prevent redisplacement.

Prevention of movement is virtually always needed in fractures of the scaphoid, ulna and femur, whereas a fractured clavicle, scapula, stable fracture of the pelvis and fractured ribs will all heal well without immobilization. Methods of immobilization include:

● A cast
● Continuous traction
● External fixation
● Internal fixation

Plaster of Paris. The plaster cast is the standard method of immobilization for most fractures. Plaster of Paris is calcium sulphate, which reacts with water to become hydrated. Plaster bandages come ready prepared and must be soaked in cold water before application. When the wet plaster is applied, the reaction takes place and the plaster feels warmer as it sets. A thin lining of stockinet is used close to the skin, for comfort and to prevent the plaster sticking, and a layer of cotton wool bandage is applied before the plaster. This allows for some swelling of the limb to take place.

There used to be no alternatives to plaster of Paris but now there are many synthetic substitutes with such advantages as lightness, radiolucency (does not interfere with radiographic procedures) and imperviousness to water.

The plaster may be applied as a normal bandage, round and round the limb, but if a lot of swelling is expected, a backslab may be applied and a full plaster used when the swelling has subsided.

Plaster is removed by the use of an electric plaster saw and plaster-cutting shears.

Observation of a cast. When a cast has been applied to a new fracture or following a manipulation there are precautions that need to be observed. There is a danger of restricting the circulation, should the limb swell. This may be sufficient to impede the arterial flow to the fingers or toes and is most likely to occur between 12 and 36 h after application of the plaster.

The clinical features of a restricted circulation are:

● Pain
● Swelling of the fingers or toes

- Numbness of the digits or pins and needles
- Change in colour − should be pink; any blue, grey or white colour should be reported
- Cold digits − this may not be a sign, especially if no other sign is present, but warm digits are more reassuring

Cast bracing. This is the application of a supportive device that allows continued function of the part. It is especially used in fractures of long bones such as the tibia and femur and allows some use of the limb. As the support is less with this type of splint, it is not usually applied until the fifth or sixth week when healing is well under way.

Traction. Sustained traction is used when it is not possible to hold the bones in place with a plaster cast, usually due to muscle contraction. It is more common in fractures of the femur, distal shaft of humerus and some fractures of the tibial shaft. The pull of the muscles is balanced by sustained traction on the distal fragment of the fracture, usually by weights. Traction is usually combined with splintage to give support to the limb and prevent angular deformity.

External fixation. The bone fragments are anchored to an external device, such as a metal bar, by pins inserted into the distal and proximal fragments of a long bone fracture. It is used especially when infection is a danger, as in an open fracture, as internal fixation would carry a greater risk of spreading infection.

Internal fixation. This involves an operation and the insertion of some form of metallic plate, intramedullary nail, screwplate or nailplate. It carries a much higher risk of introducing infection into the bone and the surgeon often has to balance this risk with the advantage of early mobilization. The age of the patient, his occupation and the site of the fracture have all to be taken into account. With the advent of improved antibiotic cover and the use of closed-suction drainage the dangers are becoming less.
Internal fixation is used:

- When the fracture cannot be maintained in an acceptable position by splintage and/or traction.
- Following an open reduction when it is usually necessary to internally fix the fragments to prevent displacement.
- To provide rapid control of limb fractures when there are other severe injuries.
- To rigidly fix the fracture for early mobility, e.g., neck of femur.

Open (compound) fractures

The big risk here is infection and the wound should be kept covered with a sterile dressing and not disturbed until the patient can urgently go to theatre.

Here, the wound can be cleaned, dead tissue removed, leaving only healthy and well-vascularized tissue able to fight off infection by microorganisms.

Most wounds will not be immediately sutured unless very recent and obviously clean and uncontaminated. Other wounds are sutured when it is certain that any infection has been prevented, often in 4 or 5 days.

The fracture itself is better treated by closed methods. Internal fixation runs the risk of spreading any infection. Antibiotics are always administered. These will be broad spectrum such as a cephalosporin (see p. 496). Tetanus prophylaxis must be given if not up to date.

The patient should be closely observed for signs of infection, especially a sustained rise in temperature.

Healing of fractures

It may take between 6 and 12 weeks for the fractured bone to heal, depending on the position and the type of fracture. Healing starts as soon as the bone is broken and usually proceeds through several stages until the break is healed. These stages include haematoma formation around the fracture, cellular proliferation by the osteoblasts, laying down of calcium to form callus and, finally, consolidation into mature bone.

Restoration of function

Rehabilitation is always necessary and should begin as soon as the fracture is treated. Patients can help themselves with the aid of the physiotherapist as active use is much better than passive movement. The physiotherapist will explain the exercises that are needed to help retain or restore function and these need to be commenced as soon as possible.

! If rehabilitation is ignored and a limb is kept immobile for long periods the muscles will waste and the joints will stiffen.

There may be permanent impairment of function.

Complications of fractures

These may be associated with the fracture itself or with the surrounding soft tissues.

Infection

Usually occurs in an open fracture but may also occur when a closed fracture is converted into an open one by operative reduction. Osteomyelitis is infection of the bone and is difficult to treat, often leading to long-term problems. The acute infection often becomes a chronic one, and part of the bone may die due to lack of blood supply. This leads to a chronic discharge of pus through a sinus and the infection often prevents or delays union of the fracture.

Prevention is by early cleaning of the wound in theatre and removal of all dead tissue. The wound should not be sutured immediately. Antibiotics are always administered.

If infection is present then free drainage is allowed and antibiotics administered. A combination of flucloxacillin plus penicillin plus fusidic acid may be appropriate but it does depend on the sensitivity of the invading organisms. Choices of antibiotic therapy in the high-risk patient may include gentamicin or ciprofloxacin instead of penicillin.

Delayed union

The fracture does not unite as quickly as expected and is freely mobile after a period of 3 or 4 months. If it persists, it will become nonunion. If healing does not occur after about 6 months, bone grafting may be considered. If callus has formed then internal fixation may be used.

Nonunion

This is a failure of the bone ends to grow together and can be diagnosed by X-ray. Healing is not going to occur and the bone ends are dense and rounded. The gap between the bones is filled with fibrous tissue and not callus.

Nonunion may be due to infection, inadequate blood supply to one or both fragments, loss of apposition between fragments, interposition of soft tissue between fragments, movement between fragments or destruction of bone by a tumour in pathologic fractures.

The treatment depends partly on the site of the fracture, as in some cases it may not affect mobility too greatly and may be left, e.g., scaphoid fracture. Bone grafting is often used. The graft is usually obtained from the patient and may come from the ilium when cancellous bone is required or from the tibia if a stronger bone is needed.

Electromagnetic stimulation may be used to encourage bone healing.

Malunion

The bone is healed but in an imperfect position. It may result in shortening or there may be some rotation or overlap of the fragments. Often occurs to a small degree but can need correcting in some instances.

Shortening

May be due to malunion, crushing or actual loss of bone as in a comminuted fracture or in children when there is interference with the growing ends of long bones (epiphyses). It is only really important in the legs and may require the raising of the shoe if more than 2 cm or an operation to correct it or shorten the other leg. It can cause backache due to tilting of the pelvis and osteoarthritis of the hip in later life.

Avascular necrosis

This is death of bone due to interference with its blood supply and may have serious consequences. It can lead to nonunion and severe osteoarthritis. It is only a problem usually when a joint is involved. The avascular bone loses its structure and eventually collapses. This may occur within a year of the injury but may take 3 or 4 years. The affected joint is likely to be arthritic whether or not union eventually occurs.

Common sites are the head of the femur following a fractured neck of femur and the scaphoid. On diagnosis, early operation may be attempted.

Blood vessel injuries

There is always some damage to soft tissues when a bone is broken but usually healing occurs without a problem. If an important artery is damaged, however, this can occasionally lead to loss of a limb. It is more likely to result in ischaemic damage such as a Volkmann's ischaemic contracture of muscle, especially common following injury to the brachial artery in a supracondylar fracture of the humerus (at the elbow), commonly seen in children.

It is vital that observation of the peripheral circulation occurs following a fracture of a long bone. The radial pulse should be checked at regular intervals following a supracondylar fracture. There may be numbness of the digits and pain due to ischaemia.

Compartment syndrome

Within a muscle compartment swelling occurs and the pressure rises. This can lead to ischaemia as a result of small vessel occlusion and the operation of fasciotomy is urgently necessary as permanent loss of function can occur in 6–8 h.

Injury to nerves

This is more common than damage to major arteries. If there is slight damage, recovery is spontaneous in a few weeks. In more severe damage recovery takes many months and may not occur without excision of the damaged section.

The nerve is often contused (bruised) by a sharp bone fragment and recovery is complete.

Injury to viscera

Examples include lung complications following fractured ribs and bladder injury following a fractured pelvis.

Tendon injuries

Tendons attach muscle to bone and if they are severed, movement is prevented. The treatment here is surgical reconstruction.

Injuries to joints

There may be dislocation, subluxation (partial displacement) or strain of the ligaments. The long-term result is often joint stiffness and osteoarthritis, from any fracture involving the joint. Adhesions may occur and the best preventive measure is early mobilization and exercise. The knee, elbow, shoulder and finger joints stiffen easily whereas the wrist usually regains its mobility. Exercises are always necessary and physiotherapy may continue long after the fracture has healed.

Osteoarthritis is likely to develop in any joint that has been involved in a displaced fracture. The risk varies according to the joint involvement at the time and the residual damage to the joint. The arthritis may occur within 6–9 months after a severe injury but may not become apparent for 15 or 20 years if the damage is slight.

Fat embolism

This is uncommon but often fatal. Globules of fat enter the venous circulation and pass through the lungs to the systemic circulation. Small blood vessels may be blocked by the fat globules and this usually occurs in the lungs (resulting in difficulty in breathing and hypoxaemia) or the brain. Fat embolism most often follows a fractured shaft of femur.

Recovery occurs if the patient can be supported over the dangerous period of hypoxia. Oxygen is given and heparin may be administered to aid capillary flow.

5.9 THE IMMUNE SYSTEM

Immunology is the study of the way in which organisms fight off disease. It includes the study of how they differentiate between self and non-self. The immune system is a defence system that will identify and destroy all substances, dead or alive, not recognized as self. It is a remarkably adaptive defence system that has evolved in vertebrates to protect them from invading pathogenic microorganisms and cancer:

- The complexity of the network rivals that of the nervous system.
- It is able to differentiate between what is foreign and what are the body's own cells and proteins.
- Once a foreign organism is recognized there are a variety of cells and molecules which will effect an appropriate response.
- Later exposure to the same foreign organism will initiate a memory response, which is characterized by heightened immune activity to eliminate the pathogen and prevent disease.

Immunity has both specific and nonspecific components:

- *Innate* immunity is nonspecific and refers to the basic resistance to disease that an individual is born with.
- *Acquired* immunity is specific and involves white blood cells called lymphocytes and antibodies.
- Innate immunity can be seen to be composed of four types of barrier:

Anatomic barriers

- Skin
- Mucous membranes

Physiologic barriers

- Temperature — body temperature inhibits the growth of some pathogens, e.g., chickens have a high body temperature which makes them immune to anthrax.
- Low pH.
- Chemical mediators — lysozyme, interferon, complement.

Phagocytic barriers — white blood cells

- Neutrophils
- Macrophages

Inflammatory barriers

- Tissue damage and infection induce leakage of vascular fluid, which contains serum proteins, and an influx of phagocytic cells occurs into the affected area.
- Inflammatory response includes vasodilatation, increase in capillary permeability and an influx of phagocytes.

Acquired immunity

This needs the presence of a functional immune system that is capable of recognizing and selectively eliminating organisms. Acquired immune responses are adaptive and display antigenic specificity and immunologic memory.

Acquired immunity involves two major populations of white blood cells:

- B lymphocytes — produce antibodies.

- T lymphocytes — produce chemicals to 'help' the B lymphocyte in antibody production.

Ageing and the immune system

- Immune function decreases with age.
- Diminished T cell function and antibody responses to antigenic challenge.
- However, circulating autoantibodies and immune complexes increase.
- Those above 60 years have decreased delayed hypersensitivity reactions, decreased T cell responses to infection and decreased T cell activity.

Hypersensitivities

The immune system is a finely tuned network that protects the host against foreign antigens, particularly infectious agents. Sometimes this network breaks down and the immune system reacts inappropriately.

Type 1 hypersensitivity is an immediate allergic response due to the production of IgE antibodies to an allergen (see Box 5.8). It is an exaggerated response to an environmental antigen — called an *allergy*. It is responsible for the severe response in anaphylaxis and for hay fever, asthma and eczema.

Hypersensitivity reactions are immediate or delayed depending on the time required for the reaction to appear after re-exposure to an antigen. *Immediate*

BOX 5.8 Common antigens associated with Type 1 hypersensitivity

Proteins	Foods
Foreign serum	Nuts
Vaccines	Seafood
Plant pollens	Eggs
Ragweed	Peas, beans
Timothy grass	Rye grass
Birch trees	**Insect products**
Drugs	Bee venom
Penicillin	Ant venom
Sulphonamides	Cockroach calyx
Salicylates	**Mould spores**
	Animal hair and dander

hypersensitivity reactions occur in a few minutes to hours. *Delayed* hypersensitivity reactions may take several hours and are at maximum severity several days after re-exposure to the antigen.

Anaphylaxis is the immediate hypersensitivity reaction (see p. 146):

- It is a rapid and severe response occurring within minutes of re-exposure to the antigen.
- It can be systemic or localized.
- Symptoms include itching, erythema, urticaria (hives), vomiting, abdominal cramps, diarrhoea and breathing difficulties.
- In severe cases, laryngeal oedema and vascular collapse may occur and result in respiratory distress, decreased blood pressure, shock and death.
- Severe anaphylaxis, when there is difficulty in breathing or collapse, is treated with adrenaline 1 in 1000, 0.5 mL, intramuscularly.
- *Chlorphenamine*, an antihistamine, and hydrocortisone are also given to reduce symptoms.

General predisposition

- Certain individuals are prone to allergies and are *atopic*.
- Atopic individuals tend to produce higher quantities of IgE.
- The airways and skin of atopic individuals are also more responsive to all types of stimuli.
- In families where one parent has an allergy, allergies develop in about 40% of the offspring.
- If both parents have allergies, the incidence in offspring is about 80%.
- Atopic individuals are more susceptible to asthma, hay fever and eczema.

Skin testing is available to determine allergies against which individuals are sensitized but can be dangerous. The allergen is injected intradermally or put onto the skin in a scratch test. A local anaphylactic response occurs within 30 min in sensitized individuals.

Localized anaphylaxis (atopy)

The reaction is limited to a particular tissue or organ, often involving the epithelial surfaces at the site of entry of the allergen.

Atopic allergies affect at least 20% of individuals in developed countries and include hay fever (allergic rhinitis), asthma, eczema and food allergies.

Eczema

This is a form of dermatitis that is nonspecific and may be acute, subacute or chronic.

Dermatitis is the name given to inflammatory conditions of the skin. They may involve the dermis or epidermis but usually involve both:

- The skin becomes red and itchy. The epidermis and superficial dermis are involved.
- There may be oedema in the acute stages.
- Tiny blisters called vesicles develop in the epidermis: fluid accumulates between the epidermal cells (*spongiosis*), eventually forming small fluid-filled collections. These burst, causing weeping and oozing of clear yellow fluid, and then crust over.
- In chronic phases, scaling and fissuring occur.
- Excoriation may lead to secondary infection.
- Intense itching and scratching cause secondary changes due to trauma to occur. This leads to chronic dermatitis.
- The skin is thickened and cracked and often covered with a thick opaque scale.
- The skin looks a bit like the bark of a tree due to its increased thickness and the underlying oedema. This is called *lichenification.*
- The dermis shows increased fibrosis.
- Dermatitis may be due to many causes, but one of the most common in childhood is atopic eczema, which usually starts in infancy. Where the disorder starts early in life, there is a good chance that it will clear in adolescence; 90% of those with infantile eczema will be clear in adulthood. A few may be able to correlate the onset of itching with dietary factors and removal of the food item, e.g., eggs, milk, from the diet will improve the condition.
- There is a tendency to dry, flaky skin (*xeroderma*) even when the eczema is not present.

Exacerbating factors

- Heat
- Humidity
- Drying of the skin
- Contact with woolly clothing may cause a flare-up

Staphylococcus aureus is found on the skin in a higher percentage of these individuals than normal and may be present in 90% of lesions.

Eczema is never present at birth but it may develop after a few weeks. Atopic eczema affects 3% of all infants.

Patterns of disease

- *Infantile eczema* — usually first appears on the facial skin at a few months of age.

- With time there is spread to other flexures.
- *Flexural or childhood dermatitis* − in toddlers or children; the skinfolds are usually involved. Some facial involvement may persist.
- *Adult dermatitis* − flexures at the neck, elbow, wrist, ankle, knee and the limbs are usually involved. Chronic eczematous changes are common on the face.
- *Seborrhoeic dermatitis* − a coarse, yellowish crust scale is seen on the scalp. May be called cradle cap or milk crust. Disappears by the age of a year.
- *Napkin dermatitis* − this is a form of contact dermatitis; 50% of babies may be affected at some time. Bright erythema is present

Treatment

- Removal of contributory factors.
- Application of emollients at least twice daily to the affected area.
- Bath and shower emollients may be used in addition.
- Topical steroids are required and the potency is dependent of the severity of the eczema.
- Infection may also be a problem.
- Other specialist treatments are available for severe refractory eczema.

Autoimmunity

In autoimmune diseases the immune system reacts against self-antigens and destroys host tissues. The exact cause is unknown but both environmental and genetic factors can trigger such a disease. Autoimmune diseases appear to be increasing in incidence globally and are often difficult to diagnose. Treatment is not usually curative but is given to manage symptoms.

Antibodies against self are called *autoantibodies* and these are sometimes produced by healthy individuals, especially the elderly, without overt auto-immune disease.

Autoimmune diseases affect 5%−7% of the population and may be:

- Organ specific (Table 5.13)
- Systemic

Systemic autoimmune diseases

- The response is directed towards a large number of target antigens and involves a number of organs and tissues.
- They reflect a generalized defect in immune regulation. The body incorrectly identifies a normal protein as a threat and autoantibodies are made.

TABLE 5.13 Some organ-specific autoimmune diseases in humans

Disease	Organ
Addison's disease	Adrenal glands
Haemolytic anaemia (autoimmune)	RBC membrane protein
Graves' disease	Thyroid
Hashimoto's thyroiditis	Thyroid cells
Idiopathic thrombocytopenic purpura	Platelets
Type 1 diabetes mellitus (IDDM)	Pancreatic beta cells
Myasthenia gravis	ACh receptor
Pernicious anaemia	Gastric parietal cells

- Tissue damage is widespread from both cell-mediated immune responses and direct cellular damage caused by autoantibodies.
- Includes SLE and RA.

Treatment of autoimmune disease

- Ideally the treatment should be aimed at reducing the autoimmune response while leaving the rest of the immune system intact. To date, this ideal has not been reached.
- Current therapies are not cures but palliatives.
- Aim to reduce symptoms to give the patient a reasonable quality of life.
- Most provide nonspecific suppression of the immune system and do not differentiate between a pathogenic immune response and a protective one.
- Immunosuppressive drugs such as corticosteroids, azathioprine and cyclophosphamide are given to slow the proliferation of lymphocytes. However, the patient is then at a much greater risk of infection and cancer.
- Removal of the thymus has been used in myasthenia where it is often abnormal.

Systemic lupus erythematosus

SLE is a complex disease that attacks connective tissue. It is an inflammatory multisystem autoimmune disease in which antinuclear antibodies occur. These may be present years before the person has symptoms. The cause of SLE is unknown but the peak incidence is in the 20s and 30s with women nine times more likely than men to be affected. The average time taken to diagnose lupus is 7 years and its prevalence is lowest in women of Northern European origin.

Some forms of lupus are drug-induced by drugs such as isoniazid and minocycline.

Presentation

There are relapses and remissions:

- The signs and symptoms are often nonspecific when the disease first arises.
- Tiredness, fever, weight loss, arthralgia, headache and skin rashes may all occur and symptoms may range from minor aches and pains to life-threatening disease.
- Major organ involvement tends to occur within 5 years of onset.
- Pulmonary involvement may be with pleurisy or bronchiolitis and there is an increased risk of pulmonary embolus.
- Cardiovascular involvement includes hypertension, pericarditis and increased risk of CHD.
- Renal involvement may be detected by proteinuria, and glomerulonephritis is common.
- Neurologic manifestations include seizures and strokes.
- Anxiety and depression are common.

Management

- Joint and muscle pains need analgesia – often NSAIDs.
- Treatment with corticosteroids is very effective but may lead to increased mortality due to infection.
- *Hydroxychloroquine*, an antimalarial drug, is the first-line treatment and helps with skin manifestations and arthralgia. It helps to suppress the inflammatory response.
- *Cyclophosphamide* is used in life-threatening disease alongside steroids.
- Patients with renal involvement have a poorer prognosis.
- Drug-induced lupus usually subsides when the drug is discontinued.

Alloimmunity

Alloimmune disease occurs when the immune system of one individual produces an immunologic reaction against the tissues of another individual. It may be observed in reactions against transfusions, grafted tissues or the fetus in pregnancy.

Preventing graft rejection

The severity of rejection is determined by certain genetic differences and whether an organ is a good match or not can be determined by *tissue typing*. Closely related individuals are likely to have similar tissue types, and grafts between identical twins are completely accepted.

Immunosuppressant drugs are given to try to suppress the immune response and graft rejection.

Immunodeficiency diseases

These are a diverse spectrum of illnesses that stem from various abnormalities of the immune system. Basic manifestations are frequent, prolonged, severe infections, which are often caused by organisms with normally low pathogenicity.

An immunodeficiency disease may result from:

- a primary congenital defect and
- a secondary cause, such as viral or bacterial infection, malnutrition or a drug treatment.

Human immunodeficiency virus and AIDS

Human immunodeficiency virus (HIV) is the cause of acquired immune deficiency syndrome (AIDS) which is the most significant immunodeficiency arising from secondary causes. AIDS is an epidemic of a retroviral disease characterized by profound immunosuppression.

HIV is a retrovirus in the lentivirus group. There are at least two types, HIV-1 and HIV-2, and HIV-2 is found mostly in West Africa and is associated with a less severe AIDS-type illness. There are two main subtypes of HIV-1 determined by DNA sequencing. These are the Group M (major) subtypes, of which there are at least 10 (denoted A–J) and Group O (outlier) subtypes of which there are only a small number found mostly in the Cameroons.

AIDS is associated with opportunistic infections, secondary neoplasms and neurologic manifestations. HIV-1 infects humans, chimpanzees, pigtailed macaques and SCID-human mice but causes immune suppression only in humans.

Transmission of HIV is possible via:

- Sexual intercourse.
- Contaminated blood products and organ donation – very rare since screening was introduced in 1985.
- Contaminated needles in IV drug users or in needlestick injuries.
- Passage of virus from infected mothers to their newborns.

Infected mothers transmit HIV by three routes:

- Transplacental, in utero.
- During delivery.
- Via breast milk – not usual.

Vertical transmission by these routes occurs in 12%–30% of infants at risk.

Although it was originally more common in homosexual males, the rate of increase of heterosexual transmission has outpaced transmission by all other means. The number of women with AIDS is increasing rapidly. The presence of any other sexually transmitted disease such as *Treponema pallidum* or herpes simplex virus increases the likelihood of transmission because of genital ulceration.

There is an extremely small but definite risk to healthcare workers, and seroconversion has been reported following an accidental needlestick injury. The risk is believed to be 0.3%. By comparison, the risk for HBV would be 30%.

Genetic variation in HIV

- HIV is capable of tremendous genetic variation with mutation occurring at rates millions of times faster than observed in human DNA.
- The influenza virus also has a high mutation rate and this has hampered the production of an effective flu vaccine.
- The rate of mutation in HIV is 65 times that of the influenza virus.
- No two AIDS patients carry an identical virus.
- HIV isolates taken from the same individual at different times can differ substantially.

Most individuals develop symptoms of AIDS 8–10 years after infection with HIV but approximately 25% of infected individuals have remained symptom-free for some 10–12 years:

- Soon after infection with HIV the virus replicates and can be detected in the serum but is only there for a few weeks and then disappears as the antibody response (seroconversion) develops.
- In most cases the time between infection and seroconversion is 6 weeks, but in some it has lasted for 3 years.
- At seroconversion antibodies to HIV can be detected in the blood (serum).
- Within a few weeks these decline and IgG appears.
- As long as the antibody to core protein remains high, an individual remains asymptomatic.
- When the antibody declines this is associated with progression from latency to infection.

Diagnosis

HIV infection is diagnosed by detecting virus-specific antibodies (anti-HIV) or identification of viral material.

Detection of IgG antibody to components of the viral envelope is the most common marker used to identify infection. It may take up to 3 months from initial infection to antibody detection. The antibodies do not protect against HIV and remain for life. The presence of antibodies cannot tell us how long the person has had the infection.

Antibody testing should only be done after a full discussion of the implications with the patient.

HIV testing is getting simpler and more rapidly available, meaning that the results could be given in hours. There are tests being developed that use the body secretions rather than plasma, e.g., semen, saliva and urine. There are special tests available to detect HIV-antibodies within 6—8 weeks of infection. Viral p24 antigen is detectable early after infection but has usually gone by 8—10 weeks following exposure.

The CD4 cell (T helper) in AIDS

- Uninfected persons have about 1100 CD4 cells per microlitre of blood.
- In AIDS this drops dramatically and may be as low as 200.
- About 40% of AIDS patients manifesting opportunistic infections have no detectable CD4 cells at all.
- The CD4 count drops very slowly over 8—10 years and then rapidly in most cases.

Clinical features

The spectrum of illnesses associated with AIDS is very broad.

Incubation

Following infection, the first 2—4 weeks are symptom free.

Acute seroconversion illness

Seroconversion may be clinically silent but nonspecific illness does develop in a proportion of patients (between 53% and 93%) about 6—8 weeks after exposure. Very few patients are correctly diagnosed in primary care at this stage because symptoms of seroconversion are nonspecific and the patient may not present themselves at this stage.

Seroconversion is a self-limiting illness with fever, myalgia (muscle aching), oral ulceration, generalized lymphadenopathy (enlarged lymph glands) and a maculopapular rash (small red spots) affecting the upper half of the body.

If diagnosis is made at this stage then treatment can be initiated before the immune system is severely damaged. There would also be less chance of spreading the infection to others before diagnosis is made.

Asymptomatic infection (clinical latency)

Most people with HIV are asymptomatic for variable lengths of time. This is a period when the number of HIV-infected lymphocytes is gradually increasing. Individuals may remain well but they are infectious. This stage lasts on average 10 years but some develop much more rapidly and some remain symptom-free much longer.

Persistent generalized lymphadenopathy with enlarged lymph nodes of more than 1 cm in diameter at two or more sites for more than 3 months does occur in a subgroup of asymptomatic patients.

Symptomatic HIV infection

The infection progresses and the viral load increases. The CD4 count goes down and the patient develops a variety of signs and symptoms. These are a result of the associated immunosuppression.

The severity of the symptoms will depend upon how immunosuppressed the patient is and how virulent are the infective organisms they encounter.

Effects of HIV infection include:

- Continuous symptoms of fever, weight loss and diarrhoea
- Neurologic disease: dementia, peripheral neuropathy, myelopathy, aseptic meningitis
- Eye disease
- Blood disorders – thrombocytopenia, anaemia
- Renal complications – HIV-associated nephropathy
- Respiratory complications

Effects of immunodeficiency

Opportunistic infections are diseases caused by organisms that are not usually pathogenic, unusual presentations of known pathogenic diseases and the occurrence of certain tumours.

CD4 T lymphocyte numbers are used as markers to predict infection risk.

Specific infections associated with HIV infection include fungal infections such as those caused by *Pneumocystis carinii* (pneumonia), cryptococcus (usually meningitis), *Candida* and *Aspergillus*. Protozoal infections such as toxoplasmosis (may cause encephalitis and cerebral abscess) and *Cryptosporidium parvum* (diarrhoea) may occur. Common viral infections include hepatitis, cytomegalovirus (CMV), herpesviruses and papovavirus. Bacterial infections include tuberculosis.

Avoidance of infection by opportunistic pathogens is important – great care with food preparation and hygiene.

Neoplasms include Kaposi's sarcoma, lymphomas and squamous cell carcinoma.

Drug treatment

There is no cure, but suppressive therapy means that HIV is now a chronic controllable condition since the advent of highly active antiretroviral therapy (HAART).

Drugs increase life expectancy but are toxic. Treatment aims to prevent mortality and morbidity whilst minimizing drug toxicity.

There are many antiretroviral drugs available in the UK now. These include reverse transcriptase inhibitors, protease inhibitors and fusion inhibitors.

Treatment of HIV is complicated and ever-changing. It should always be initiated by a specialist. The patient has to be committed to adhere to the strict regimen.

The British HIV Association (BHIVA) has produced guidelines for the treatment of HIV.

5.10 CANCER

Known since the time of the ancient Egyptians, cancer occurs in most plants as well as animals. *Neoplasia* means new growth. *Neoplasms* are often referred to as tumours, and the study of tumours is called *oncology*.

Malignant tumours are collectively referred to as cancers, from the Latin for 'crab'. The lesion can invade and destroy adjacent structures and spread to distant sites (*metastasize*) to cause death.

Benign tumours

- May affect any tissue.
- Grow locally but do not spread or invade.
- Damage tissues by pressure.
- Resemble the tissue of origin and, if endocrine, are likely to produce hormones.
- Usually have a capsule of connective tissue.

Malignant tumours

- Cellular abnormalities are present and there may be invasion of the surrounding tissues.
- Local increase in cell number and increased mitotic activity.
- Loss of normal regular arrangement.
- Variation in cell size and shape.
- Increase in nuclear size and density of staining.
- No well-defined capsule.

Carcinoma in situ is a small tumour that remains localized in the epithelial layer, usually on the cervix or skin but can be the bladder and other organs. There is no invasion of underlying tissue; the cancer remains where it began — in situ.

The only definite evidence of malignancy is invasion of the underlying tissues and metastases:

- Sometimes the tissue of origin can be identified and the tumour is *differentiated.*
- Other tumours may follow a very undifferentiated growth pattern and be classed as *poorly differentiated.*
- Malignant neoplasms composed of undifferentiated cells are said to be *anaplastic.* This is the most extreme disturbance in cell growth and structure of the tissue is lost.
- The rate of growth of malignant tumours correlates in general with their level of differentiation.
- *Dysplasia* is a term used to describe disorderly but nonneoplastic proliferation which exhibits loss of uniformity and architectural orientation. This is seen in epithelial tissue and if marked and involving the entire thickness of the epithelium, the lesion is known as *carcinoma* in situ.

Naming tumours

The generic name, which describes the tissue of origin and whether the tumour is benign or malignant, is qualified by the specific tissue of origin and this may be further qualified by further terms describing the cell of origin and the pattern of growth. Benign tumours tend to be named by adding *-oma* to the cell type from which the tumour arises.

Tumours of the epithelium

Epithelial tissue is constantly dividing and the majority of cancers occur in this type of tissue.

Benign tumours

- May be papillary (warty) or solid.
- Glandular tissue — adenomas and may be solid or papillary.

Malignant tumours

- Generic name is carcinoma.
- Can qualify as squamous cell or basal cell if the skin is involved.
- Glands — adenocarcinoma but can also describe the cell type, e.g., columnar cell.

Tumours of the mesenchyme

- Benign tumours — named from the cellular tissue from which they arise: fibroma (fibrous tissue), osteoma (bone), angioma (blood vessels), etc.

- Malignant tumours — generic name is sarcoma and as with carcinoma, this is qualified by the cell of origin and growth type, e.g., osteosarcoma — tumour of bone, osteogenic sarcoma — tumour of bone-forming cells.
- Most sarcomas grow rapidly.

Tumours of the reticuloendothelial system

This is a complicated field. Benign tumours do exist but are difficult to distinguish. There are two main types:

- Those arising from blood-producing cells — leukaemias.
- Solid tumours — lymphomas.

Tumours of the nervous system

- Benign and malignant but malignant very rarely spread outside the nervous system.
- Tumours of nerve cells proper — neurons — only arise in the embryo or shortly after birth — neuroblastomas and retinoblastomas.
- Almost all tumours are either gliomas that arise from the supporting connective tissues within the brain, or meningiomas, that arise from the membranes surrounding the brain (see also p. 396).

Tumours of mixed tissues

Very rarely tumours which contain a whole range of different tissues may be found — teratomas. They are thought to arise from primitive cells of embryonic type and are usually found in the testes or ovary. Sometimes they are benign but often malignant changes occur.

Carcinogenesis

This is a multistage process that is still not completely understood. There is an evolving process causing changes to the genetic material (DNA) within the nucleus of the cell. The tumour appears to be derived from a single stem cell.

Theories suggest that there is an initiation stage, such as contact with a carcinogen, which does not lead to the immediate development of a tumour but is rapid and essential for development to occur. The initiated cells may be dormant for very long periods or even the whole lifespan of the individual and several further independent accidents may have to occur to the same cell for tumour development to continue. This would explain why most forms of cancer increase in incidence as we get older, i.e., the chances of cumulative accidents to the cell increase with time. Examples of carcinogens include cigarette smoke, viruses, radiation and certain chemicals in foods named *xenobiotics*.

Cancers in humans can be divided into three groups depending on age and incidence:

- Embryonic:
  - Neuroblastoma (tumours of embryonic nerve cells)
  - Wilms' tumours (embryonal tumours of the kidney)
  - Retinoblastomas.
- Those occurring predominantly in the young: Some leukaemias
  - Tumours of the bone and testes.
- Those with an increasing incidence with age: Prostate, colon, breast, skin, salivary glands, etc.

There are at least three possible explanations for age-related tumour incidence:

- Continuous exposure throughout life to low levels of carcinogens.
- Hormonal changes occur with age and these allow neoplastic changes to occur.
- Age-associated changes in some cells increase susceptibility to neoplastic transformation.

Metastases

Cancers grow into surrounding tissues by progressive infiltration, invasion, destruction and penetration of the tissue. This is local spread. The danger is that they can also spread further:

- Via the lymphatic system
- Via the bloodstream
- By seeding within body cavities

Basal cell carcinomas of the skin and primary tumours of the central nervous system are highly invasive in their primary sites but only rarely metastasize. At the other extreme are osteogenic sarcomas that have usually metastasized to the lungs before discovery.

Approximately 30% of newly diagnosed patients with solid tumours are present with metastases. An additional 20% have occult (hidden) metastases at the time of diagnosis:

- When local invasion occurs, tumours may penetrate the lymphatics and be carried to the regional lymph nodes where they may be arrested. Some are destroyed but some grow.
- If tumour cells get into the bloodstream they can be carried to any organ in the body. Many are destroyed but others grow into secondary tumours.
- Arteries are less readily penetrated than veins.

- All portal drainage flows to the liver and all caval blood flows to the lungs. This means these two organs are often targeted by metastases from the primary cancer.
- Carcinomas often involve the lymph nodes, sarcomas do not.
- Metastases are common in the lungs, liver and bone but rare in muscle and spleen.

Breast cancer

Approximately one in eight women in England will be diagnosed with breast cancer and may develop breast cancer during their lifetime, and about 11,400 women died of this disease in 2014. The death rate from breast cancer is falling due to better treatment and earlier detection using mammography.

The risk for breast cancer increases with advancing age and the peak incidence is between 65 and 69 years (Cancer Research UK, 2018).

Risk factors

- Age — risk increases with age.
- Having a sister or mother with breast cancer.
- Reproductive — the younger a woman has her first full-term pregnancy, the lower the risk of breast cancer.
- Hormonal — late menarche and early menopause reduce the risk. Removal of the ovaries is protective. Increasing oestrogen levels may be a risk.
- Hormone replacement therapy (HRT) has been linked to an increased incidence of breast cancer but this is with prolonged use of HRT (more than 8 years) and the risk is lost as soon as the HRT is discontinued.
- Environmental — high-dose radiation.
- Diet perhaps — results of research are mixed but there may be a higher risk with a high-fat diet. There is a low incidence in Japan that could be related to diet.
- Some studies show that there may be a correlation between alcohol consumption and breast cancer.
- Viral factors have been suspected following research with mice.
- Trauma is not thought to have any effect.
- Familial — 7% of breast cancers are familial. Autosomal dominant gene with 90% penetration by the age of 50.
- Breast feeding for longer than a year may be protective.

Screening

In the UK, screening is commenced at the age of 50 years and is offered until the age of 70 years, once every 3 years. Regular screening can reduce breast cancer mortality by up to 25%. Mammography has a 90% accuracy but is less accurate premenopausally due to the density of breast tissue.

Screening should begin earlier for those at high risk, and regular breast self-examination should be practised by all women.

Diagnosis

The patient may present with a breast lump, nipple retraction, breast pain, a discharge from the nipple, inflammation or an axillary lump. Mammography, ultrasound, examination and cytology or needle biopsy may all be involved in the diagnosis.

Pathogenesis

Most cancers arise from the ductal epithelium. There are two classes of breast cancer.

Carcinoma in situ — noninvasive

- Growth is confined to the basement membrane of the duct or gland.
- Difficult to detect because there may be no fibrous lump; the cancer does metastasize, although.
- The usual treatment consists of complete local excision with radiotherapy and/or tamoxifen.
- Paget's disease of the nipple is an intraduct carcinoma, which presents as a red scaly lesion of the nipple.

Infiltrating carcinoma — invasive

- Most breast cancers are of this type.
- Infiltrating ductal carcinomas account for 75% of all tumours.
- Invasive lobular carcinoma — 10%.
- Other types include tubular, medullary and mucinous; these carry a better prognosis usually.
- Sixty per cent of tumours occur in the upper, outer aspect of the breast because most glandular tissue is found here.

Presentation

- Early signs are insidious.
- A nontender lump, most often in the upper, outer quadrant of the breast.
- At first the lump is mobile and pain is usually absent until the later stages.
- Dimpling or retraction of the skin over the lump — peau d'orange appearance. This is due to oedema caused by blockage of the small lymphatic ducts.
- Retraction of the nipple, due to a shortening of the ducts.

- Asymmetry of the breasts may be noted on mirror examination. The affected breast appears more elevated.
- The lump appears fixed to the chest wall at a later stage.
- Nodular axillary lumps may be present. These are enlarged lymph nodes.
- In the late stages ulceration may occur, and occasionally elderly patients may still present with a fungating mass.

Treatment of invasive breast cancer

- Treatment is individual and depends on staging and receptor status (many cancers are oestrogen-dependent).
- Staging is from Stage 0 for a carcinoma in situ that is not invasive through to Stage IV where distant metastases are present. The stage depends on the size of the tumour and its spread into the lymphatics or beyond. This is called TNM Staging as it is based on Tumour size, Nodal spread and Metastases.
- If surgery is offered it is likely to be wide excision of the lump or lumpectomy but in some cases a mastectomy (removal of the breast) may be preferable.
- Dissection of axillary lymph nodes is necessary as histology of the lymph nodes is vital to determine if the cancer has spread.
- Adjuvant hormonal therapy with an oestrogen antagonist such as ***tamoxifen*** is required for 5 years if the tumour is positive for oestrogen receptors. There are newer agents available now. These are selective oestrogen receptor modulators (SERMs) such as ***anastrozole.***
- ***Trastuzumab (Herceptin)*** is used if the cancer overexpresses a gene called the HER2 gene.
- Adjuvant chemotherapy with multiple agents may be used.
- Radiotherapy can reduce local recurrence and also increase survival.

Routes of spread
Locally

- Involving a progressive amount of breast tissue.
- Eventually results in skin involvement and ulceration or attachment to the muscle and chest wall.

Via the lymphatic system

- To axillary nodes at an early stage; many of those with operable cancer have axillary nodes.
- To internal mammary lymphatics.

- Skin lymphatics — leads to multiple tumour nodules. The skin becomes stiff and board-like.
- Mediastinal and abdominal nodes later in the disease.

Via the blood

- Very common and present in virtually all fatal cases.
- Most frequent metastases occur in the lungs, liver, bones and brain.
- The patient may first present with a pathologic fracture or bony pain.

Cancer of the prostate gland

This is a disease of older men and is now the most common male cancer. It is the second most common cause of death from cancer in men (cancer of the lung is the first). One in eight men will develop prostate cancer in their lifetime.

The prostate gland is situated around the upper end of the urethra just below the bladder. It is involved in the secretion of prostatic fluid that nourishes sperm.

Most cancers of the prostate are adenocarcinomas.

Risk factors

- Age. Prostate cancer mainly occurs in men above 50 years of age. At postmortem 30% of men above 75 years have prostate cancer. Two-thirds of those who die from prostate cancer are above 75 years of age.
- Diet may be important. Red meat and saturated fats increase the risk whilst lycopene (an antioxidant found in tomatoes) appears to have a protective effect.
- Some forms are familial.
- As with all cancers, a balanced and healthy diet together with exercise may help to prevent health issues.

Clinical features

- May be asymptomatic and found following operation for benign prostatic hyperplasia.
- Routine screening may show raised serum prostate-specific antigen (PSA).
- Difficulty in passing urine is usually the first symptom — poor stream, hesitancy, terminal dribbling, frequency and nocturia.
- May present with a UTI.
- Perineal pain may be present in advanced disease.
- Often metastasizes to bone and pathologic fracture may be the first sign.

Investigations

- Rectal examination usually reveals a hard irregular prostate.
- FBC and biochemical profile.
- Serum PSA and acid phosphatase.
- Transrectal ultrasound and biopsy.
- MRI, CT scan and bone scan — looking for metastases to stage the disease.

Treatment

- This depends on staging and other factors.
- Localized tumour that is well differentiated may be left untreated in an elderly man, especially if other pathologies are present. Watchful waiting may be appropriate.
- Localized tumours can be treated with radical prostatectomy or local radiotherapy. Complications may include erectile dysfunction or incontinence.
- Hormone therapy to reduce circulating testosterone levels (androgen suppression) can prolong survival.
- Palliative radiotherapy is very effective in the management of bone metastases.

Cancer of the testes

This is the most common malignancy in men aged 20–30 years. There are about 2300 new cases annually (Cancer Research UK, 2015) in the UK and the incidence is rising.

More than 95% of tumours are testicular germ cell tumours. They are classified as seminomas, teratomas or yolk sac tumours.

Clinical features

- Unilateral testicular swelling — all men should self-examine for this. A painless lump is usually the first sign, but it is sometimes associated with pain.
- Some present with a dragging sensation.
- As the disease progresses there may be weight loss, lethargy and respiratory symptoms if associated with lung metastases.
- Headache from cerebral metastases may occur.
- Back pain from glandular involvement retroperitoneally.

Investigations

- Testicular ultrasound.

- Various blood tests for hormone levels.
- Chest X-ray, CT scan of thorax, abdomen and pelvis and brain scan if cerebral metastases are suspected.

Treatment

- This depends very much on the type of tumour as seminomas are radio-sensitive but teratomas are not.
- Surgery — inguinal orchidectomy.
- May be followed by radiotherapy to lymph nodes.
- Chemotherapy with agents such as *cisplatin, etoposide* and *bleomycin.*
- Postorchidectomy surveillance is monthly for the first year and approximately 20%–25% relapse, usually within the first year.
- In more than 96% of cases, a stage I seminoma may be disease-free following orchidectomy and low-dose radiotherapy.
- In metastatic teratoma all patients receive chemotherapy.

Cancer of the ovary

This is the fifth most common carcinoma in women (around 7300 new cases in the UK in 2015) and the fourth most common cause of death (4128 deaths in UK in 2014). Most patients do not present until the disease is advanced and 35% survive ovarian cancer for 10 or more years (Cancer Research UK, 2018).

Incidence is most common between 75 and 79 years of age and in nulliparous women. Oral contraceptives appear to reduce the risk for up to 10 years following their use.

Clinical features

- Early disease is normally asymptomatic and the onset of symptoms is insidious.
- Early symptoms are vague and may include abdominal bloating, urinary frequency, fatigue, anorexia and depression.
- More advanced disease presents with abdominal pain, distension of the abdomen, ascites (common), occasionally vaginal bleeding.

Investigations

- CA-125 test. If raised above 35 IU/mL, further investigations.
- Pelvic and abdominal ultrasound, laparoscopy, aspiration of ascites for cytology, CT scan.
- Many cases are diagnosed at laparotomy.

Treatment

Staging is done and treatment is based on this.

Stage I ovarian cancer is limited to the ovaries, Stage II has extended to the pelvis, Stage III has peritoneal implants of the tumour outside the pelvis and Stage IV has distant metastases.

Surgery is the mainstay of treatment and the aim is to remove as much of the tumour as possible. A total abdominal hysterectomy with bilateral salpingo-oophrectomy and examination of all peritoneal surfaces, biopsy of lymph nodes and peritoneal washings are usual.

Further management depends upon the staging of the tumour. Intraperitoneal chemotherapy may be used.

NICE have issued guidelines for the use of chemotherapy. Some tumours are sensitive to platinum-based drugs such as ***cisplatin*** or ***carboplatin.*** Response can be measured by CT scan.

Radiotherapy is occasionally used in early disease.

The overall survival at 5 years is less than 35%. Most women (70%) do not present until Stage III or IV and the survival rates at 5 years for these stages are 17% and 5%. At Stage I and II, survival is between 80% and 100% at 5 years.

Cancer of the cervix

Around 3200 women are diagnosed with cervical cancer in the UK each year (Cancer research UK, 2018). The average age for detection of a precancerous lesions is 33—38 years and for invasive disease is between 50 and 60 years.

Invasive carcinoma has decreased over the years due to the cervical screening programme. Abnormal cervical smears have increased, especially in those under 25 years of age.

Risk factors

- Associated with human papilloma virus (HPV), especially types 16 and 18. These are sexually transmitted viruses. The immune system usually (but not always) clears them within 2 years.
- Women with multiple sexual partners or who are partners of promiscuous males are at higher risk.
- Often associated with chronic cervicitis and cervical dysplasia.
- More common in lower socioeconomic groups.
- Nonattendance at cervical screening programmes.

Pathogenesis

It is a progressive disease and premalignant lesions occur 10—12 years before the development of invasive carcinoma.

Virtually all cases of cervical cancer are linked to HPV infection.

There are now vaccines to prevent HPV infection. Since 2008, all girls aged 12 or 13 are routinely offered this vaccine at school. The vaccine is not effective against all types of HPV so screening is still important.

Progressive changes

Cervical intraepithelial neoplasia (CIN). Also called cervical dysplasia. The disease is confined to the epithelium and some of the cervical cells are replaced by abnormal neoplastic ones. It does not always progress to cancer and many will spontaneously return to normal. This is carefully followed by smears. CIN I is confined to the lower third of the epithelium, CIN II is the lower and middle third of the epithelium and CIN III affects the full thickness of the epidermis.

Invasive carcinoma. There is invasion into adjacent tissues and spread to distant organs such as the lungs via the lymphatics.

Cervical cancer is staged from 0 (carcinoma in situ preinvasive) to IVb with distant metastases.

Clinical features

- Regular screening by cervical (Papanicolaou) smear is needed as the early disease is asymptomatic.
- Vaginal discharge that may be intermittent or continuous.
- Vaginal bleeding that may be spontaneous or may follow intercourse. Postmenopausal bleeding may also occur.
- Vaginal discomfort and urinary symptoms.

Investigations

- Colposcopy is examination of the cervix by the use of a light and a small microscope. This is done as an outpatient and a biopsy is taken.
- Cone biopsy − If all the abnormal cells cannot be seen at colposcopy. A cone-shaped piece of tissue is removed from the cervix to be examined under the microscope.
- CT scanning of pelvis and abdomen is used to aid staging of the disease.
- MRI to give a clear picture of the tumour and any local invasion or lymph node involvement.

Management

- This depends on the stage of the disease.
- Premalignant and early cancer is treated with loop diathermy usually but cryosurgery or laser therapy can also be used.

- Cone biopsies remove a small amount of tissue and may be all that is needed to treat an early cancer. Pregnancy is still possible if the internal os is not damaged.
- For invasive carcinoma the treatment depends upon the stage and may include radical trachelectomy, hysterectomy, pelvic lymphadenectomy and more extensive pelvic surgery where necessary.
- Radiotherapy and platinum-based chemotherapy (***cisplatin***) may be used in some cases. This improves survival for high-risk patients following radical hysterectomy.

Radiotherapy

- Radiotherapy uses high-energy rays, usually X-rays, to kill cancer cells. It is a highly potent cytotoxic agent and reacts with both normal and malignant cells to induce the production of free radicals, which damage the intracellular DNA. The cell can function as usual, but is unable to complete cell division. Normal cells are better able to repair the damage caused by sublethal doses of radiation than cancer cells. This difference in repair capacity is exploited in radiotherapy.
- The total dose of radiation to be administered is divided into fractions and the time interval between fractions is calculated to allow maximum repair of normal tissue but only limited repair of malignant tissue.
- Not all cancers are sensitive to radiotherapy. The toxic effects of radiotherapy require oxygen and so tumours that are hypoxic due to a poor blood supply are less sensitive.
- Some cancers can be cured with radiotherapy alone, e.g., Hodgkin's disease, but often radiotherapy is given in addition to other treatments. It may be given before surgery to reduce the size of a tumour and this is called neoadjuvant radiotherapy. Radiotherapy following surgery is adjuvant radiotherapy.
- Radiotherapy may be used when a patient is medically unfit for surgery or a tumour is anatomically not resectable.
- Radiotherapy may also be used to control the cancer when a cure is not possible or it may be used palliatively to ease the symptoms of the cancer, e.g., to relieve bone pain.
- Radiotherapy should not be administered at any stage of pregnancy.

Administration of radiotherapy

External radiotherapy − The source of radiation comes from a machine outside the body. External beam therapy (*teletherapy*) may be produced at a lower voltage from an X-ray source. This could be used to treat superficial skin lesions such as basal cell carcinomas. It may be produced at a higher voltage by a gamma-emitting source or by a linear accelerator. This is suitable for deep-seated tumours.

Internal radiotherapy is where the radiation comes from implants inside the body. *Brachytherapy* is ionizing radiation emitted from a sealed source placed close to the tumour, e.g., caesium needles or iridium wires.

Radioactive iodine can be taken orally to treat cancer of the thyroid gland.

Determining dosage

The course of treatment is planned by an MDT and the total dose of radiation needed to treat the cancer is carefully worked out. It is administered in many fractions or small doses.

The maximum dose is given when the intention is curative. It is influenced by:

- The radiosensitivity of the tumour. Lymphomas are more sensitive than carcinomas, for instance.
- The radiosensitivity of the normal tissue within the radiation field.
- The volume of the normal tissue unavoidably irradiated.
- In palliative radiotherapy the aim is symptom relief with the minimum side effects possible.

Radiotherapy is usually given as an outpatient and most patients attend for several weeks from Monday to Friday, although some may only attend once or twice a week.

Side effects

Technology has vastly increased over the last few years, and it has become possible to target the tumour much more effectively whilst sparing healthy tissue. This is aided by MRI and CT scans that can define the position of the tumour much more accurately than used to be the case. This has led to more effective treatment with radiotherapy and less side effects.

Most side effects are temporary and their extent depends on the area being treated and the dose of radiation given. Many people have no problems at all.

Skin reactions

These occur less often these days as the machines are more sophisticated and the maximum effect of the radiation is below the skin.

The extent of damage will depend on the total dose of radiation administered and the dose in each fraction, the area of skin in the treatment field and how fair-skinned the patient is.

The skin is especially sensitive where two skin surfaces come into contact, where there has been recent trauma and where the epidermis is thin and smooth.

There are four types of skin reaction:

- Inflammation — Skin colour turns pink to red and may be slightly oedematous. Rather like sunburn. The skin may be sore or itchy.
- Dry desquamation — The skin becomes dry and scaly as the sebaceous glands are destroyed but this is not permanent.
- Moist desquamation — There is blistering and peeling of the epithelial layers. This is reversible but treatment should stop for a while.
- Long-term effects will result if the sweat or sebaceous glands are destroyed. Side effects may occur up to 5 years later with atrophy of the skin.

The hair follicles are especially sensitive to radiotherapy and alopecia (hair loss) may occur. The hair loss is usually temporary.

The skin may be gently washed using a mild unperfumed soap and patted dry. No deodorants, perfumes or lotions should be applied to the area except those provided. Some research supports the use of aloe vera.

Tiredness and fatigue

This is quite common, especially towards the end of the treatment, and it may last for some time after the treatment has stopped.

Radiotherapy to the head and neck

- Soreness of the mouth and throat due to drying of the mucous membranes. These consist of epithelial cells that are sensitive to radiotherapy.
- Taste may change as some taste buds will be destroyed. Ability to eat may be affected and small, frequent meals should be taken.
- Extra fluids should be taken, and Complan or Build-up may help to prevent weight loss.
- Alcohol and tobacco may irritate the mouth, and it is best to avoid them during treatment.
- Oral hygiene is very important and the teeth may be brushed but a very soft toothbrush should be used. A mouthwash may help to keep the mouth clean and moist but only one prescribed should be used.
- Soluble paracetamol may help.

Radiotherapy to the abdomen and pelvis

- Nausea and vomiting. Antiemetics will be prescribed.
- Diarrhoea as the lining of the intestine is affected — antidiarrhoeal tablets may be prescribed.
- Antimicrobials may be needed to prevent bacterial superinfection.
- Cystitis and sexual dysfunction may occur.

Cancer BACUP (www.cancerbacup.org.uk) provides helpful leaflets for the patients and their families on radiotherapy.

There is a freephone helpline (telephone number available on the website) where information and support are provided by specialist nurses. All information provided aims to be high quality and up to date.

Chemotherapy

This is the treatment of cancer with cytotoxic drugs that destroy dividing cells. The aim of chemotherapy is to destroy the abnormal cancer cell, shrinking the primary tumour and also killing metastasized cells, while the normal body cells are spared.

The difference between the cancer cell and other body cells is the rate at which it reproduces and divides. Chemotherapy drugs attack the cell at different stages in the cell cycle when it is preparing for division or actually dividing.

The duration of the cell cycle varies from tissue to tissue. Some tissues are subject to much wear and tear, e.g., skin and cells lining the gastrointestinal tract. Others such as liver cells lie dormant unless damaged. The cell cycle can be as short as a few hours and as long as a number of years! Healthy cells that need to divide frequently, such as blood cells, can also be damaged by cytotoxic drugs but these cells are better able to repair themselves than cancer cells.

Often two or more drugs are used at the same time and this is called *combination therapy*.

Chemotherapy may be used to:

● cure cancer,
● control cancer and prevent it from spreading,
● relieve symptoms.

It may be used in addition to surgery or radiotherapy.

There are three distinct groups of cytotoxic drugs:

● Cell cycle nonspecific drugs that bind to DNA and disable cell division, attacking the tumour cells whether they are dividing or dormant.
● Cycle-specific drugs that must be administered when cells are proliferating.
● Tissue-specific agents that deprive tissue of a substance needed for division.

Treatment with chemotherapy in cancer is complex and confined to specialists in oncology.

Cell-cycle nonspecific drugs
Alkylating agents

These are among the most widely used of cancer chemotherapy agents. They act by inserting an alkyl group into the DNA and damaging it, thus interfering with cell replication.

Cyclophosphamide

- Used in chronic lymphatic leukaemia, lymphomas and some solid tumours.
- May be given orally or intravenously.
- A urinary metabolite may cause haemorrhagic cystitis: 3–4 L of extra fluids a day should be given to prevent this.

Chlorambucil

- Chronic lymphatic leukaemia, non-Hodgkin's lymphoma, ovarian cancer and Hodgkin's.
- Extra side effects are rashes and marrow suppression.

Melphalan

- Myeloma, lymphomas, solid tumours.
- Given at intervals of 3–4 weeks.

Busulfan

- Chronic myeloid leukaemia.
- Frequent blood counts are needed as irreversible bone marrow aplasia may occur.

Lomustine (nitrosurea)

- Hodgkin's and solid tumours.
- Can cross the blood–brain barrier due to lipid solubility.

Cytotoxic antibiotics

These are derived from soil fungi, a variety of *Streptomyces* species that are too toxic to be used as antimicrobials. All bind to DNA and they are widely used. They may act as radiomimetics so should not be given alongside radiotherapy.

Doxorubicin

- One of the most successful, well-used antitumour drugs.
- Acute leukaemias, lymphomas and solid tumours.
- Given by fast running infusion at 21-day intervals.
- May have toxic effects on the heart.
- Acts by intercalating the DNA.

Bleomycin

- Lymphomas, squamous cell carcinoma and solid tumours.
- Causes little marrow suppression.
- By injection only.

Cell-cycle-specific

These are mostly antimetabolites. They mimic a normal metabolite and become incorporated into new nuclear material but do not function. Often combine irreversibly with vital cellular enzymes.

Folate antagonists

Folate is needed for the synthesis of DNA.

Methotrexate

- Causes myelosuppression.
- Damages the epithelium of the GI tract.
- In high doses can be toxic to the kidney — not given in renal disease.
- Used in combination regimens.
- May be given orally, intravenously, intramuscularly or intrathecally.
- Used as maintenance in childhood acute lymphatic leukaemia, choriocarcinoma, lymphomas, some solid tumours.
- Resistance may develop in tumour cells.
- High-dose therapy may be used for periods up to 12–36 h. This could be lethal if doses of folate were not given to rescue the normal body cells, which recover better than the tumour cells.

Pyrimidine antagonists

- Cytarabine — mostly used to induce remission in myeloid leukaemia.
- Fluorouracil — used to treat solid tumours of the breast and colon. Can be used topically for malignancies of the skin.

Purine antagonists

- Mercaptopurine — maintenance for acute leukaemias.
- Tioguanine — given by mouth for acute leukaemias.

Mitotic poisons

Vinca alkaloids

- From the periwinkle plant.
- Interfere with microtubule assembly and cause metaphase arrest.

- Given by injection.
- Relatively nontoxic but vincristine can cause peripheral neuropathy.
- Vincristine, vindesine, etoposide — can be given orally.
- Vinblastine — not neurotoxic but more myelosuppressive.

Taxanes

- Derived from the yew tree.
- Paclitaxel (Taxol) and docetaxel (Taxotere) act by spindle promotion.
- They are active against breast and ovarian cancers and are also used in small cell lung cancers.

Platinum compounds

- Cisplatin, carboplatin and oxaliplatin block DNA replication.
- Cause nausea and vomiting.
- Needs hydration therapy before administration.
- Transformed the treatment of testicular cancer.
- Major role in other tumours, e.g., lung, ovarian, head and neck cancer.

Tissue-specific agents

A number of tumours of the endocrine system require hormones for their growth. Oestrogens and progestins are essential for some breast and endometrial tumours and prostatic tumours may need androgens.

Both hormones and hormone antagonists can be useful in the treatment of cancers of the reproductive system and their metastases.

Hormones

Medroxyprogesterone acetate is a progestogen that is used as the second- or third-line management of breast cancer. It is also used for endometrial cancer.

Diethylstilbestrol is an oestrogen that used to be widely employed in the treatment of prostate cancer but its role is declining due to its side effects.

Androgens are occasionally used as the second- or third-line treatment in breast cancers. They are testosterone esters and examples are Primoteston and Virormone.

Hormonal antagonists

Tamoxifen

- An antioestrogen that is effective against oestrogen-dependent breast cancers.
- It is an oestrogen receptor antagonist and is the drug of choice in post-menopausal women with metastatic disease.

- Overall 30% of patients with metastatic disease respond to hormonal manipulation.
- Oestrogen receptor-positive tumours respond in 60% of cases.
- Tumours that are nonoestrogen dependent only respond in 10% of cases.
- Not all breast cancers are oestrogen dependent and some may be progesterone dependent.

Cyproterone acetate (Cyprostat) An antiandrogen used in cancer of the prostate.

Trastuzumab (Herceptin) Licensed for the treatment of breast cancer and metastases that overexpresses human epidermal growth factor receptor-2 (HER2).

Disruption of pituitary function

The pituitary controls the secretion of sex hormones. Antiluteinizing hormone analogues act on the pituitary to reduce secretion of gonadotrophic hormones. They reduce secretion of androgens in males and are as good as orchidectomy in cancer of the prostate. Examples are *buserelin*, *goserelin*, *leuprorelin* or *triptorelin.*

Combination chemotherapy

Courses are known by the first letters of the drugs they contain. For example, an ICE course used in the treatment of acute myeloid leukaemia is a combination of the anticancer drugs idarubicin, cytarabine and etoposide:

- Different drugs exert their influence at different points in the cell cycle and so may be synergistic, e.g., cisplatin and 5-fluorouracil.
- Decreases the chances of drug resistance developing in the tumour.
- NICE have issued guidance for the use of many anticancer drugs and this can be found on their website.

Adverse effects of chemotherapy

These depend very much on the drug given. Some effects are immediate and some are delayed. As the drugs attack dividing cells, some of the side effects are similar to those of radiotherapy.

Immediate effects may include nausea and vomiting, mouth ulcers and anorexia.

Delayed effects may include alopecia and suppression of bone marrow cells.

Thrombocytopenia, agranulocytosis, anaemia and leucopenia can occur. The reduced white cell count means lowered immunity and this itself may make it more difficult for the body to fight the cancer.

Regular blood counts are done and if the white cell count falls too low the treatment may have to be delayed.

Drug administration

Extreme care has to be taken when these drugs are administered parenterally. Should extravasation occur, the accidental leakage of the irritant drug into the tissues can lead to severe local necrosis (death) and permanent tissue damage. The drugs are usually given via a Hickman line to avoid this risk.

Those giving the drugs have to take precautions to avoid contact with the drug, and gown and gloves are worn when preparing and giving these drugs. Direct contact with the skin can lead to dermatitis, inflammation, blistering and other allergic responses.

Written guidelines are provided to cover the preparation, administration and disposal of these drugs. Should any spillage or contamination of yourself or others occur, the guidelines must be followed and help sought immediately.

Chemotherapy is given in cycles, and toxicity is monitored carefully. The World Health Organization has produced a grading for toxicity.

Drug resistance

This is a major obstacle in cancer chemotherapy:

- Some tumours have a low level of resistance, e.g., childhood acute leukaemia.
- Some tumours appear to respond but then patients relapse with resistant disease, e.g., small cell lung cancer.
- Some tumours are resistant from the start, e.g., melanoma.

5.11 SURGERY

Operations are classified according to a scale of magnitude, which relates broadly to the risks involved and the physiologic disturbance:

- *Minor surgery* — This may sometimes be done in the community and may only involve a local anaesthetic, e.g., skin lesions. It may also be carried out in a day surgery unit, e.g., needle biopsy.
- *Intermediate surgery* — This is usually done in a day surgery unit and would include operations such as a hernia repair.
- *Major surgery* — Much abdominal surgery falls into this category, e.g., cholecystectomy.
- *Complex major surgery* would include another aspect, e.g., cholecystectomy with anastomosis.
- *Complex major plus* includes heart surgery.

Complications of surgery

- Early — within 24 h.
- Intermediate — up to 3 weeks postoperative.
- Late — any time after, may be up to years on occasions.

Complications may be:

- Local — at the operation site.
- General — affecting other systems, e.g., respiratory system.

Section 6

Pharmacology

Section Outline

6.1 DRUGS AND THE LAW

There are two main Acts of Parliament that control the prescription and administration of many drugs. These are the Medicines Act 1968 and the Misuse of Drugs Act 1971.

The Medicines Act 1968

This was the first comprehensive legislation on medicines in the United Kingdom, and the act regulated the manufacture, distribution and importation of all medicines for human or animal use. European Community (EC) legislation now takes precedence over the 1968 Act, which is amended from time to time to fall in line with new EC requirements.

The Medicines and Healthcare Regulatory Agency was set up in 2003 to ensure that medicines and medical devises work and are safe. They have a website at www.mhra.gov.uk. They assess the quality and safety of medicines and authorize their sale in the United Kingdom.

The Misuse of Drugs Act 1971

The act relates to drugs which are liable to cause dependence if misused. These drugs are referred to as 'controlled drugs' and known as CDs. Accurate records of all purchases, amounts of drug issued and dosages given have to be kept. There must be special labels on the containers of these drugs to make them clearly recognizable.

A nurse's survival guide to the ward. https://doi.org/10.1016/B978-0-7020-7831-6.00006-1

The penalties for offences involving these drugs are graded according to the potential for harm the drug may have, and for this purpose the rugs are put into one of the following three classes:

- Class A includes cocaine, diamorphine and fentanyl.
- Class B includes cannabis, barbiturates and oral amphetamines
- Class C includes most benzodiazepines

The Controlled Drugs (Supervision of Management and Use) Regulations 2006 were introduced in response to the Shipman Inquiry, which found that ineffective monitoring had allowed Dr. Harold Shipman to use diamorphine to kill at least 15 patients and possibly many, many more, over a period of time, without being detected.

The Care Quality Commission is responsible for ensuring that healthcare providers are creating a safer environment for the management of CDs and further information is available on their website at www.cqc.org.uk.

In hospitals the following are regulations for controlling these drugs:

- They are stored in a double-locked cupboard of their own.
- The key must be carried by the nurse in charge.
- There is a special Controlled Drugs Order Book for those drugs in frequent use which can be kept as stock. The sister in charge must sign each order.
- Each administration of these drugs has to be recorded in the Controlled Drug Book with the patient's name, the dose of the drug, the time it was given and the signature of the nurse who administers the drug and another who has checked all these details.

The content of the CD cupboard is checked regularly by the pharmacist against the contents of the CD Book and any discrepancies are fully investigated.

There are nice guidelines for CD use available on their website at www. nice.org.uk.

The Misuse of Drugs Regulations 1985 divides drugs into five schedules, each with its own requirements governing supply, prescribing and record-keeping.

Schedule 1 are drugs that are not used medicinally, and possession and supply are prohibited. An example would be lysergic acid diethylamide.

Schedule 2 includes drugs subject to full CD requirements. Examples include:

diamorphine (heroin)	morphine
pethidine	methadone
amphetamine	cocaine
fentanyl	remifentanil

Schedule 3 drugs are subject to the same special prescription requirements (except phenobarbital) but not to the safe custody requirements (except buprenorphine and diethylpropion). They do not need a special register, but invoices must be retained for 2 years. Examples include buprenorphine and midazolam.

Schedule 4 drugs are subject to minimal control and include most benzo-diazepines, an example being diazepam.

Schedule 5 includes those drugs which, because of their strength, are exempt from virtually all CD regulations other than retention of invoices for 2 years. An example would be low doses of codeine present in combined preparations.

6.2 MEDICINES MANAGEMENT

In 2007, The Nursing and Midwifery Council (NMC) published their 'Standards for Medicines Management'. These have been updated in 2018 and are available on the NMC website (www.nmc.org.uk). The standards replaced the NMC's 'Guidelines for the Administration of Medicines' (2004), and continue to emphasize the importance of the trained nurse using thought and professional judgement when administering medication and so going beyond the mechanistic delivery of the prescribed dose on the treatment sheet. They describe the importance of using local expertise regarding medicine management and refer to the importance of the pharmacist in the role of advisor.

The administration of medicines

As a registered nurse, the administration of medicines is an important aspect of your professional practice.

Safety is of prime importance in the administration of medicines, and the effects of any medication should be assessed and evaluated. Any side-effects should be reported to the medical team without delay.

The 'five rights' act as a simple and basic reminder of some of the essential points of care as follows:

- Right client.
- Right drug.
- Right dose.
- Right time.
- Right route.

Who can administer medicines in a hospital setting?

The NMC standards state that prescribed medications should only be administered by registered practitioners who are competent for the purpose and aware of their personal accountability. If the registrant delegates any part of the administration, they are accountable to ensure that the patient, carer or care assistant is competent to carry out the task. Students must never administer or supply medicinal products without direct supervision.

Two registrants should check drugs to be administered intravenously and one of those two registrants should administer the drug.

Important points

- The nurse should never administer a medication without knowing its therapeutic use, normal dosage, side-effects, precautions and contraindications. There should always be a copy of the British National Formulary (BNF) available when medicines are administered so that any unfamiliar drugs can be looked up.
- The nurse must be certain of the identity of the patient to whom the medication is to be administered and should also have knowledge of his planned care.
- Always check that the patient is not allergic to the medicine before administration.
- The prescription must be very clear and legible. Doctors are asked to print the drug name and in hospital must always use the generic name of the medication and not the trade name. The label on the medicine dispensed should be clear and unambiguous.
- The expiry date of the medicine (if available) should be checked.
- If there is any ambiguity or query regarding the drug, the dose or the route of administration, which should all be very clear on the prescription sheet, the nurse must refuse to administer the medication and should contact the prescriber.
- If any contraindications to the prescribed medicine are discovered or where the patient develops a reaction, the prescriber should be contacted without delay.
- When a medication has been administered, this must be recorded at the time in a clear and accurate manner and with a signature which is legible. If the patient refuses his medication, this should also be recorded and the nurse in charge should assess the situation and contact the prescriber.
- A medicine must never be charted before it is given. When you sign for that drug you are saying that the client has actually taken it.
- Always check that the client understands the medication that she or he is receiving and is aware of any important side-effects. Emphasize the importance of the treatment and explain its mode of action in simple terms.
- If an error is made in the administration of a medicine, this should immediately be reported to the nurse in charge, who will inform the prescriber.
- Evaluate the action of the prescribed medication and record any positive or negative effects, informing the prescriber of these.

6.3 NURSE PRESCRIBING

The Medicines Act of 1968 allowed only doctors, dentists and veterinary surgeons to prescribe, but this has been rapidly changing within the National Health Service (NHS) in recent years. Nonmedical prescribing is rapidly expanding in the United Kingdom, and nurse prescribing has been extremely successful. Nurses in the United Kingdom have some of the widest prescribing powers in the profession worldwide, and evidence suggests that the standard of care provided by nurse prescribers is high, alongside patient satisfaction. There are different categories of prescribers, including independent nurse prescribers and supplementary prescribers.

Prescribing by certain groups of nurses began in October 1994 and permitted some nurses with a health visiting and district nursing qualification to prescribe certain drugs and dressings from a nurse prescribers' formulary. The primary legislation allowing nurse prescribing was set out in the Medicinal Products: Prescription by Nurses Act of 1992.

In 2002 registered nurses and midwives with additional training were allowed to prescribe from the Nurse Prescribers' Extended Formulary, a limited list that included over 120 prescription-only medications.

From May 2006, independent prescribing for nurses from a full formulary was permitted by legislation. Independent nurse prescribers could now prescribe any medicine for any condition within their competence. Thirteen CDs were also included for specific conditions. Changes in legislation in 2009 allowed nurses to prescribe unlicensed medicines and from 2012 nurses have been allowed to prescribe almost any CD. In 2016 over 10% of the total workforce of qualified nurses are nurse prescribers. The nurse prescribers must be first-level registered nurses or midwives and have passed the appropriate university course in order to meet the 'Standards of Proficiency for Nurse Prescribers' first produced by the NMC in 2006.

Pharmacists, optometrists, chiropodists, podiatrists, physiotherapists and therapeutic radiographers can also qualify as independent prescribers but may be subject to slightly different rules and regulations.

6.4 PHARMACOLOGY IN PRACTICE

Pharmacology is the study of drugs and their actions. It includes absorption, metabolism and elimination of the drug, as well as the mode of action of the drug. Drug absorption will vary depending on the route of administration.

Drug administration

The aims of administration are as follows:

- To establish optimal drug concentration at the target site.
- To maintain optimal concentration for the required period of time.
- To minimize adverse drug reactions due to general distribution.

Routes of administration

Oral

This is usually the most convenient route. Medication for oral administration may come in several of the following forms:

Tablets. The drug has been diluted, powdered and compressed by a tabletting machine into a shape that will be easy to swallow. Tablets are often coated with sugar or some colouring material.

Some tablets have an *enteric coating*, which is usually shiny in nature and has an acid-resistant layer to prevent dissolution in the stomach. This is used for drugs that may irritate the stomach lining.

Some oral medications may be specially formulated for *slow release* and will have SR after their name.

Capsules. These usually contain oily or nauseous preparations in an envelope made of gelatine or a similar substance. Examples are ampicillin and cod liver oil. The medication is liberated when the outer capsule is digested in the stomach or intestine.

Mixtures. These are liquid preparations in water or other solvent base which usually contain a number of ingredients. An example is magnesium trisilicate mixture, which is used as an antacid. Bottles containing mixtures **should be shaken** before administration as ingredients may separate out during storage.

Linctus. Used as a cough suppressant and made with a strong syrup base and flavouring agents. An example is linctus codeine.

Oral drug absorption. This is the passage of the drug from the gut lumen, through the gut mucosa and into the bloodstream. Although some absorption takes place in the stomach, the surface area here is much less than the small intestine, where most of the absorption takes place.

The absorption of oral medication is influenced by many factors.

Food in the stomach. Drugs are usually absorbed more quickly if the stomach is empty and in the case of most antibiotics, the client is instructed to take the medication 1 h before food for this reason.

Drugs which may irritate the stomach should be given with or after food, and this instruction will usually be on the container. An example is aspirin.

Interactions with other drugs. Drugs that inhibit gastric emptying, e.g., atropine, amphetamine, morphine, may reduce the rate of absorption of other drugs.

Diseases of the gastrointestinal (GI) tract, e.g. ulcerative colitis, may lead to poor absorption of the medication.

Transit time. The time taken for passage through the small intestine. The longer the medication is in the gut, the more of it will usually be absorbed.

GI movement aids the absorption of a drug, and as the drug passes through the intestine, it is fragmented and dissolved. If there is excessive peristalsis, as in diarrhoea, the drug will not have time to be absorbed.

Laxatives also decrease absorption.

Acid in the stomach. This will destroy some drugs, e.g., acid-sensitive penicillins, so they have to be given by injection.

Enzymes. These will break down proteins and amino acids such as insulin, which therefore has to be given by injection.

Metal ions and tetracycline. Tetracycline forms a complex with either calcium or iron and if either of these is given with tetracycline, a large molecule is formed that cannot be absorbed and the patient will not get the benefit of either drug. As there is calcium in milk, tetracycline should not be taken with a drink of milk. Magnesium and aluminium also complex and may be found in antacids.

The concentration of a drug in the intestine depends on the:

- amount ingested,
- rate with which it is released from the formulation,
- volume of GI contents with which it is mixed.

Sublingual/buccal

The drug is administered under the tongue or sprayed into the mouth. This route is used for drugs that are destroyed rapidly by the liver, e.g., glyceryl trinitrate (GTN). If GTN is taken orally and swallowed, it is absorbed and passes into the hepatic portal vein, reaching the liver and being metabolized before it can have any vasodilatory action. When given sublingually, it is absorbed directly into the systemic circulation, thus bypassing the liver.

This route is also useful if the patient is not allowed fluids or feels sick. Examples include the analgesic buprenorphine which may be given sublingually and the antiemetic prochlorperazine given buccally.

Rectal

Drugs may be given rectally for local or systemic action. For local action, a suppository or an enema may be given when the patient is constipated to promote a bowel action. Glycerin suppositories are the most common. Glycerol is a mild irritant to the rectal mucosa and thus stimulates the defecation reflex.

Steroid enemas are administered for local action on an inflamed bowel in ulcerative colitis.

Normally the rectum is empty and a suppository will melt and be absorbed via the rectal mucosa into the bloodstream, making this a good route for systemic drug administration.

The rectal route is especially useful when:

- a drug is irritating the stomach mucosa,
- the patient is vomiting or nauseated,

- there is difficulty in swallowing,
- the patient is drowsy or unconscious.

Examples of drugs given rectally are as follows:

- Paracetamol.
- Diazepam — for convulsions.

Transdermal (via the skin)

It is usually in the form of a patch that releases the drug through a rate-controlling membrane. The drug is absorbed through the skin and into the blood supply. Hormone replacement therapy, fentanyl (an opioid) and GTN may be administered this way.

Topical application

This is for local effect on the skin and mucous membranes as follows:

- Creams — these are emulsions of oil and water that are well absorbed into the skin and may be used for dry and scaly skin or as the base for other drugs, such as steroids in eczema.
- Eye drops — sterile preparations for instillation into the eye. This could be for an infection, e.g., chloramphenicol drops, or to have an effect on the pupil or the drainage system.
- Ear drops — these are for application to the external auditory meatus, e.g., Cerumol, which helps to dissolve wax in the ear.
- Vaginal pessaries or cream — for local action.

An advantage of topical application is that a high local concentration can be achieved, usually without a systemic effect. A disadvantage is that absorption can occasionally occur with serious effects.

Inhalation

This route is used for drugs that are absorbed via the respiratory mucosa for systemic action, e.g., volatile anaesthetics, and for drugs acting on the respiratory system.

The drug may be administered as follows:

- A gas, as in anaesthetics.
- An aerosol, as in salbutamol inhalers used to treat asthma. Aerosols contain particles dispersed in a gas and small enough to remain suspended for a long time.
- A powder dispensed from a rotary inhaler as in sodium cromoglicate (Intal) for the treatment of asthma.
- A nebulizer — the machine converts a solution of the drug into an aerosol. These are used in respiratory conditions, e.g., salbutamol for asthma.

Injection

Injections may be given as follows:

- Intradermally — into the skin. Used for allergy testing and diagnostic tests. Less than 0.1 mL may be given.
- Subcutaneously — under the skin. Used for insulin and heparin administration where slow and steady release is needed. Up to 2 mL may be administered. Sites for subcutaneous injection are shown in Fig. 6.1. Absorption of the drug does depend on local blood supply and may be more rapid with exercise. The needle was traditionally inserted at a 45° angle but with the advent of shorter specialist needles the recommendation for insulin injection is an angle of 90°.
- Intramuscularly — into a muscle. Up to 4 mL may be given into well-developed muscle. The sites used are shown in Fig. 6.2 and detailed in the following section. Again absorption is variable depending on the site and the state of the circulatory system.
- Intravenously — into the venous circulation. This route may only be used by doctors and registered nurses who have done a course in intravenous drug administration.
- Intrathecally — into the spinal theca.

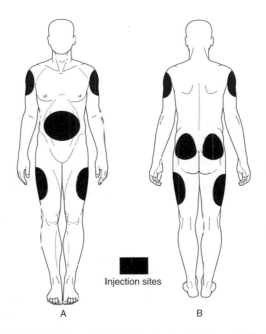

FIGURE 6.1   Sites used for subcutaneous injection. A. Anterior aspect. B. Posterior aspect. *From Jamieson/Clinical Nursing Practices, third ed., reproduced with permission.*

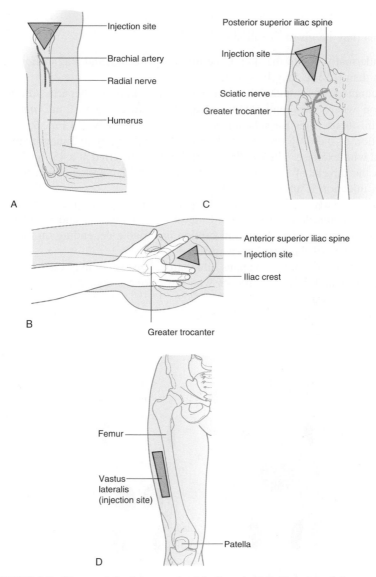

FIGURE 6.2   Sites used for intramuscular injection. A. Deltoid region of the arm. B. Ventrogluteal site. C. Dorsogluteal site. D. Vastus lateralis site. *Adapted from Rodger, M.A., King, L., 2000, with permission. Original illustration by Alison Tingle.*

- Intraosseous — into the bone marrow cavity. A route more commonly used in paediatrics but also in adults when intravenous access cannot be obtained.
- Into various body cavities, e.g., the peritoneum and the pleura.

The administration of any injection is an aseptic procedure, and great care should be taken with handwashing technique.

Care must also be taken to avoid needle-stick injury to yourself as there is a danger of transmitting blood-borne viruses such as hepatitis B and human immunodeficiency virus (HIV).

Some advantages of intravenous administration

- The drug is delivered into the bloodstream and so is able to act immediately.
- There is no reliance on absorption, and the whole dose of the drug reaches the bloodstream, enabling better calculation of the amount the patient actually receives.
- A continuous infusion allows the rate of administration to be controlled and the action of the drug thus modified.

Some disadvantages of intravenous administration

- Once the drug is given it cannot be removed from the body.
- Any allergic response is likely to be more severe.
- There is danger of infection if rigorous asepsis is not applied.
- Only those with special training can administer the drug.

Intramuscular injection sites Drugs are less frequently given by this route than in years gone by.

The mid-deltoid site in the upper arm is easily accessible but due to the small area available a limited number of injections can be given here.

The vastus lateralis site on the anterolateral aspect of the thigh is part of the quadriceps muscle group and is easily accessible when sitting or lying. The middle third of the muscle is used, and there are no major blood vessels or nerves in danger here. Absorption is slower than the arm but more rapid than the buttocks.

The ventrogluteal site is the site of choice and is often used. Up to 2.5 mL may be safely injected.

The dorsogluteal site is very occasionally used for deep intramuscular (IM) injections but has the lowest absorption rate and does become atrophied in the elderly or emaciated patient. There is also a risk of hitting the sciatic nerve or the superior gluteal arteries with the needle.

6.5 CLASSIFICATION OF DRUGS

Anaesthetics

- Drugs that produce a loss of sensation.
- In local anaesthesia, sensory nerve impulses are blocked and the patient remains alert. An example of a local anaesthetic is lidocaine (lignocaine) hydrochloride.

- In general anaesthesia there is loss of consciousness and the patient is unaware of, and unresponsive to, painful stimulation.
- The most widely used general anaesthetic given intravenously is propofol. It can be used for both induction and/or maintenance of anaesthesia.
- General anaesthesia may also be maintained by inhalation anaesthetics, and an example is isoflurane.

Analgesics

- Drugs that relieve pain.
- Paracetamol is a nonopioid drug that does not irritate the stomach and of similar efficacy to aspirin but has no anti-inflammatory action. When simple analgesia is needed, it is usually the drug of first choice. The dose is 1 g every 4—6 h. It is dangerous in overdosage and can cause acute liver failure. It can also be given intravenously.
- Codeine and dihydrocodeine are mild opioids that are stronger than paracetamol but also cause more side-effects, such as constipation. Dihydrocodeine may also cause nausea and vomiting.
- Compound analgesic preparations usually contain paracetamol with a low dose of an opioid analgesic. Examples are co-codamol (paracetamol 500 mg plus codeine phosphate 8 mg) and co-dydramol (paracetamol 500 mg and dihydrocodeine 10 mg).
- Nonsteroidal anti-inflammatory drugs (NSAIDs) such as aspirin and ibuprofen are used for chronic pain of an inflammatory nature but are also useful in the treatment of mild to moderate pain, especially if it is musculoskeletal in origin.
- They irritate the stomach mucosa and also reduce the thickness of the mucous lining of the gut.
- Ibuprofen causes the least problems. Diclofenac has a higher incidence of gastric erosion.
- Opioid analgesics are the strongest and are reserved for severe visceral pain or analgesia in palliative care. Examples include morphine sulphate, diamorphine, pethidine and fentanyl. These drugs may produce dependence if used over a period of time.
- Morphine given for acute pain over a short period does not produce serious problems with dependency. MST Continus, which is a modified-release formulation of morphine, is not suitable for acute pain.

Side-effects of morphine include:

- drowsiness,
- nausea,
- dizziness,

- constipation,
- respiratory depression that is dose-dependent.

Diamorphine is more soluble and has a faster action than morphine. It may produce nausea and an antiemetic such as metoclopramide (10 mg) may be used to counteract this.

In cases of chronic pain, the doctor may prescribe mild analgesia to start with but if this does not control the pain, a stronger drug should be prescribed from further along the 'analgesic ladder' (see Box 6.1).

Analgesia in palliative care

- The aim where treatment of a disease is not curative is to keep the patient as comfortable and pain-free as possible.
- The number of drugs given should be as few as necessary to obtain symptom control and oral or transdermal medication is usually satisfactory.
- Analgesics are always more effective in preventing the development of pain than in the relief of established pain and so need to be given regularly.
- Nonopioid analgesics may be well sufficient in some cases if administered regularly. These would include paracetamol and/or NSAIDs.
- NSAIDs are especially useful in the control of bone metastases and some may be given by suppository, e.g., naproxen.

Morphine is the most useful of the opioid analgesics as it not only relieves pain but also promotes a state of euphoria and mental detachment. Morphine may be given by mouth as an oral solution, four-hourly, and the doctor should increase the dose if pain is occurring between doses.

Modified-release tablets of morphine, such as MST Continus, are an alternative and have the advantage that they only need to be taken every 12 h.

Fentanyl given via the transdermal route is useful when analgesic requirements are stable but not if they are changing rapidly.

The BNF gives detailed dose regimens that the doctor may use for prescribing.

BOX 6.1 The analgesic ladder

Step 1	Nonopioids — paracetamol, aspirin and other NSAIDs
Step 2	Mild opioids and combinations — tramadol, codeine, dihydrocodeine, co-codamol, co-dydramol.
Step 3	Strong opioics — morphine, diamorphine, fentanyl, etc.

Alongside regular analgesic drugs in palliative care, muscle spasm can be helped by a muscle relaxant such as diazepam or baclofen.

Chronic pain is a complex area, and neuropathic (nerve) pain is difficult to control. Adjuvant medications such as tricyclic antidepressants, e.g., amitriptyline, or antiepileptic-like drugs such as gabapentin are used in addition to analgesia.

Modified-release morphine should never be given more frequently than every 12 h.

Other routes of administration include rectally as a suppository or trans-dermally as a patch applied to the skin surface.

Morphine is not usually given by repeated administration of IM injections as this is both inconvenient and uncomfortable for the terminally ill patient as follows:

- If morphine cannot be taken orally, a syringe driver may be used to administer the drug by slow continuous subcutaneous infusion.
- Diamorphine rather than morphine is used as this has a higher solubility, enabling larger doses to be given in a small volume.
- Symptoms can be controlled with the minimum of discomfort to the patient.

Always remember that all opioid analgesics can cause constipation, and this may be the source of much distress for the patient. If the patient is not able to tolerate a high-fibre diet, laxatives may have to be used.

- Larger doses of opioids may cause respiratory depression and hypotension. Other side-effects include nausea, vomiting and drowsiness.
- Repeated administration does cause dependence and tolerance, but this should not be a deterrent to pain control in the terminally ill.

Antacids

- Drugs that neutralize the acidity of the gastric juice.
- They may be given in dyspepsia, gastritis, peptic ulcers and oesophageal reflux.
- Examples are magnesium trisilicate and aluminium hydroxide.

Anthelmintics

- Drugs which destroy or eliminate intestinal worms.
- Examples are mebendazole and piperazine for threadworm and roundworm and niclosamide for tapeworm infections.

Antiarrhythmics

- Drugs given to prevent or reduce irregularities of cardiac rhythm.
- Examples are digoxin, adenosine, amiodarone and lidocaine.

Digoxin was originally derived from the foxglove. It is still sometimes used in the treatment of heart failure, atrial fibrillation and atrial flutter. Digoxin slows the heart rate and increases the force of contraction (it is a positive inotrope).

It is toxic in doses only just above therapeutic and the patient may suffer from digoxin toxicity. Signs are:

- isturbed vision,
- pulsus bigeminus (coupling),
- abdominal pain,
- confusion.

Adenosine is a naturally occurring compound within the body. It can be used in the treatment of supraventricular arrhythmias. It is given by rapid intravenous injection as the body destroys it very quickly.

Side-effects may include severe bradycardia, flushing, dyspnoea and bronchospasm, but these are usually short-lived.

Amiodarone is a valuable antiarrhythmic drug used in both ventricular and atrial tachyarrhythmias. It is used in the treatment of rapid atrial fibrillation. The drug has a very long half-life and when given regularly over a period of time stays in the body for months after it has been discontinued.

Side-effects include hypotension. With long-term administration, micro-deposits in the cornea, pulmonary fibrosis and discoluoration of the skin in sunlight (*photosensitivity*) may occur.

Lidocaine (lignocaine) is a local anaesthetic but is also an antiarrhythmic drug. It is occasionally used in ventricular arrhythmias and is usually given by intravenous infusion in this case.

Side-effects can include anxiety, restlessness, dizziness and tremors, as well as nausea and occasionally seizures.

Antibiotics

- Antibacterial substances are originally derived from other living organisms such as fungi.
- Antibiotics are given for bacterial infections. They do not kill viruses, and viral infections should not be treated with these drugs.
- Duration of therapy depends on the nature of the infection and the response to treatment. It is most important that a course of treatment is completed even if the patient feels better, and it is also important that the drugs are taken at the correct time to maintain the necessary level of drug in the blood.

- Examples of antibiotics are penicillin, amoxycillin, erythromycin, cephalosporins, gentamicin, metronidazole, trimethoprim and vancomycin.
- *Penicillin* was one of the first antibiotics. It is bactericidal (kills bacteria) and interferes with the synthesis of the bacterial cell wall. It is used in a wide variety of bacterial diseases such as:
- throat infections,
- pneumonia,
- meningitis,
- syphilis.

It is effective against many gram-positive cocci such as streptococci, meningococci and gonococci and also some anaerobic (can live in the absence of oxygen) bacteria.

Penicillin G (benzylpenicillin) has to be given by injection as the acid in the stomach destroys it, but penicillin V is a derivative that can be given orally.

Side-effects are rare, but some people are dangerously allergic to penicillin and anaphylaxis may result. The nurse should always check if the patient is allergic to penicillin before starting a course of the drug.

Amoxycillin is derived from penicillin but is a broad-spectrum antibiotic (kills both gram-negative and gram-positive bacteria). It may be given orally or intravenously.

Erythromycin is effective against a wide range of organisms and may be used if the patient is allergic to penicillin. It may be given orally or intravenously but is always well diluted, as it is an irritant to the veins. It is also an irritant to the GI tract and may cause nausea and diarrhoea.

Cephalosporins include first-generation drugs such as cefalexin, second-generation such as cefuroxime and cefaclor and third-generation drugs such as cefotaxime. The spectrum of activity of the drugs is different, and the third-generation drugs are more active against gram-negative bacteria. They are less susceptible to bacterial destruction than penicillin. Cefotaxime can penetrate the central nervous system (CNS) and so is very useful in meningitis. There is a danger of antibiotic-associated colitis with broad-spectrum antibiotics and superinfection with resistant bacteria may occur.

Gentamicin is a bactericidal antibiotic used in the treatment of septicaemia, meningitis and other CNS infections; biliary tract infections and many other instances. It can only be given by injection, as it is not absorbed in the GI tract. Plasma concentration monitoring is needed to ensure neither excessive nor subtherapeutic levels of the drug. The level should be checked after 3 or 4 doses of gentamicin, before administration to ensure that the trough dose is sufficient and approximately 1 h after intravenous or IM administration to ensure that the peak concentration is not too high. This is because gentamicin is toxic to the kidneys and the auditory nerve at high concentration.

Metronidazole is effective against anaerobic bacteria and protozoa. Surgical sepsis, leg ulcers, pressure sores and pseudomembranous colitis can all be treated. The drug is used prophylactically in gut and dental surgery. It can be used to treat trichomoniasis, an infection due to the protozoan *Trichomonas vaginalis* that often infects the vagina and causes inflammation of the genitalia with vaginal discharge. The drug may be given orally, rectally or intravenously and has a half-life of about 8 h.

Side-effects include GI disturbances, headache, dizziness, ataxia and occasionally seizures. Alcohol should be avoided while taking metronidazole.

Trimethoprim is a bacteriostatic drug (prevents bacteria multiplying). It is usually used in urinary tract infections. Adverse effects include nausea and other GI disturbances.

Vancomycin is valuable in multiresistant staphylococcal infections and in those allergic to penicillin and cephalosporins. It can be given orally or intravenously and side-effects include ototoxicity (damage to hearing) and nephrotoxicity (damage to the kidney). It is contraindicated in renal failure as dangerously high levels of the drug can be reached.

Anticoagulants

- These are drugs that prevent or reduce the formation of thrombi in the blood vessels.
- They may be given prophylactically to prevent a deep vein thrombosis occurring postoperatively, for example, or may be given when a thrombosis has already occurred, as in pulmonary embolism.
- Heparin has to be given by injection but acts immediately. It is now usually given as fractionated or low-molecular-weight heparin, which does not require monitoring and may be given in the community.
- Warfarin is an oral anticoagulant for long-term therapy. It interacts with many other drugs and foods and the patient's International normalised ratio (INR) has to be monitored whilst they are taking this drug. This is a comparison of the patient's prothrombin time to a control.
- Newer oral anticoagulants include dabigatran and rivaroxaban. These are used after hip or knee replacement surgery and are replacing warfarin in other areas. This is because they are safer and do not require monitoring via regular blood samples.
- The main side-effect of anticoagulants is bleeding.

Antidepressants

- Drugs that help to relieve depression.
- These include the following:
- Tricyclics such as amitriptyline and imipramine. These are dangerous in overdose, causing arrhythmias and convulsions.
- Monoamine oxidase inhibitors (MAOIs) which interact with several types of food such as cheese, yeast extracts and food that is 'going off'. The

patient is given a card with instructions, and failure to adhere to these may lead to a dangerous rise in blood pressure (BP). The drugs are only prescribed by a specialist.

- Selective serotonin reuptake inhibitors (SSRIs) that are less dangerous in overdose situations and less sedative in action. Examples are fluoxetine (Prozac) and citalopram.

Antiepileptics (anticonvulsants)

- Drugs which control epilepsy.
- The aim of treatment with these drugs is to prevent the occurrence of seizures. Ideally this should be with only one drug and the combination of antiepileptic drugs is to be avoided where possible because of the complex interactions that may occur.
- Abrupt withdrawal of the drug may precipitate rebound seizures and individual doses should not be missed.
- Examples of antiepileptic drugs are carbamazepine, phenytoin, sodium valproate and vigabatrin.

Antiemetics

- Drugs that reduce nausea and vomiting.
- They should only be used when the cause of the vomiting is known as they may cause symptom relief that could delay diagnosis.
- Examples are prochlorperazine (Stemetil), metoclopramide (Maxolon), domperidone and ondansetron.

Antifungals

- Drugs given for fungal infections. Sometimes fungal infections are associated with a defect in host resistance.
- Nystatin is used for *Candida albicans* infections of the skin and mucous membranes (thrush) but is too toxic to be taken orally.
- Amphotericin is active against most types of fungi and may be taken orally to treat intestinal candidiasis and systemic fungal infections.

Antihistamines

- Drugs which reduce some of the effects of released histamines.
- Histamine is released by the mast cells in an allergic reaction, and antihistamines are given for allergies such as hay fever where they reduce the rhinitis, sneezing and rashes due to allergies.

- They are also used for insect bites and stings to reduce the irritation and inflammation.
- Often make the patient drowsy as a side-effect.
- Examples are chlorphenamine (Piriton) and promethazine hydrochloride (Phenergan).
- Nonsedative antihistamines are available, e.g., loratadine. Some non-sedating antihistamines such as terfenadine have occasionally caused fatal arrhythmias and have been discontinued.

Antihypertensive drugs

- Drugs that reduce BP.
- Examples are β-adrenergic antagonists (β-blockers) such as atenolol, ACE inhibitors such as ramipril, calcium channel blockers such as amlodipine and diuretics such as bendroflumethiazide.

Antiplatelet drugs

- Decrease platelet aggregation and so reduce the incidence of myocardial infarction and thrombotic stroke.
- Examples are aspirin, dipyridamole and clopidogrel.
- Aspirin is given to reduce the incidence of cerebrovascular disease and myocardial infarction in those at risk. Only a small dose is needed daily (75 mg).

Antipsychotics

- They are also known as neuroleptics and used in the treatment of psychoses such as schizophrenia or acute behavioural disturbance.
- They may also be used to alleviate acute anxiety.
- Sometimes they are given in the form of depot injections.
- Over a period of time they may give parkinsonian side-effects such as a tremour and movement disorders.
- Examples are haloperidol, flupentixol and risperidone.

Antipyretics

- Drugs that reduce the body temperature.
- Examples are aspirin and paracetamol.
- Aspirin is not given to children under the age of 16 years because of an association with Reye's syndrome.

Antispasmodics

- Drugs that relax smooth muscle as found in the gut.
- They are useful in abdominal colic or distension as in irritable bowel disorder.
- Examples are mebeverine hydrochloride (Colofac), hyoscine butylbromide (Buscopan) and peppermint oil.

Antivirals

- Combat viral infections.
- Aciclovir (Zovirax) is active against the herpesvirus and may be used as a topical application for cold sores (herpes simplex) or shingles (herpes zoster).
- Aciclovir may be given intravenously in herpes encephalitis and may be given by mouth to the immunocompromised in chickenpox. It does not eradicate the virus, which lies dormant in the body but may flare up again when conditions are suitable.
- Antivirals are used for the treatment of HIV disease.

Anxiolytics

- Drugs given to reduce anxiety.
- An example is diazepam.
- These drugs are used for alleviating definite acute and severe anxiety states, and the lowest possible dose is given for the shortest possible time as they produce dependency.
- Diazepam does have other uses and may be given rectally or intravenously to halt status epilepticus or febrile convulsions.

β-blockers

- Block the β-adrenergic receptor and so reduce the effect of noradrenaline (norepinephrine) and adrenaline (epinephrine) on the body.
- Used as treatment for angina and are also given post-MI.
- Some of them are cardioselective, e.g., atenolol, which reduces side-effects.
- They are also used in migraine, anxiety, hyperthyroidism and certain arrhythmias but should not be given to those with asthma as they may induce an asthma attack.
- Propranolol is a nonselective β-blocker, which will block the β receptors in the lungs and so is more likely to cause an asthma attack than atenolol.

Bronchodilators

- Relax bronchial smooth muscle and thus cause dilatation of the air passages.
- Examples are salbutamol (Ventolin), a β-2 receptor agonist and ipratropium bromide (Atrovent), an anticholinergic drug.
- Salbutamol and ipratropium can both be given by inhaler or by nebulizer.

Corticosteroids

- Steroid hormones are synthesized by the adrenal cortex, and cortisol is the naturally occurring hormone.
- Corticosteroids are anti-inflammatory and suppress the immune system. They have many uses in inflammatory conditions, allergic responses and autoimmune diseases but also have many side-effects, especially with long-term use.
- They are usually given in the form of an inhaler in asthma — beclometasone and budesonide are examples. Steroids may also be given orally, usually as prednisolone, and intravenously as hydrocortisone.

Cytotoxics (chemotherapeutic agents)

- They are toxic to dividing cells and used in the treatment of cancer.
- Examples are methotrexate and vincristine.
- The drugs are toxic to all dividing cells and thus have side-effects such as a fall in the white cell count and hair loss.

Diuretics

- They cause the patient to pass more urine. They are best given in the morning if possible. Examples are furosemide, bendroflumethiazide and spironolactone.
- Diuretics are given to reduce the circulating blood volume in heart failure and in hypertension. Salts such as potassium are also lost in the urine and to prevent this, a potassium-sparing diuretic such as amiloride may need to be given with the diuretic.
- Spironolactone is an aldosterone antagonist commonly used in heart failure and also causes potassium retention.

Fibrinolytics

- Drugs that digest fibrin in blood clots.
- These drugs are used to dissolve the blood clot and restore the circulation following a myocardial infarction or a thrombotic stroke. In the case of

myocardial infarction, angioplasty is now the first-line treatment where possible.
- An example is tenecteplase.

Hypnotics
- Induce sleep. An example is zolpidem.
- These drugs may produce dependency and are becoming less frequently prescribed. They are only prescribed for very short periods.

Immunosuppressives
- They suppress the immune system and are used in autoimmune disorders or following organ transplantation to reduce rejection of the donor organ.
- An example is azathioprine.

Hypoglycaemic agents
- These are drugs that are given in diabetes mellitus to lower blood glucose.
- Insulin is given by subcutaneous injection to people with Type 1 diabetes and those patients with Type 2 diabetes whose blood glucose cannot be adequately controlled by diet and tablets.
- There are many different types of oral medication and these are shown in Table 5.11. Included are gliclazide and metformin.

Inotropes
- They affect the contraction of the heart muscle.
- Drugs such as digoxin have a positive inotropic action and increase the force of the heartbeat.
- Some drugs such as β-blockers have a negative inotropic effect and decrease the force of the heartbeat.

Laxatives
- They are drugs used to promote a softer or bulkier stool or to encourage a bowel action.
- They are given for constipation.
- Examples are lactulose and senna.

Miotics

- They are rugs which constrict the pupil of the eye.
- They are used in glaucoma to open up the drainage channels in the trabecular meshwork resulting from spasm of the ciliary muscle, and constriction of the pupil is a side-effect.
- An example is pilocarpine.

Muscle relaxants

- They are used in conjunction with general anaesthesia to produce complete muscle relaxation, especially in abdominal surgery.
- As they prevent muscles contracting, they also stop respiration and the patient has to be ventilated.
- Examples are atracurium and vecuronium.

Mydriatics

- They dilate the pupil of the eye.
- An example is homatropine.
- They may be used when the doctor needs to have a clear view of the retina as in examination of the eye in diabetes.

Nonsteroidal anti-inflammatory drugs

See analgesics.

Vaccines

These are preparations of antigenic material that can be given to stimulate the production of antibodies and thus confer immunity to a disease. They consist of the following:

- A live attenuated form of the infective agent, as in rubella vaccine.
- An inactivated preparation of the virus, as in influenza vaccine, or the bacterium, as in typhoid vaccine.
- Detoxified exotoxins produced by the microorganism, as in tetanus vaccine.

6.6 POISONING

A poison is any substance which, when introduced into a living organism, destroys life or injures health.

Accidental poisoning

This may be encountered at any age, but the causes differ.

Neonatal poisoning

This is usually a result of therapeutic doses of drugs or self-poisoning in the late stages of labour. It could be due to the miscalculation of doses.

Children

Accidental poisoning is the common between the ages of 1 and 5 years when children like to explore the environment with their mouths as well as their eyes and fingers!

Older children and adults

This is usually a result of a mishap at school or at work, e.g., inhalation of gases or fumes from organic solvents.

The elderly

Especially if confused, the person may forget they have taken a dose of their drug or make mistakes with doses.

Deliberate self-poisoning

This is the most common form of poisoning in adults. It accounts for at least 95% of all poisoning admissions to hospital. The peak age is between 20 and 35 years, but it is not uncommon below the age of 15.

Symptoms and signs

Usually poisoned adults are able to tell us what they have taken, but the presence of signs and symptoms may help us to see how severe the poisoning is.

Coma

This is one of the common signs of poisoning and is usually due to depression of the CNS by:

- hypnotics,
- antidepressants,
- anticonvulsants,
- tranquillizers,
- opioid analgesics,
- alcohol.

Loss of consciousness does not occur with paracetamol poisoning unless another drug or alcohol has been taken as well.

Convulsions

These are caused by CNS stimulation by anticholinergics, sympathomimetics, tricyclic antidepressants and MAOIs.

Single convulsions may not require treatment, but if they recur frequently, a benzodiazepine such as lorazepam or diazepam may be given intravenously.

Respiratory features

- Cough, wheezing and breathlessness often occur after inhalation of irritant gases such as ammonia, chlorine and smoke from fires.
- Cyanosis may be due to a combination of factors in the unconscious patient. It can also be due to methaemoglobinaemia caused by poisons such as chlorates, nitrates, nitrites, phenol and urea herbicides.
- Hypoventilation is common with any CNS depressant.
- Respiration often becomes shallower rather than slower, and a marked reduction in rate is likely to be due to opioids.
- Hyperventilation is most commonly due to salicylate (aspirin) poisoning and occasionally to CNS stimulant drugs and cyanide.
- Pulmonary oedema may follow inhaled poisons and paraquat poisoning (contained in some weed killers).

Cardiovascular features

- Tachycardia may be due to anticholinergics, sympathomimetics and salicylates.
- Bradycardia may be caused by digoxin and β-blockers.
- Arrhythmias and conduction deficits may be caused by a variety of drugs, including tricyclic antidepressants, some antipsychotics and some antihistamines.
- Hypotension is common in severe poisoning, for example, with CNS depressants that may lower the systolic BP to 70–80 mmHg. The BP falls lower as the coma gets deeper. A systolic BP of less than 70 mmHg may lead to irreversible brain damage or renal tubular necrosis.
- Diuretics lower the BP by depleting the blood volume.
- Hypertension is less common than hypotension in overdosage but occurs with sympathomimetic drugs such as amphetamines and cocaine.

Pupil changes

- Very small and pinpoint pupils, especially if the respiratory rate is slowed, suggest opioid analgesics.

- Dilated pupils suggest tricyclic antidepressants or other anticholinergics or antihistamines.

Body temperature

- Hypothermia may occur, especially if the patient has been unconscious for any length of time.
- Hyperthermia can occur if CNS stimulants have been taken or in serotonin syndrome.
- Antidotes
- Most important here is naloxone, which is the antidote to morphine and other opioids. When given intravenously, it may completely reverse a coma within 1–2 min and will counteract the respiratory depression seen in an opioid overdose. It may be given by continuous intravenous infusion if necessary.
- Flumazenil is the antidote for severe benzodiazepine poisoning but is not always used in less severe cases.
- *N*-acetylcysteine (Parvolex) is given in paracetamol poisoning and can prevent liver failure if given soon enough after the overdose.

Screening for poisons

- It may not be possible to establish the identity of the drug or the size of the dose taken.
- The purpose of screening is to identify and quantify poisons amenable to treatment. There is no point in doing an emergency screening if the result has no bearing on the treatment that will be given.
- Paracetamol is the drug that is most likely to be screened for.

Management of the patient

About 90% of adults and children have minimal symptoms and require little medical care. Half of the remainder is seriously ill and recovery depends upon good care as follows:

- Patients who have features of poisoning should usually be admitted to hospital.
- Ensure that the airway, breathing and BP are adequate.
- Assess the level of consciousness.
- Contact the poisons information services if there is any uncertainty about the toxicity of the substance or the management of the poison.
- Consider whether an antidote is available or necessary.
- Consider the need to prevent absorption of the poison.

TOXBASE and the UK National Poisons Information Service

No one can expect to know all the constituents of the drugs, household products, agricultural and industrial preparations that may be taken. Toxic effects and appropriate treatment may not be known either. The UK National Poisons Information Service gives specialist information and advice and is available day and night by calling 0844 892 0111. They provide information on the diagnosis, treatment and management of poisoning.

TOXBASE is the database of the National Poisons Information Service, and information is available to registered users at www.toxbase.org.

Minimizing the absorption of ingested poisons

Gastric lavage is very rare and only used when a life-threatening amount of poison has been taken within the previous hour. It should never be attempted without intubation, and an anaesthetist should be present if the patient is very drowsy or comatose as follows:

- It should never be attempted when a corrosive material has been ingested.
- There is danger of inhalation of stomach contents.

Activated charcoal

This is given by mouth to bind poisons in the GI tract as follows:

- Charcoal is not absorbed and combines with some drugs in the GI tract to prevent their absorption.
- Most useful when poisons are toxic in small doses, e.g., tricyclic antidepressants.
- The sooner it is given, the more effective it will be.
- It is best given within the first hour of ingestion but may be effective up to 2 h after ingestion and longer if modified-release preparations are taken.
- It is a black, gritty slurry and patients do not like to take it. It can be mixed with soft drinks to mask the taste.

Repeated doses of charcoal are sometimes given to increase the elimination of certain drugs.

There is a good section on the emergency treatment of poisoning in the front of the BNF where there are short sections on some individual drug categories such as antidepressants, calcium channel blockers and hypnotics.

References

ACAS, 2014. Bullying and Harassment at Work: A Guide for Employees. Available at: m.acas.org.uk/media/pdf/r//l/Bullying-and-harrassment-at-work-a-guide-for-employees.pdf.

BHF, 2018. Cardiovascular Disease Statistics. https://www.bhf.org.uk/what-we-do/our-research/heart-statistics/heart-statistics-publications/cardiovascular-disease-statistics-2018.

Borgert, M.J., Goossens, A., Dongelmans, D.A., 2015. What are effective strategies for the implementation of care bundles in ICUs: a systematic review. Implement. Sci. 10 (119). https://doi.org/10.1186/s13012-015-0306-1.

British Heart Foundation, 2017. Cardiovascular Disease Statistics. https://www.bhf.org.uk/research/heart-statistics. Accessed 3rd August 2018.

British Thoracic Society, 2017. BTS guidelines for oxygen use in adults in healthcare and emergency settings. Thorax 72 (Suppl. 1), 1−100.

Cancer Research UK, 2015. Lets beat cancer sooner. Testicular cancer statistics. https://www.cancerresearchuk.org/health-professional/cancer-statistics/statistics-by-cancer-type/testicular-cancer. Accessed 3rd August 2018.

Cancer Research UK, 2016. Lets beat cancer sooner. Lung cancer statistics. www.cancerresearchuk.org/health-professional/cancer-statistics/statistics-by-cancer-type/lung-cancer#heading-Two. Accessed 3rd August 2018.

Cancer Research UK, 2018. Thyroid cancer Survival. https://www.cancerresearchuk.org/about-cancer/thyroid-cancer/survival. Accessed 3rd August 2018.

Carper, B., 1978. Fundamental patterns of knowing in nursing. Advances in Nursing Science 1 (1), 13−23.

Department of Health & Social Care, 2018. Department of Health and Social Care Single Departmental Plan. DH, London.

Department of Health, 2002. Comprehensive Critical Care: A Review of Adult Critical Care Services. DH, London.

Dougherty, L., Lister, S., 2015. The Royal Marsden Manual of Clinical Nursing Procedures, ninth ed. John Wiley & Sons, Chichester.

Driscoll, J., 2007. Practicing Clinical Supervision: A Reflective Approach for Healthcare Professionals, second ed. Bailliere Tindall, Edinburgh.

Duffy, K., McCallum, J., McGuinness, C., 2016. Mentors in waiting. Nurse Educ. Pract. 16, 163−169.

Edwards, S.L., 2002b. Nursing knowledge: defining new boundaries. Nurs. Stand. 17 (2), 40−44.

Edwards, S.L., 2003. Critical thinking at the bedside: a practical perspective. Br. J. Nurs. 12 (19), 1142−1149.

Edwards, S.L., 2007. Critical thinking: a two-phase framework. Nurse Educ. Pract. 7 (5), 303−314.

Edwards, S., 2017. What nursing students reveal about and learn from mentors when using story of clinical practice. Nurs. Manag. 23 (10), 32−39.

Edwards, S.L., 2017a. Reflecting differently. New dimensions: reflection-before-action and reflection-beyond-action. Int. Pract. Dev. J. 7 (1), 1–14.

Edwards, S.L., 2017b. What student nurses reveal about and learn from mentors when using stories of clinical practice. Nurs. Manag. 23 (10), 32–39.

Edwards, S.L., O'Connell, C.F., 2007. Bullying in nursing practice and education. Nurse Educ. Pract. 7, 26–35.

Elia, M., 2003. The MUST Report. Nutritional Screening for Adults: A Multidisciplinary Responsibility. BAPEN, Redditch.

Gailbraith, A., Bullock, S., Manias, E., Hunt, B., Richards, A., 2007. Fundamentals of pharmacology: an applied approach for nursing and health, second ed. Pearson Prentice Hall, Harlow.

Garretson, S., Malberti, S., 2007. Understanding hypovolaemic, cardiogenic and septic shock. Nurs. Stand. 21 (50), 46–55.

Gibbs, G., 1988. Learning by Doing: A Guide to Teaching and Learning Methods. Oxford Polytechnic FEU, Oxford.

Johns, C., 1994. Guided reflection. In: Palmer, A., Burns, S., Bulman, C. (Eds.), Reflective Practice in Nursing. Blackwell Science, London.

Kozier, B., Erb, G., Berman, A., Snyder, S., 2012. Fundamentals of Nursing: Concepts, Process and Practice, second ed. Pearson, Harlow.

Lavallee, J.F., Gray, T.A., Dumville, J., Russell, W., Cullum, N., 2017. The effects of care bundles on patient outcomes: a systematic review and meta-analysis. Implement. Sci. 12 (1), 142.

McCarron, K., 2011. Understanding care bundles. Nurs. Made Incred. Easy 9 (2), 30–33.

National Institute for Clinical Excellence, 2012. Incident Reporting Procedure. NICE, London.

National patient Safety Agency, 2012. Release of organization patient safety incident reports. accessed at: http://www.nrls.npsa.nhs.uk.

NHS choices, 2015. Coronary artery bypass graft. https://www.nhs.uk/conditions/coronary-artery-bypass-graft-cabg/. Accessed 3rd August 2018.

NICE, 2013. Hypertension in Adults, Quality Standard, updated 2017. https://www.nice.org.uk/guidance/qs28. Accessed 1st April 2018.

NICE, 2014. Chronic kidney disease in adults: assessment and management. Clinical Guideline CG182. https://www.nice.org.uk/guidance/cg182/chapter/1-Recommendations. Accessed 3rd August 2018.

Nursing and Midwifery Council, 2004. Guidelines for the Administration of Medicines. NMC, London.

Nursing, Midwifery Council, 2015. The Code: Professional Standards of Practice and Behaviour for Nurses and Midwives. NMC, London.

Professional Standards Authority, 2015. Right-Touch Regulation, Revised. PSA, London.

Public Health England, 2017. Tuberculosis in England, 2017 Report. http://assets.publishing.service.gov.uk/government/uploads/system/uploads/attachment_data/file/686185/TB_Annual_Report_2017_v1.1.pdf. Accessed 3rd August 2018.

Public Health England, 2017a. Combating High Blood Pressure. https://www.gov.uk/government/publications/health-matters-combating-high-blood-pressure/health-matters-combating-high-blood-pressure.

Public Health England, 2017b. Tuberculosis in England: 2017 Report. https://assets.publishing.service.gov.uk/government/uploads/system/uploads/attachment_data/file/686185/TB_Annual_Report_2017_v1.1.pdf.

Purvis, Y., Edwards, S., 2005. Initial needs of bereaved relatives following sudden and unexpected death. Emerg. Nurse 13 (7), 28–34.

Richards, A., Edwards, S., 2014. Essential Pathophysiology for Nursing and Healthcare Students. Elsevier, Edinburgh.

Rolfe, G., 2000. Research, Truth Authority: Post Modern Perspectives in Nursing. MacMillan Press Limited, London.

Royal College of Nursing, 2016. Standards of Infusion Therapy. RCN, London.

Royal College of Physicians, 2017. National Early Warning Score (NEWS) 2. RCP, London.

Royal College of physicians, 2017. National early warning score (NEWS) 2, accessed at: https://www.rcplondon.ac.uk/projects/outputs/national-early-warning-score-news-2. [Accessed 01/08/18].

Schon, D.A., 1983. The Reflective Practitioner: How Professionals Think in Action. Basic Books, New York.

Shuvy, M., Atar, D., Steg, P.G., Halvorsen, S., Jolly, S., Yusuf, S., Lotan, C., 2013. Oxygen therapy in acute coronary syndrome: are the benefits worth the risk. Eur. Heart J. 34, 1630—1635.

Smith, G.B., 2012. Acute life-Threatening Events Recognition and Treatment. Intensive Care Society, Portsmouth.

Smith, G.B., Osgood, V.M., Crane, S., 2002. ALERT a multiprofessional training course in the care of the acutely ill adult patient. Resuscitation 52, 281—286.

Stroke Association, 2015. Together we can conquer stroke. Stroke association Strategy 2015-2018. www.stroke.org.uk/sites/default/files/stroke_association_strategy_2015-2018.pdf. Accessed 3rd August 2018.

Stroke Association, 2018. State of the Nation Stroke Statistics Together we can conquer stroke www.stroke.org.uk/system/files/sotn_2018.pdf. Accesses 3rd August 2018.

The Stroke Association, 2015. Together We Can Conquer Stroke, Stroke Association Strategy 2015—2018. www.stroke.org.uk/sites/default/files/stroke_association_strategy_2015_to_2018.pdf.

The Stroke Association, 2017. State of the Nation Stroke Statistics, 2017. www.stroke.org.uk/sites/default/files/state_of_the_nation_2017_final_1.pdf.

WHO, 2013. A Global Brief on Hypertension, World Health Day 2013. http://www.who.int/cardiovascular_diseases/publications/global_brief_hypertension/en/. Accessed 1st April, 2018.

WHO, 2015. Q & As on hypertension. Online Q & A. http://www.who.int/features/qa/82/en/. Accessed 3rd August 2018.

WHO, 2015. Q & As on Hypertension. Available at: http://www.who.int/features/qa/82/en/. Accessed 3rd August 2018.

WHO, 2017. Diabetes Key facts. Fact Sheet. http://www.who.int/news-room/fact-sheets/detail/diabetes.

WHO, 2017. Diabetes Fact Sheet, Media Centre. Available at: http://www.who.int/mediacentre/factsheets/fs312/en/.

Further Reading

British Epilepsy Association. Online. www.epilepsysociety.org.uk.

British Heart Foundation, Public Health England, Stroke Association, Royal College of General Practitioners, Primary Care Leadership Forum, Blood Pressure UK, British and Irish Hypertension Society, 2016. High Blood Pressure: How Can We Do Better? Data collated and visualised by the National Cardiovascular Intelligence Network (NCVIN).

Edwards, S.L., 2001. Shock: types, classifications and exploration of their physiological effects. Emerg. Nurse 9 (2), 29–38.

Edwards, S.L., 2001. Using the glasgow coma scale: analysis and limitations. Br. J. Nurs. 10 (2), 92–101.

Edwards, S.L., 2002. Physiological insult/injury: pathophysiology and consequences. Br. J. Nurs. 11 (4), 263–274.

Edwards, S.L., 2004. Compartment syndrome. Emerg. Nurse 12 (3), 32–38.

Edwards, S.L., 2006. Tissue viability: understanding the mechanisms of injury and repair. Nurs. Stand. 21 (13), 48–57.

Edwards, S.L., 2008. Pathophysiology of acid base balance: the theory practice relationship. Intensive Crit. Care Nurs. 24 (1), 28–40.

European Association of Urology, 2007. Guidelines on Renal Cell Carcinoma. European Association of Urology, Arnheim.

Galbraith, A., Bullock, S., Manias, E., Hunt, B., Richards, A., 2007. Fundamentals of Pharmacology. Addison Wesley, London.

Hinchliff, S., Montague, S., Watson, R., 2005. Physiology for Nursing Practice, second ed. Baillière Tindall, London.

Joint British Diabetes Societies Inpatient Care Group, 2012. The Management of the Hyperosmolar Hyperglycaemic State (HHS) in Adults With Diabetes. Available at: https://diabetes-resources-production.s3-eu-west-1.amazonaws.com/diabetes-storage/migration/pdf/JBDS-IP-HHS-Adults.pdf.

Marieb, E., 2015. Human Anatomy and Physiology. Pearson.

McCance, K., Huether, S., 2014. Pathophysiology. Elsevier.

Motor Neurone Disease Association, 2018. Get the Facts You Need. Online. Available: www.mndassociation.org (accessed April 2018).

National Institute of Health, Clinical Excellence, 2011. Hypertension Flow Chart and Guidelines. https://pathways.nice.org.uk/pathways/hypertension#path¼view%3A/pathways/hypertension/hypertension-overview.xml&content¼view-index.

National Institute of Clinical Excellence. Tuberculosis, NICE Clinical Guideline (2016); clinical diagnosis and management of tuberculosis, and measures for its prevention and control. www.nice.org.uk/guidance/ng3 (accessed April 2018).

National Institute for Clinical Excellence, 2012. The Diagnosis and Management of the Epilepsies in Adults and Children in Primary and Secondary Care. NICE Clinical Guideline. https://www.nice.org.uk/guidance/cg137 (accessed April 2018).

National Institute for Clinical Excellence, 2017a. Parkinson's Disease in Adults: Guidance and Guidelines. https://www.nice.org.uk/guidance/ng71 (accessed April 2018).

National Institute for Clinical Excellence, 2017b. Stroke and Transient Ischaemic Attacks. www.nice.org.uk/guidance/cg68 (accessed April 2018).

Neal, M., 2015. Medical Pharmacology at a Glance. Wiley Blackwell.

Office for National Statistics, 2018. Cancer Statistics Registrations: Registrations of Cancer Diagnosed in 2016. www.ons.gov.uk/peoplepopulationandcommunity/healthandsocialcare/conditionsanddiseases/bulletins/cancerregistrationstatisticsengland/final2016.

Parkinson's UK, 2018. Online. www.parkinsons.org.uk/ (accessed April 2018).

Willmott, H., 2015. Trauma and Orthopaedics at a Glance. Wiley Blackwell.

Appendix 1

Units of measurement

UNITS (SI), THE METRIC SYSTEM AND CONVERSIONS

The International System of Units (SI) or Système International d'Unités is the measurement system used for scientific, medical and technical purposes in most countries. In the United Kingdom, SI units have replaced those of the imperial system, e.g., the kilogram is used for mass instead of the pound (in everyday situations, both mass and weight are measured in kilograms although weight, which varies with gravity, is really a measure of force).

The SI comprises seven base units with several derived units. Each unit has its own symbol and is expressed as a decimal multiple or submultiple of the base unit by using the appropriate prefix, e.g., millimetre is one thousandth of a metre.

Base units

Quantity	Base unit and symbol
Length	Metre (m)
Mass	Kilogram (kg)
Time	Second (s)
Amount of substance	Mole (mol)
Electric current	Ampere (A)
Thermodynamic temperature	Kelvin (°K)
Luminous intensity	Candela (cd)

Derived units

Derived units for measuring different quantities are reached by multiplying or dividing two or more base units.

Quantity	Derived unit and symbol
Work, energy, quantity of heat	Joule (J)
Pressure	Pascal (Pa)
Force	Newton (N)
Frequency	Hertz (Hz)
Power	Watt (W)
Electrical potential, electromotive force, potential difference	Volt (v)
Absorbed dose of radiation	Gray (Gy)
Radioactivity	Becquerel (Bq)
Dose equivalent	Sievert (Sv)

Factor, decimal multiples and submultiples of SI units

Multiplication factor	Prefix	Symbol
10^{12}	Tera	T
10^{9}	Giga	G
10^{6}	Mega	M
10^{3}	Kilo	k
10^{2}	Hecto	h
10^{1}	Deca	da
10^{-1}	Deci	d
10^{-2}	Centi	c
10^{-3}	Milli	m
10^{-6}	Micro	μ
10^{-9}	Nano	n
10^{-12}	Pico	p
10^{-15}	Femto	f
10^{-18}	Atto	a

Rules for using units and writing large numbers and decimals

- The symbol for a unit is unaltered in the plural and should not be followed by a full stop except at the end of a sentence: 5 cm not 5 cm. or 5 cms.
- Large numbers are written in three-digit groups (working from right to left) with spaces, not commas (in some countries the comma is used to indicate a decimal point): fifty thousand is written as 50 000; five hundred thousand is written as 500 000.
- Numbers with four digits are written without the space, e.g., four thousand is written as 4000.

- The decimal sign between digits is indicated by a full stop positioned near the line, e.g., 50.25. If the numerical value of the decimal is less than 1, a zero should appear before the decimal sign: 0.125 not .125.
- Decimals with more than four digits are also written in three-digit groups but this time working from left to right, e.g., 0.000 25.
- 'Squared' and 'cubed' are expressed as numerical powers and not by abbreviation: square centimetre is cm^2 not sq. cm.

Commonly used measurements requiring further explanation

- Temperature — although the SI base unit for temperature is the kelvin, by international convention temperature is measured in degrees Celsius (°C).
- Energy — the energy of food or individual requirements for energy are measured in kilojoules (kJ); the SI unit is the joule (J). In practice, many people still use the kilocalorie (kcal), a non-SI unit, for these purposes.
- 1 calorie = 4.2 J
- 1 kilocalorie (large calorie) = 4.2 kJ
- Volume — volume is calculated by multiplying length, width and depth. Using the SI unit for length. the metre (m), means ending up with a cubic metre (m^3), which is a huge volume and is certainly not appropriate for most purposes. In clinical practice, the litre (L or l) is used. A litre is based on the volume of a cube measuring $10 \times 10 \times 10$ cm. Smaller units still, e.g., millilitre (mL) or one thousandth of a litre, are commonly used in clinical practice.
- Time — the SI base unit for time is the second (s), but it is acceptable to use minute (min), hour (h) or day (d). In clinical practice, it is preferable to use 'per 24 h' for the excretion of substances in urine and faeces: g/24 h.
- Amount of substance — the SI base unit for amount of substance is the mole (mol). The concentration of many substances is expressed in moles per litre (mol/L) or millimoles per litre (mmol/L), which replaces milliequivalents per litre (mEq/l). Some exceptions exist and include haemoglobin and plasma proteins in grams per litre (g/L); and enzyme activity in international units (IU, U or iu).
- Pressure — the SI unit of pressure is the pascal (Pa) and the kilopascal (kPa) replaces the old non-SI unit of millimetres of mercury pressure (mmHg) for blood pressure and blood gases. However, mmHg is still widely used for measuring blood pressure. Other anomalies include cerebrospinal fluid, which is measured in millimetres of water (mmH_2O), and central venous pressure, which is measured in centimetres of water (cmH_2O).

MEASUREMENTS, EQUIVALENTS AND CONVERSIONS (SI OR METRIC AND IMPERIAL)

Length

1 kilometre (km)	= 1000 metres (m)
1 metre (m)	= 100 centimetres (cm) or 1000 millimetres (mm)
1 centimetre (cm)	= 10 millimetres (mm)
1 millimetre (mm)	= 1000 micrometres (μm)
1 micrometre (μm)	= 1000 nanometres (nm)

Conversions

1 metre (m)	= 39.370 inches (in)
1 centimetre (cm)	= 0.3937 inches (in)
30.48 centimetres (cm)	= 1 foot (ft)
2.54 centimetres (cm)	= 1 inch (in)

Volume

1 litre (L)	= 1000 millilitres (mL)
1 millilitre (mL)	= 1000 microlitres (μL)

N.B. The millilitre (mL) and the cubic centimetre (cm^3) are usually treated as being the same.

Conversions

1 litre (L)	= 1.76 pints (pt)
568.25 millilitres (mL)	= 1 pint (pt)
28.4 millilitres (mL)	= 1 fluid ounce (fl oz)

Weight or mass

1 kilogram (kg)	= 1000 grams (g)
1 gram (g)	= 1000 milligrams (mg)
1 milligram (mg)	= 1000 micrograms (μg)
1 microgram (μg)	= 1000 nanograms (ng)

N.B. To avoid any confusion with milligram (mg), the word microgram (μg) should be written in full on prescriptions.

Conversions

1 kilogram (kg)	= 2.204 pounds (lb)
1 gram (g)	= 0.0353 ounce (oz)
453.59 grams (g)	= 1 pound (lb)
28.34 grams (g)	= 1 ounce (oz)

Temperature conversions

To convert Celsius to Fahrenheit:
multiply by 9, divide by 5, and add 32 to the result:
e.g., 368°C to Fahrenheit:
$36 \times 9 = 324 \div 5 = 64.8 + 32 = 96.8°F$
therefore $36°C = 96.8°F$

To convert Fahrenheit to Celsius:
subtract 32, multiply by 5, and divide by 9:
e.g., 104°F to Celsius:
$104 - 32 = 72 \times 5 = 360 \div 9 = 40°C$
therefore $104°F = 40°C$

Temperature comparison

°Celsius	°Fahrenheit
100	212
95	203
90	194
85	185
80	176
75	167
70	158
65	149
60	140
55	131
50	122
45	113
44	112.2
43	109.4
42	107.6
41	105.8
40	104
39.5	103.1
39	102.2
38.5	101.3
38	100.4
37.5	99.5
37	98.6

36.5	97.7
36	96.8
35.5	95.9
35	95
34	93.2
33	91.4
32	89.6
31	87.8
30	86
25	77
20	68
15	59
10	505
41	
0	32
−5	23
−10	14

N.B. Boiling point $= 100°C = 212°F$
Freezing point $= 0°C = 32°F$

Appendix 2

Normal values

The values below represent an 'average' reference range, in adults, for blood, cerebrospinal fluid, urine and faeces. These ranges should be used as a guide only. Reference ranges vary between individual laboratories and readers should consult their own laboratory for those used locally. This is especially important where reference values depend upon the analytical equipment and temperatures used.

BLOOD (HAEMATOLOGY)

Test	Reference range
Activated partial thromboplastin time (APTT)	30—40 s
Bleeding time (Ivy)	2—8 min
Erythrocyte sedimentation rate (ESR)	
Adult women	3—15 mm/h
Adult men	1—10 mm/h
Fibrinogen	1.5—4.0 g/L
Folate (serum)	4—18 µg/L
Haemoglobin	
Women	115—165 g/L (11.5—16.5 g/dL)
Men	130—180 g/L (13—18 g/dL)
Haptoglobins	0.3—2.0 g/L
Mean cell haemoglobin (MCH)	27—32 pg
Mean cell haemoglobin concentration (MCHC)	30—35 g/dL
Mean cell volume (MCV)	78—95 fL
Packed cell volume (PCV or haematocrit)	
Women	0.35—0.47 (35%—47%)
Men	0.4—0.54 (40%—54%)
Platelets (thrombocytes)	150—400 × 10^9/L
Prothrombin time	12—16 s
Red cells (erythrocytes)	
Women	3.8—5.3 × 10^{12}/L
Men	4.5—6.5 × 10^{12}/L

Reticulocytes (newly formed red cells in adults)	$25-85 \times 10^9$/L
White cells total (leucocytes)	$4.0-11.0 \times 10^9$/L

BLOOD-VENOUS PLASMA (BIOCHEMISTRY)

Test	Reference range
Alanine aminotransferase (ALT)	10–40 U/L
Albumin	36–47 g/L
Alkaline phosphatase	40–125 U/L
Amylase	90–300 U/L
Aspartate aminotransferase (AST)	10–35 U/L
Bicarbonate (arterial)	22–28 mmol/L
Bilirubin (total)	2–17 mmol/L
Caeruloplasmin	150–600 mg/L
Calcium	2.1–2.6 mmol/L
Chloride	95–105 mmol/L
Cholesterol (total)	ideally below 5.2 mmol/L
High-density lipoprotein cholesterol	
Women	0.6–1.9 mmol/L
Men	0.5–1.6 mmol/L
$PaCO_2$ (arterial)	4.4–6.1 kPa
Copper	13–24 mmol/L
Cortisol (at 08.00 h)	160–565 nmol/L
Creatine kinase (total)	
Women	30–150 U/L
Men	30–200 U/L
Creatinine	55–150 mmol/L
γ-glutamyltransferase (γGT)	
Women	5–35 U/L
Men	10–55 U/L
Globulins	24–37 g/L
Glucose (venous blood, fasting)	3.6–5.8 mmol/L
Glycosylated haemoglobin (HbA$_1$)	4%–6%
Hydrogen ion concentration (arterial)	35–44 nmol/L
Iron	
Women	10–28 µmol/L
Men	14–32 µmol/L
Total iron-binding capacity (TIBC)	45–70 µmol/L
Lactate (arterial)	0.3–1.4 mmol/L
Lactate dehydrogenase (total)	230–460 U/L
Lead (adults, whole blood)	<1.7 µmol/L
Magnesium	0.7–1.0 mmol/L
Osmolality	275–290 mmol/kg
PaO_2 (arterial)	12–15 kPa
Oxygen saturation (arterial)	>97%
pH	7.36–7.42
Phosphate (fasting)	0.8–1.4 mmol/L

Potassium (serum)	3.6—5.0 mmol/L
Protein (total)	60—80 g/L
Sodium	136—145 mmol/L
Transferrin	2—4 g/L
Triglycerides (fasting)	0.6—1.8 mmol/L
Urate	
Women	0.12—0.36 mmol/L
Men	0.12—0.42 mmol/L
Urea	2.5—6.5 mmol/L
Uric acid	
Women	0.09—0.36 mmol/L
Men	0.1—0.45 mmol/L
Vitamin A	0.7—3.5 μmol/L
Vitamin C	23—57 μmol/L
Zinc	11—22 μmol/L

CEREBROSPINAL FLUID

Test	Reference range
Cells	0—5 mm^3
Chloride	120—170 mmol/L
Glucose	2.5—4.0 mmol/L
Pressure (adult)	50—180 mm/H_2O
Protein	100—400 mg/L

URINE

Test	Reference range
Albumin/creatinine ratio	<3.5 mg albumin/mmol creatinine
Calcium (diet dependent)	<12 mmol/24 h (normal diet)
Copper	0.2—0.6 μmol/24 h
Cortisol	9—50 μmol/24 h
Creatinine	9—17 mmol/24 h
5-Hydroxyindole-3-acetic acid (5HIAA)	10—45 μmol/24 h
Magnesium	3.3—5.0 mmol/24 h
Oxalate	
Women	40—320 mmol/24 h
Men	80—490 mmol/24 h
pH	4—8
Phosphate	15—50 mmol/24 h
Porphyrins (total)	90—370 nmol/24 h
Potassium (depends on intake)	25—100 mmol/24 h

Protein (total)   no more than 0.3 g/L
Sodium (depends on intake)   100–200 mmol/24 h
Urea   170–500 mmol/24 h

FAECES

Test	Reference range
Fat content (daily output on normal diet)	<7 g/24 h
Fat (as stearic acid)	11–18 mmol/24 h

Appendix 3

Drug measurement and calculations

The International System of Units is used for drug doses and concentrations and patient data (including weight and body surface area), drug levels in the body and other measurements (see Appendix 1 for more information).

WEIGHT

Grams (g) and milligrams (mg) are the units most often encountered in drug dosages. Doses of less than 1 g should be expressed in milligrams, e.g., 250 mg rather than 0.25 g. Similarly, doses less than 1 mg should be expressed in micrograms, e.g., 200 micrograms rather than 0.2 mg. Whenever drugs are prescribed in microgram dosages, the units should be written in full, e.g., digoxin 250 micrograms, as the use of the contracted terms µg or mcg may in practice be mistaken for mg and, as this dose is 1000 times greater, disastrous consequences may follow.

Drug dosages are often described in terms of unit dose per kg of body weight, i.e., mg/kg, µg/kg, etc. This method of dosage is frequently used for children and allows dosages to be tailored to the individual patient's size.

VOLUME

Litres (L or l) and millilitres (mL or ml) account for almost all measurements expressed in unit volume for the prescription and administration of drugs.

CONCENTRATION

When expressing concentration of dosages of a medicine in liquid form, several methods are available as follows:

- Unit weight per unit volume − describes the unit of weight of a drug contained in unit volume, e.g., 1 mg in 1 mL, 40 mg in 2 mL. Examples of drugs in common use expressed in these terms: pethidine injection 100 mg in 2 mL; chloral hydrate mixture 1 g in 10 mL; phenoxymethylpenicillin oral solution 250 mg in 5 mL.

- Percentage (weight in volume) — describes the weight of a drug expressed in grams (g) which is contained in 100 mL of solution, e.g., calcium gluconate injection, 10% of which contains 10 g in each 100 mL of solution or 1 g in each 10 mL or 100 mg (0.1 g) in each 1 mL.

- Percentage (weight in weight) — describes the weight of a drug expressed in grams (g) which is contained in 100 g of a solid or semisolid medicament, such as ointments and creams, e.g., fusidic acid ointment, 2% of which contains 2 g of fusidic acid in each 100 g of ointment.

- Volume containing '1 part' — a few liquids and to a lesser extent gases, particularly those containing drugs in very low concentrations, are often described as containing 1 part per 'x' units of volume. For liquids, 'parts' are equivalent to grams and volume to millimetres, e.g., adrenaline injection 1 in 1000 which contains 1 g in 1000 mL or expressed as a percentage (w/v) — 0.1%.

- Molar concentration — only very occasionally are drugs in liquid form expressed in molar concentration. The mole is the molecular weight of a drug expressed in grams, and a one molar (1 M) solution contains this weight dissolved in each litre. More often the millimole (mmol) is used to describe a medicinal product, e.g., potassium chloride solution 15 mmol in 10 mL indicates a solution containing the molecular weight of potassium chloride in milligrams × 15 dissolved in 10 mL of solution.

BODY HEIGHT AND SURFACE AREA

Drug doses may be expressed in terms of microgram, milligram or gram per unit of body surface area. This is frequently the case where precise dosages tailored to individual patients' needs are required. Typical examples may be seen in cytotoxic chemotherapy or in drugs given to children. Body surface area is expressed as square metres or m^2 and drug dosages as units per square metre or units/m^2, e.g., cytarabine injection 100 mg/m^2.

FORMULAE FOR CALCULATION OF DRUG DOSES AND DRIP RATES

Oral drugs (solids, liquids)

Amount required = {Strength required × Volume of stock strength/Stock strength}

Parenteral drugs

1. Solutions (IM, IV injections)
   Volume required = {Strength required × Volume of stock strength/Stock strength}
2. Powders
   It is essential to follow the manufacturer's directions for dilution, then use the appropriate formula.
3. IV infusions
   Rate (drops/min) = {Volume of solution (mL) × Number of drops per mL/Time (min)}
   Macrodrip (20 drops/mL) − clear fluids
   a. Rate (drops/min) = {Volume of solution (mL) × 20/Time (min)}
   b. Macrodrip (15 drops/mL) − blood
   Rate (drops/min) = {Volume of solution (mL) × 15/Time (min)}
4. Infusion pumps
   Rate (mL/h) = Volume (mL) ÷ Time (h)
5. IV infusions with drugs
   Rate (mL/h) = {Amount of drug required (mg/h) × Volume of solution (mL)/Total amount of drug (mg)}

N.B. After selecting the appropriate formula, ensure that all strengths are in the same units, otherwise convert.

1% solution contains 1 g of solute dissolved in 100 mL of solution.

1:1000 means 1 g in 1000 mL of solution, therefore 1 g in 1000 mL is equivalent to 1 mg in 1 mL.

Other useful formulae

Children's dose (Clarke's Body Weight Rule)
   Child's dose = {Adult dose × Weight of child (kg)/Average adult weight (70 kg)}
   Children's dose (Clarke's Body Surface Area Rule)
   Child's dose = {Adult dose × Surface area of child (m^2)/Surface area of adult (1.7m^2)}

ACKNOWLEDGMENTS

The measurement section was adapted from Henney, C.R., et al., 1995. Drugs in Nursing Practice, fifth ed. Churchill Livingstone, Edinburgh, with permission; and the formulae from Havard, M., 1994. A Nursing Guide to Drugs, fourth ed. Churchill Livingstone, Edinburgh, with permission.

Glossary

Acidosis Abnormally high acidity of body fluids and tissues.

Albumin A protein found in the blood plasma and important in maintaining plasma volume.

Allogenic Pertaining to grafted tissue derived from a donor of the same species.

Anaemia Reduction in the quantity of oxygen-carrying haemoglobin in the blood.

Anastomosis Artificial connection or joining between two tubular body parts, usually small intestine.

Angiography Demonstration of blood vessels after an injection of contrast medium.

Angiopathy Disorder of the blood vessels.

Anion Negatively charged ion, e.g., bicarbonate.

Anthropometry Measurement of parts of the body.

Anuria Failure of the kidneys to produce urine.

Aplasia Total or partial failure of development of an organ or tissue.

Arthropathy Joint disease.

Ascites Fluid in the peritoneal cavity.

Atelectasis Failure of part of the lung to expand.

Atheroma Deposition of lipid material in the intimal layer of arteries.

Blast cells Formative, immature cells.

Catecholamines A group of chemicals secreted by the body that includes adrenaline, noradrenaline, dopamine and some other neurotransmitters.

Cation A positively charged ion, e.g., sodium and potassium.

Cholecystitis Inflammation of the gall bladder.

Coagulopathy Disorder of blood clotting.

Colloid Substances which are unable to pass through the cell membrane; diffusible but not soluble in water. Used to describe some intravenous fluids, e.g., Haemaccel.

Crystalloid Organic salts that will pass through the cell membrane. Used to describe intravenous fluids such as saline 0.9%.

Cytokine Secretions of the lymphoid system that act as signals to other lymphoid cells.

Dysphagia Difficulty in swallowing.

Dysphasia Disorder of language following brain damage, e.g., a stroke.

Dysplasia Abnormal development or formation of tissue.

Empyema Pus in the pleural cavity.

Enteritis Inflammation of the small intestine often resulting in diarrhoea.

Epigastrium Upper central region of the abdomen.

Erythema Flushing of the skin due to dilatation of the blood capillaries.

Erythropoietin Hormone released by the kidney that stimulates the formation of red blood cells.

Euthyroid Having a thyroid gland that functions normally.

Exacerbation Increased severity of symptoms.

FEV_1 Forced expiratory volume in the first second of exhalation in a respiratory function test. Is usually 80% of the total FEV.

Gastrin Hormone released into the bloodstream by the stomach and stimulating the production of gastric juice.

Glucocorticoids Any steroid hormone that promotes gluconeogenesis, e.g., cortisol.

Gluconeogenesis Synthesis of glucose by the body from noncarbohydrate sources, e.g., protein.

Gynaecomastia Breast enlargement in the male.

Haematemesis Vomiting blood.

Haematocrit Volume of red cells in the blood expressed as a percentage of the total blood volume.

Haematuria Blood in the urine.

Haemodilution Decrease in the proportion of red cells relative to plasma, brought about by an increase in total volume of the plasma.

Haemoptysis Coughing up blood.

Haemothorax Blood in the pleural cavity.

Halitosis Bad breath.

Hepatocyte Liver cell.

Hepatomegaly Enlargement of the liver that is palpable.

Hirschsprung's disease Congenital intestinal disease of nervous tissue leading to intractable constipation.

Hypercalcaemia Excessive calcium in the blood.

Hypercarbia Raised carbon dioxide in arterial blood.

Hypersplenism Depression of blood cell counts by an enlarged spleen in the presence of an active bone marrow.

Hyperuricaemia Excessive uric acid in the blood; characteristic of gout.

Hypokalaemia Abnormally low potassium level in the blood.

Hyponatraemia Abnormally low sodium level in the blood.

Hypovolaemia Diminished quantity of total blood.

Hypoxaemia Diminished amount of oxygen in arterial blood.

Hypoxia Diminished amount of oxygen in the tissues.

Idiopathic Condition of unknown or spontaneous origin, e.g., some forms of epilepsy.

Ileus Intestinal obstruction — term usually restricted to paralytic rather than mechanical obstruction.

Ischaemia Deficient blood supply to any part of the body.

Ketoacidosis Acidosis due to accumulation of ketone bodies.

Leucocytosis Increase in the number of white blood cells in the blood.

Leukaemia Malignant disease in which increased numbers of any type of white blood cell are produced.

Lipolysis Fat breakdown into fatty acids by the enzyme lipase.

Lymphoid Tissue responsible for the production of lymphocytes and antibodies.

Macrocytic Describing an abnormally large red blood cell.

Mallory-Weiss syndrome Tearing of the tissues around the junction of the oesophagus and stomach as a result of violent vomiting.

Methaemoglobin Form of oxidized haemoglobin that cannot carry oxygen.

Microcytic Describing abnormally small red blood cells.

Mineralocorticoids Hormonal secretion of the adrenal cortex — aldosterone mainly.

Myopathy Disease of the muscles.

Neoplasm New growth that may be cancerous or noncancerous.

Nephroureterectomy Removal of the kidney along with part or the whole of the ureter.

Neutropenia Reduced number of neutrophils (type of white blood cell) in the blood.

NSAID Nonsteroidal anti-inflammatory drug, e.g., aspirin.

Oliguria Production of an abnormally small volume of urine. May be due to sweating, dehydration, blood loss or kidney disease.

Pancreatitis Inflammation of the pancreas.

Papilloedema Swelling of the optic disc.

Petechiae Small haemorrhagic round flat dark red spots caused by bleeding into the skin or beneath the mucous membrane.

Pneumothorax Air in the pleural cavity.

Polycythaemia Increase in the number of circulating red blood cells.

Polydipsia Excessive thirst leading to the drinking of large quantities of fluids.

Polyuria Passing excessive amounts of urine.

Proteolysis Protein breakdown.

Queckenstedt's test Performed during a lumbar puncture. Compression of the internal jugular vein produces a rise in CSF pressure if there is no obstruction to circulation of fluid in the spinal region.

Remission Period of abatement of a disease.

Resection Surgical excision.

Salpingitis Inflammation of the fallopian tubes.

SCID Severe combined immune deficiency — genetic disorder affecting 1 in 25,000 babies. The baby has no resistance to infection and has to be enclosed in a protective plastic bubble from birth.

Septicaemia The persistence and multiplication of living bacteria in the bloodstream.

Splenomegaly Enlargement of the spleen.

Steatosis (hepatic) Infiltration of hepatocytes with fat.

Subphrenic abscess A collection of pus in the space below the diaphragm.

Supine Lying on the back with the face upwards.

Thrombocytopenia Reduction in the number of platelets in the blood.

Tinnitus Any noise, often buzzing, thumping or ringing in the ears.

Toxaemia Blood poisoning caused by the products of bacteria.

Toxoplasmosis Disease due to the protozoan *Toxoplasma gondii*. Often spread from cats.

Transferrin Protein that acts as a carrier for iron in the bloodstream.

Uraemia Excessive amounts of urea and nitrogenous waste in the bloodstream.

Index